Patient Centred Care in Medical Imaging and Radiotherapy

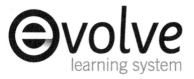
learning system

Evolve Learning Resources for Students and Lecturers.
See the instructions on the inside cover for access
to the web site. http://evolve.elsevier.com/Vosper/patient/

Think outside the book...**evolve**

Content Strategist: *Claire Wilson*
Senior Content Development Specialist: *Catherine Jackson*
Project Manager: *Sruthi Viswam*
Designer/Design Direction: *Christian Bilbow*
Illustration Manager: *Jennifer Rose*

Patient Centred Care in Medical Imaging and Radiotherapy

Edited by

Aarthi Ramlaul MA BTechRad NDipRad

Principal Lecturer, Diagnostic Radiography and Imaging, University of Hertfordshire, Hatfield, UK

Martin Vosper MSc PGDip BSc(Hons) HDCR(R)

Senior Lecturer, Diagnostic Radiography and Imaging, University of Hertfordshire, Hatfield, UK

Foreword by

Richard C. Price MSc, PhD, FCR

Dean of School of Health and Social Work, University of Hertfordshire, Hatfield, UK

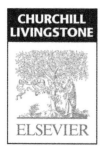

CHURCHILL LIVINGSTONE

ELSEVIER

Edinburgh   London   New York   Oxford   Philadelphia   St Louis   Sydney   Toronto   2013

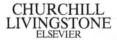

CHURCHILL
LIVINGSTONE
ELSEVIER

ISBN 978-0-7020-4613-1

British Library Cataloguing in Publication Data
A catalogue record for this book is available from the British Library

Library of Congress Cataloging in Publication Data
A catalog record for this book is available from the Library of Congress

Notices
Knowledge and best practice in this field are constantly changing. As new research and experience broaden our understanding, changes in research methods, professional practices, or medical treatment may become necessary.

Practitioners and researchers must always rely on their own experience and knowledge in evaluating and using any information, methods, compounds, or experiments described herein. In using such information or methods they should be mindful of their own safety and the safety of others, including parties for whom they have a professional responsibility.

With respect to any drug or pharmaceutical products identified, readers are advised to check the most current information provided (i) on procedures featured or (ii) by the manufacturer of each product to be administered, to verify the recommended dose or formula, the method and duration of administration, and contraindications. It is the responsibility of practitioners, relying on their own experience and knowledge of their patients, to make diagnoses, to determine dosages and the best treatment for each individual patient, and to take all appropriate safety precautions.

To the fullest extent of the law, neither the Publisher nor the authors, contributors, or editors, assume any liability for any injury and/or damage to persons or property as a matter of products liability, negligence or otherwise, or from any use or operation of any methods, products, instructions, or ideas contained in the material herein.

ELSEVIER
your source for books, journals and multimedia in the health sciences
www.elsevierhealth.com

ELSEVIER

Book Aid
International

Working together to grow libraries in developing countries

www.elsevier.com • www.bookaid.org

The Publisher's policy is to use
paper manufactured from sustainable forests

Contents

Section 1: Communication

Section 2: Psychosocial aspects of patient care

Contents

Section 3: Radiation hazards and safety

Section 4: Physical and medical aspects of patient safety

Section 5: Infection control

Section 6: Medical imaging procedures

Section 7: Cancer therapy procedures

Section 8: Performance and ethico-legal aspects of care

Contents

Foreword

Both medical imaging and radiotherapy utilise science and technology applied to patients. This means that to ensure each imaging event or radiotherapy treatment meets required standards, radiographers need extensive knowledge and understanding of the radiation sciences, anatomy, physiology and pathology, image interpretation and on the safe and effective use of available technologies. There are many texts that focus on these subjects but a successful examination or treatment outcome is dependent on the integration of each element of the process into a whole which means adaptation to unique patient circumstances.

Edited by Aarthi Ramlaul and Martin Vosper, both senior lecturers at the University of Hertfordshire *Patient Centred Care in Medical Imaging and Radiotherapy* puts the patient firmly in the centre. Both editors also contribute chapters in their own right but in putting the book together they are to be commended on their choice of other expert contributors. The choice of topics and the order in which they appear have clearly been well thought out. Divided into 8 sections with a total of 29 chapters the reader can easily work their way through from start to finish or alternatively easily locate a section or chapter to which they wish to refer. The format of each chapter is consistent; each beginning with an outline; subsections are clearly delineated and key points highlighted in boxed sections.

The book begins with a strong section on communication consisting of 4 chapters. Regrettably, we all hear accounts of instances where communication is not at its best but effective communication is a skill that no practitioner can be without. The text treats the topic with the importance it clearly deserves and is a message for all not just for some. All would do well to reflect on this key aspect of practice, even those who pride themselves on their communication skills are well advised to do so and avoid the danger of complacency. What better prompt for reflection than this book? Other sections cover psychosocial aspects of patient care, radiation hazards and safety, physical and mental aspects of patient safety, infection control, medical imaging procedures, cancer therapy procedures and performance and ethical legal aspects of care. All of these essentials put together provide the most comprehensive text of its kind in imaging and radiotherapy. Furthermore, if the reader wants to explore and read further they will be assisted by extensive reference and bibliography sections.

Publication of this book is timely in today's world of high expectations where patients and the public are better informed about medical imaging and radiotherapy. Practitioners surely realise that patients have different needs and that they have to be fully equipped to deal with a range of situations and expectations as well as the questions that will inevitably be asked. Sometimes expectations are unreasonably high but nevertheless practitioners have to handle such situations sensitively. Ultimately, it is for patients to decide and consent to whatever examination and/or treatment is recommended. Radiographers are part of that process of providing clear information on what can be expected at all stages of the particular procedure. In particular, practitioners have responsibility for a patient's safety when within their care; sections of the book deal comprehensively and without compromise on this important aspect of care.

A criticism that could be levelled at our profession is that we have focused for far too long on the technical aspects of an examination or treatment procedures. The book successfully addresses this issue and presents a clear message that it is time to give an equal hearing to the knowledge, understanding and skills necessary for interacting with the patient at the centre. It does not mean that technical and other skills are relegated in importance but it does mean that the ability to communicate with patients and their carers to assure a safe and effective examination or treatment is equally important. Overall the book delivers a strong message to would-be practitioners and practitioners alike. It reinforces the inescapable fact that a duty of care is owed to patients, their carers, the public and colleagues to deliver to the expected standard of care. Such responsibility gives rise to accountability for practice for which we all have to answer; consequences of failing to meet appropriate standards are explored in the final chapters.

Patient centred care is universal and there will be a demand for the book far beyond the United Kingdom. It will surely cater for the needs of students, learners and practitioners of all ages. For both undergraduate and post graduate students alike the book will be a must on reading lists. It will surely find its way onto the shelves of libraries and learning resource centres of colleges and universities wherever radiography education is delivered. The 29 chapters written by experts in their field will provide that vital underpinning knowledge so essential for both students at the start of their career and for practitioners wishing to revisit and reflect on their practice.

This new book fills a gap in the array of texts available to support radiography practice. It rightly puts the patient at the heart of medical imaging and radiotherapy. It provides thoughtful and deep consideration of a whole range of key topics and questions concerning care with the patient at the centre.

Professor Richard C. Price
Hatfield, UK

Introduction

What is *patient centred care*? Patient centred care is health service delivery which is focused on the needs and wishes of patients or clients. Both in medical imaging and radiotherapy, evaluation of service performance in the last century dwelt heavily on scientific measures, such as radiation doses, treatment volumes or objective image quality. There may have been a tendency in some quarters to regard patients as technical challenges rather than living consumers of healthcare with individual perspectives. Patient centred care entails working with people to identify their values, needs and expectations regarding their own health and social care; communicating with them providing the necessary information in an accessible manner; enabling shared decision-making; enabling informed consent; and permitting participation in the evaluation of their care. This has to have a positive impact on their overall care pathway and ultimate outcomes.

Recent government initiatives and publications have highlighted the need for practitioners to review service delivery, taking into account the needs of patients. In the UK, Lord Darzi, in his 2008 *NHS Next Stage Review*, noted that: *'if quality is at the heart of everything we do, it must be understood from the perspective of patients'*. The expectations of the government and the public have also changed – requirements are now higher than ever, with increasingly well-informed patients demanding greater service and accountability from the healthcare sector. However, workforce remodelling and changes in the economic climate have meant that practitioners face fresh challenges in providing care. Closure of some facilities and consolidation of others has meant that practitioners are faced with increasingly high workloads. This might result in a production line system of working, with limited time for patient communication and reassurance.

Service providers are being tasked with providing patient centred care. However, it is appreciated that not all users of the services we provide are patients: some are clients who use health promotion and health screening services, while others are carers and families of patients and clients. In this text however, for the purposes of providing material in an accessible manner, the term 'patient' has been used in a holistic sense for most parts of the text. Where the term 'patient' is used, this refers to users of the service we provide as practitioners.

The practice of medical imaging and radiotherapy is two-fold: one aspect involves a complex integration of technical skills and abilities in providing a diagnostic or therapeutic service. The other lies in providing high quality individual care to the patient. It is important that we as practitioners are able to fully meet the needs of the diverse patient population in our care. We have to ensure that we adhere to safe and ethical working practices, so that patients benefit from the services we provide. All too often, unnecessary lapses in communication, poor teamworking and failure to follow standard protocols have, in the past, led to patient harm. Patient safety is the cornerstone of high quality healthcare. It is said that sometimes making a small change can bring about a huge difference.

The aim of the text is to provide a broad coverage of care quality perspectives in all aspects of medical imaging and radiotherapy, within a single volume. Nursing procedures, except those relevant to the procedures detailed within the chapters, are outside the remit of this text and therefore have not been covered. The term 'practitioner' is used throughout the text in place of 'radiographer', 'radiotherapist' or 'radiologic technologist', except for explanatory purposes. All chapters begin by providing a brief outline of the chapter content and end with a list of key points made. References that contributors have used in the writing up of their chapters and their suggested further reading can be sought from the list of information sources in the 'Bibliography' and 'References' sections. A list of abbreviations and a glossary have also been provided for reference.

The text begins with a section on communication, opening with the principles that govern this. Student practitioners need to understand the philosophy and principles that underpin good communication in care. Communication with specific patient groups details the requirements for good practitioner–patient interaction when dealing with the elderly, children and adolescents, to mention only a few. The following chapter on communication with patients with disabilities and additional needs, gives key guidance on working with patients who have sensory impairments and learning disabilities, among others. The last chapter in this section gives an overview on the importance of inter-professional communication and collaboration in the work environment.

Section two has been written to take into account the psychosocial aspects of patient care, considering cultural and social diversity issues as well as issues following the diagnosis of cancer. End-of-life care has in the past been overlooked by many authors, and has been included in this section, as it is of the utmost importance that the patient and their relatives are afforded special care and considerations throughout any medical imaging or treatment procedure.

Sections three and four are concerned with the physical and scientific basis of safety in medical imaging and radiotherapy. There is coverage of the potential effects and hazards of ionising radiations, sound, magnetic fields, drugs and contrast agents. The side-effects of radiotherapy are included. Additionally, the safety aspects of patient moving and handling are explored.

Section five takes into account the commonly encountered pathogens that present risks to patients and the methods of infection prevention that can be applied by practitioners. Guidance on the correct use of protective clothing, hand-washing and gloving techniques is provided.

Sections six and seven cover patient care issues pertinent to specific branches of medical imaging and cancer therapy. Expansion in technologies has brought about an increasing number of specialist areas with their own considerations.

Section eight explores available means of measuring and validating care quality, as well as the professional ethico-legal principles which underpin medical imaging and radiotherapy practice. The Code of Conduct and Ethics has been included within the chapter in its entirety for ease of reference.

This book is aimed particularly at radiography students working in medical imaging or radiotherapy and is intended as a handbook of good practice in patient care. It should also be relevant to allied health practitioners who wish to maintain and update their knowledge. We hope you find this text a useful resource and wish you well in your studies and careers.

Aarthi Ramlaul and Martin Vosper
April 2013

Acknowledgements

The editors would like to thank all contributors for their creative energies during the production of this text. This includes a number of colleagues from the University of Hertfordshire.

In addition we would like to thank the following persons for the development of the online materials accessible through *Evolve:*

- Selina Fowler, Senior Lecturer at the University of Hertfordshire; and Sarah Mercer, Reporting Radiographer, for the medical imaging patient care case study scenarios

- Marie McCabe, Consultant Radiographer at the Edinburgh Cancer Centre; and Maureen Thomson & Karen Moore, Consultant Radiographers at the Beatson West of Scotland Cancer Centre, for the radiotherapy patient care case study scenarios.

Contributors

Segun S. Adeyemi, MA RT(R)
Senior Lecturer, Diagnostic Radiography and Imaging, University of Hertfordshire, Hatfield, UK

Naomi Brown, MSc BSc(Hons) PGCert
Senior Lecturer and Ultrasound Course Leader, University of Hertfordshire, Hatfield, UK

Hilary Bungay, PhD MA HDCR PGCLT
Senior Lecturer, Allied Health & Medicine, Anglia Ruskin University, Cambridge, UK

Louisa Clark, MSc BSc(Hons)
Senior Lecturer, Radiotherapy and Oncology, University of Hertfordshire, Hatfield, UK

Suzanne Easton, MSc PGCertEd PGCert BSc(Hons)
Senior Lecturer in Diagnostic Imaging, University of the West of England, Bristol, UK

Andrew England, MSc PGCert BSc(Hons)
Lecturer in Medical Imaging, University of Liverpool, Liverpool, UK

Terri Gilleece, MSc PgD PgCHEP DCR(T)
Lecturer, Radiotherapy & Oncology, School of Health Sciences, University of Ulster, Newtownabbey, UK

Samantha Glendinning, PGCert BSc(Hons) FHEA
Senior Lecturer, Radiotherapy and Oncology, University of Hertfordshire, Hatfield, UK

Tracey A. Gregory, MA PGCert Ed BSc(Hons)
Senior Lecturer in Radiography, University of Derby, Derby, UK

Laureen Hemming, PGCEA Bphil BA(Open) RGN DipN RCNT
Senior Lecturer and Specialist Tutor, Oncology Nursing and Palliative Care, University of Hertfordshire, Hatfield, UK

Suzanne M. Henwood, PhD MSc PGCE HDCR DCR
Associate Professor, Department of Medical Imaging, Faculty of Social and Health Sciences, Unitec, Auckland, New Zealand

Johnathan Hewis, PgDip PGCert BSc(Hons) FHEA
Senior Lecturer, Medical Imaging, School of Medical and Applied Sciences, Faculty of Sciences, Engineering and Health, Central Queensland University, Queensland, Australia

Ciara M. Hughes, PhD MMedSc BSc
Lecturer in Clinical Physiology, School of Health Sciences, University of Ulster, Newtownabbey, UK

Pauline Humphrey, MSc DCR(T)
Consultant Radiographer for Brachytherapy, Bristol Haematology and Oncology Centre, Bristol, UK

Jenny Lorimer, MA HDCR(R) DCR(R)
Senior Lecturer, Diagnostic Radiography and Imaging, University of Hertfordshire, Hatfield, UK

Melanie Mansfield, MA PGCert PGCHE BSc(Hons)
Senior Lecturer, Diagnostic Radiography and Imaging, University of Hertfordshire, Hatfield, UK

Paula McClean, BSc(Hons)
Senior Lecturer, Radiotherapy and Oncology, University of Hertfordshire, Hatfield, UK

Stephanie R. McKeown, PhD MA CBiol, FSB
Emeritus Professor of Cancer Biology, University of Ulster, Newtownabbey, UK

Toni Meyer, MA BSc(Hons)
Senior Lecturer, Diagnostic Radiography and Imaging, University of Hertfordshire, Hatfield, UK

Pauline Mitchell, MUS MA PGDip BSc(Hons) DCR(R)
Senior Lecturer, Sheffield Hallam University, Sheffield, UK

Leonie Munro, MA PgDip ND:DiagRad(SA) Pub Admin Cert for Trainers
MarLeo's Communication Services CC, South Africa; Retired Radiographer

Elaine Parry-Jones, PGCert BSc(Hons)
Senior Lecturer and Radiotherapy Clinical Lead, University of Hertfordshire, Hatfield, UK

F.I. Peer, ND:Rad(Diag) ND:Rad(Nuc Med) NHD:Rad (Nuc Med) BTech:Rad MTech:Rad DTech:Rad
Manager, Nuclear Medicine, Inkosi Albert Luthuli Central Hospital, Durban, South Africa

Bridget Mary Porritt, PGDip BSc(Hons)
University Teacher, Radiotherapy, University of Liverpool, UK

Aarthi Ramlaul, MA BTechRad NDipRad
Principal Lecturer, Diagnostic Radiography and Imaging, University of Hertfordshire, Hatfield, UK

Pauline J. Reeves, PhD MSc PGDip PGCert TDCR
Associate Lecturer in Diagnostic Radiography, Sheffield Hallam University, Sheffield, UK

Murray Schofield, PGCert BSc
Specialist Radiographer, York District Hospital, and Lecturer, Sheffield Hallam University, UK

Sindy Singh, DCR(T)
Education and Training Supervisor, Radiotherapy, Charing Cross Hospital, London, UK

Aladdin Speelman, MAppSci: Med Imaging/CT BTech Rad (D) NHDip: PSE ND: Rad (D)
Lecturer: Radiography Education (Diagn), Cape Peninsula University of Technology, Cape Town, South Africa

Martin Vosper, MSc PGDip BSc(Hons) HDCR(R)
Senior Lecturer, Diagnostic Radiography and Imaging, University of Hertfordshire, Hatfield, UK

Patsy Whelehan, MSc DCR
Senior Research Radiographer, University of Dundee Ninewells Hospital and Medical School, Dundee, UK

Kimberly Williamson, BSc(Hons)
Practice Educator, Oncology, Northampton General Hospital, Northampton, UK

Saminah Yunis, MSc PGCert DCR(R)
Trainee Consultant Radiographer, Gastrointestinal/Fluoroscopy, Mid-Yorkshire NHS Trust, West Yorkshire UK

List of abbreviations

3D—three dimensional (volume)
4D—four dimensional (moving volume)
5-FU—5-fluorouracil
5-HT—5-hydroxytryptamine
A&E—accident and emergency department
ACE—angiotensin converting enzyme
AEC—automatic exposure control
ALARA—as low as reasonably achievable
ALARP—as low as reasonably practicable
ANTT—aseptic non-touch technique
AP—antero-posterior
ASTRAL—angioplasty and stent for renal artery lesions
BCG—Bacillus Calmette – Guérin
BMUS—British Medical Ultrasound Society
BPM—best practical means
BSL—British sign language
CAM—complementary and alternative medicine
CAS—coronary artery stent
CBD—common bile duct
CD—cluster of differentiation (for example in CD52 antigen)
C-diff—*Clostridium difficile*
CHART—continuous hyper-fractionated accelerated radiotherapy
CIN—contrast-induced nephropathy
CKD—chronic kidney disease
CPD—continuing professional development
CR—computed radiography
CRF—cancer related fatigue
CSF—cerebrospinal fluid
CT—computed tomography
CTC—common toxicity criteria
CTU—computed tomographic urography
CTZ—chemoreceptor trigger zone
CVS—chorionic villus sampling
dB—decibels
DCBE—double contrast barium enema
DDA—Disability Discrimination Act
DDR—direct digital radiography
DES—drug eluting stent
DMSA—dimercaptosuccinic acid

DNA—deoxyribonucleic acid
DoH/ DH—Department of Health
DPD—dihydropyrimidine
DRL—diagnostic reference level
DSM IV—Diagnostic and Statistical Manual, 4th edition
DTPA—diethylene triamine pentaacetic acid
DVT—deep vein thrombosis
EBRT—external beam radiotherapy
ECG—electrocardiogram
EMF—electromagnetic field
EoLC—end-of-life care
EORTC—European Organisation for Research and Treatment
ER—Estrogen receptor
ErbB2—erythroblastic leukemia viral oncogene homologue 2
ERCP—endoscopic retrograde cholangiopancreatogram
ESUR—European Society for Urogenital Radiology
FDG—fluorodeoxyglucose
FNA—fine needle aspiration
FNAB—fine needle aspiration biopsy
GFR—glomerular filtration rate
GABA—gamma-aminobutyric acid
GI—gastro-intestinal
GP—general practitioner
GTN—gliceryl trinitrate
GU—genito-urinary
Gy—gray
HCAI—healthcare associated infections
HCC—hepatocellular carcinoma
HCP—healthcare professional
HDR—high dose rate
HIDA—hepatobiliary iminodiacetic acid
HIV—human immunodeficiency virus
HMPAO—hexamethylpropylene amine oxime
HOCM—high osmolar contrast medium
HPA—Health Protection Agency
HCPC—Health Care Professions Council
HPV—Human papilloma virus
HSG—hysterosalpingogram

ICNIRP—International Commission on Non-Ionising Radiation Protection
ICRP—International Commission on Radiological Protection
ICRU—International Commission on Radiation Units and Measurements
ICU—intensive care unit
IEC—International Electrotechnical Commission
IMRT—intensity modulated radiotherapy
IOFB—intraocular foreign body
IR—interventional radiology
IR(ME) R—Ionising Radiations (Medical Exposure) Regulations
IRR—Ionising Radiations Regulations
IUD—intrauterine device
JOL—justification, optimisation and limitation
kHz—kilohertz
kV—kilovolts
LDL—low density lipoproteins
LDR—low dose rate
LFT—liver function test
LH—luteinising hormone
LH—luteinising hormone releasing hormone
LOCM—low osmolar contrast medium
mA—milliamps
MAA—macroaggregated serum albumin
MAb—monoclonal antibody
MAG3—mercaptoacetylglycylglyclglycine
MARS—Medicines (Adminstration of Radioactive Substances) Regulations
MDA—medical devices agency
MDCT—multidetector computed tomography
MDRD—modification of diet in renal disease equation
MDP—methylene diphosphonate
MDT—multidisciplinary team
mg—milligram
mGy—milligray
MIBG—metaiodobenzylguanidine
mL—millilitre
MLC—multileaf collimator
MHRA—Medicines and Heathcare products Regulatory Agency
MHz—megahertz
MI—mechanical index
MMR—measles, mumps and rubella
MPI—myocardial perfusion imaging
MR—magnetic resonance and also modified release of drugs
MRI—magnetic resonance imaging
mRNA—messenger ribonucleic acid
MRSA—methicillin-resistant *Staphylococcus aureus*
MS—multiple sclerosis
MSK—musculoskeletal
mSv—milliSievert

mT—milliTesla
MUGA—multigated acquisition
NCSI—National Cancer Survivorship Initiative
NHS—National Health Service
NHSBSP—National Health Service Breast Screening Programme
NICE—National Institute for Clinical Excellence
NLP—neurolinguistic programming
NPSA—National Patient Safety Agency
NRPB—National Radiological Protection Board
NSAID—non steroidal anti-inflammatory drug
NSF—nephrogenic systemic fibrosis
NTC—normal tissue complication rate
OAR—organ at risk
P53—a tumour suppressor gene
PA—postero-anterior
PACS—picture archiving and communication system
PAD—peripheral artery disease
PCA—patient-controlled analgesia
PCN—percutaneous nephrostomy
PEG—percutaneous endoscopic gastrostomy
PES—post-embolisation syndrome
PET—positron emission tomography
PGD—patient group direction
PIE—percutaneous ethanol injection
POPUMET—protection of patients undergoing medical examination or treatment
PRG—percutaneous radiological gastrostomy
PTA—percutaneous transluminal angioplasty
PTBD—percutaneous transhepatic biliary drainage
PTC—percutaneous transhepatic cholangiogram
PTV—planned target volume
QA—quality assurance
RBC—red blood cell
RBE—relative biological effectiveness
RCT—randomised controlled trial
RES—reticuloendothelial system
RF—radiofrequency
RIDDOR—Reporting of Injuries, Diseases and Dangerous Occurrences Regulations
RIG—radiologically inserted gastrostomy
RIS—radiology information system
RNA—ribonucleic acid
RNID—Royal Institute for the Deaf (now Action on Hearing Loss)
RPA—radiation protection advisor
RPS—radiation protection supervisor
RTA—road traffi c accident
RTOG—radiation oncology / toxicity grading
SA—*Staphylococcus aureus*
SAR—specific absorption rate
SARS—severe acute respiratory syndrome
SCr—serum creatinine
SNR—signal to noise ratio
SCoR—Society and College of Radiographers

List of abbreviations

SPECT—single photon emission computed tomography
SPIO—superparamagnetic iron oxide
Sv—Sievert
SWL—safe working load
T1 —longitudinal relaxation time in MRI
T2 —transverse relaxation time in MRI
TA—transactional analysis
TB—tubercle bacillus
TCP—tumour cure probability
TD—transdermal, also tolerance dose
TDS—time, distance and shielding
TI—thermal index
TLD—thermoluminescent dosimetry

TNF—tumour necrosis factor
TPA—tissue plasminogen activator
TSH—thyroid stimulating hormone
UAE—uterine artery embolisation
UK—United Kingdom
UKAS—United Kingdom Association of Ultrasonographers
µmol—micromoles
US—ultrasound
UTI—urinary tract infection
VF—ventricular fibrillation
WBC—white blood cell
WHO—World Health Organisation

Section | 1 |

Communication

Chapter | 1 |

Principles of communication

Suzanne M. Henwood, Leonie Munro

INTRODUCTION

The main role of healthcare professionals is to deliver high quality services to patients, often in difficult and emotive situations. Communication is a central and fundamental part of achieving this[1] and there has been much recent emphasis on patient centred communication and care,[2-4] as well as on the role of relationships in patient care.[5]

It is well documented that communication between some health professionals and patients can be poor, for a range of reasons, including lack of the necessary skills.[6-11] It is claimed that health professionals often do not revisit communication training following qualification, despite the fact that communication skills training shows a positive impact on behaviours[12] and that relational skills may decline post-qualification.[13]

The fast interaction times of emergency departments and some other specialty doctors, which are similar to the interaction times of medical imaging, pose particular problems;[14-15] it is clear from the literature that there is no one 'magic bullet' to solve all communication problems.

Effective communication is vital between healthcare professionals and patients.[6] There is a need for an effective patient–professional relationship and hence, there should be an understanding of the principles and role of verbal and non-verbal communication. The latter can be divided into paralinguistics, proxemics and kinesics. These will now be explained:

Paralinguistics refer to voice, pitch, stresses and pauses during verbal communication. *Proxemics* refers to the perception of use of personal, social and public space during person-to-person interactions. *Kinesics* refers to body movements, gestures, posture, etc. during communication.[6] Patient needs are both physical and psychological, and other aspects, such as patient compliance and outcomes, should be taken into account.[11,16-19]

Verbal and non-verbal communication[11,18,20] help to foster openness, rapport and trust between practitioner and patient, and that is vital to effective patient care.

If we look specifically at radiography, practitioners need to consider communication with patients, before, during and after undertaking the required examinations or treatments. For example, patients are asked to confirm their personal details prior to the examination or treatment; they are also informed of what to expect during any examination or treatment and are instructed on any breathing or positional requirements. Following the completion of the examination, the practitioner informs the patient of the expected time of the results. Increasingly, practitioners are also expected to offer an opinion on findings. There is an assumption within such interactions, that the practitioner and the patient interacted with full understanding of each other. However, evidence suggests that this is not always the case, with communication complaints across healthcare being well publicised.[21-23] In fact, communication complaints are more common than complaints about technical issues.[24] Communication failings are also often a common reason for safety errors, which can result in medical mistakes.[25-26]

Greater understanding of the range and types of communication used in patient and staff interactions, together with an appreciation of the factors which influence those interactions, would reduce the chance of any misunderstanding and increase the effectiveness of healthcare communication.

WHAT IS COMMUNICATION?

There are numerous definitions of communication but to date, there has not been an agreed universal one, despite the large amount of research into healthcare communication, which has emerged in the last 30 years.[28] Some authors have attempted to define communication within the differing contexts of the workplace,[18,29-30] while others have offered communication frameworks, which contain four key components: (1) the interaction; (2) the people; (3) the process and (4) the environment.[31-32] Modern communication may include verbal, non-verbal, written or digital elements. Also, health professionals must adjust their own communication style to that of the patient in order to improve efficiency and satisfaction for both.[34] Good communication is necessary to create therapeutic relationships, manage health problems and gain clients' confidence. It is also true that patients both 'need to know' and 'need to be known'.[35]

Communication is a complex, dynamic process that involves creating, exchanging and sharing thoughts, ideas, emotions and information;[6,37] it needs to be unambiguous.[38] For our needs, we need a definition that is flexible and appropriate within a complex and rapidly changing health context.

What is clear, is that communication is individual in nature and will change depending on: the age of a patient;[39-41] speaking, hearing or visual impairments;[42] educational background;[43] cultural history;[44-45] language[46] and any specific situations[41,47-49] including abusive backgrounds,[50] end-of-life[33] or mental health.[51] Each interaction has to be tailored specifically to the patient; which often is not the case.[47] Patient preferences in communication also have to be considered.[48] Communication can be described as being socially constructed and evolving in use, specific to the people and the context in which it emerges.[47]

Communication can also be with oneself. When one holds a mental conversation with oneself, such as meditating or day-dreaming, planning or decision-making, this is termed 'intra-communication'. Intra-communication is a vital, but often overlooked aspect in a practical healthcare context. The words we say, the pictures we create and the meaning we assign to signals, determine our behaviour and therefore cannot be overlooked.

Inter-communication involves two or more persons and uses concepts such as sender and receiver. A 'sender' is a person using words, signs and symbols to interact with the 'receiver', in order to share and exchange ideas, thoughts, etc. The interchange between sender and receiver becomes a 'dance', as each interacts with the response of the other and 'shared meaning' is hopefully created. This is where strong internal views and poor listening become evident, as each person involved may dance 'in solo' and, misunderstandings can occur when each party assumes the other has fully understood the signs and symbols being shared, although in reality a very different internal representation of those signs and symbols has been created. We may not take the time to check out our interpretations with the person with whom we are communicating.

Another consideration is that, increasingly, mass communication is being used to portray health-related information and this includes media: radio, printed and online press, mobile communications, e-mail and social networking sites, television, etc.[52-53] The presence of huge numbers of receiving viewers or listeners, along with the technology involved, further complicates the communication process and increases the chances for miscommunication. Even within the relatively simple face-to-face and one-to-one context, there is no one simple process that fully explains the enormously complex, individual and dynamic process that is communication. Having said that, there are some well researched, clearly defined components of communication which are important to explain and which impact on communication effectiveness, some of which we will now consider.

Verbal and non-verbal communication

We use verbal and non-verbal communication in both formal and informal situations. From the moment of birth, an infant interacts and expresses itself by using vocal cords to cry and make noises.[54-55] The child then progresses to using simple words to communicate, based on the language spoken within the family. Verbal communication refers to the use of our vocal cords to produce sound and spoken words. Words on their own are meaningless however, unless we can interpret their meaning; this requires sharing the same language and internal references as the speaker.[54] Shared meaning is not guaranteed in communication, especially between people with different backgrounds and cultures. Language is not always verbal and can also include sign language or written forms of communication.[54]

Non-verbal communication can include, e.g. gestures, facial expressions, tone of voice, dress code and posture.[6] Each element acts as a 'filter' through which communication is interpreted. While some cultural groups share some of those filters, there is controversy in the literature as to whether some gestures are truly pancultural[57] or culture specific;[37,58] also whether gestures are learned or innate behaviour.[37] It would seem there is some agreement that all infants instinctively point to things, indicating that some shared gestures are cross-cultural, but in complex, adult communication, there is much which remains unknown.

This is further complicated by any impairment to normal communication, such as deafness, blindness or mental incapacity, or those under sedation[51] (see also Chapter 5, Cultural and social diversity issues in patient care).

It is suggested that humans use gestures more than spoken language to communicate and that the actual words contribute to only a small percentage of the meaning of any communication, alongside tone of voice and non-verbal behaviour.[59] Also, as we all know, there may be a difference between 'what is said' and 'how it is said' and this can be especially important in a healthcare setting.[60] Patients may pick-up on a tone of voice and suffer anxiety or misapprehension, e.g. during the narration of news or results. It would thus be good practice for a patient to have both a verbal explanation, as well as written information to reinforce the meaning of what is being conveyed to them.[11]

Demonstrations can also be useful; practitioners often use practise sessions to demonstrate breathing requirements[61] to those patients who, for a range of reasons, fail to follow verbal instructions. This also involves checking that such an instruction has been correctly interpreted by the patient.[11] We now extend this discussion to the use of some common signs and symbols and their use as communication codes.

Signs, symbols and codes

Some authors do not make a distinction between the meaning of signs and symbols[62] but they are usually taken to mean different things.[62-63] Signs are used in all communication. A sign can be anything: a colour, a frown, a punctuation mark, a mathematical formula, etc., but does not have an innate 'meaning' of its own because it signifies something else.[54-62] Let us consider the colour green, which comprises the alphabet letters of 'g-r-e-e-n' that on their own do not signify anything. Green as a sign can stand for many things: as a traffic signal, it is the colour that indicates when a driver can proceed; in nature, it is a signal of growth; it could be a figure of speech to indicate feeling nauseous ('he looked really green') or to signal inexperience, such as the new intake of radiography students are still 'green'.

Signs can be considered as two-part entities, with a physical part, the 'signifier', and a conceptual part, the 'signified'.[54] It is clear that what is signified might not be the same to all people. For example a nod of the head can mean 'yes' in some cultures and 'no' in others, with potential confusion. Signs can also be thought of as three-part in nature: the physical sign itself, the object or event being signified and the mental interpretation of the consequence of that linkage. There can be considered to be three types of signs: icons, indexes and symbols.[54] An icon resembles the item being signified, e.g. a drawing or photograph. A sign is an index when there is causal connection between the signifier and signified. A doctor, for example, could on clinical examination of a patient who presents with a right-sided abdominal pain – signifier – interpret this as possible appendicitis – signified. Clearly, there needs to be agreement between healthcare staff as to the meaning of indexes.

A sign is a symbol when it can be encoded based on an agreement or convention. There are many examples of symbols on the control panels in medical imaging or radiotherapy rooms. Misinterpretation of symbols could have unfortunate consequences when staff examine patients' medical records or use equipment.

Signs do not function in isolation, they require a system to be encoded and decoded. As communication requires encoding and decoding, it is obvious that creating and interpreting messages require the use of codes. A code system comprises an agreed structure. When we speak, we use language as a code which requires the signs to be used in a specific order for encoding and decoding to occur. A code is learned and shared by members of a communicating group. When student health professionals commence their training they have to learn to decode and encode signs used by healthcare personnel who share and use the signs of the hospital code.[64] Examples of communication codes include: dress codes, pictorial codes, social codes, tactile codes, Morse code and language. We now turn to meaning in communication, based on some communication models.

Communication models

Various models are used to discuss human communication, depending on the field of research. Shannon and Weaver's signs of the hospital[36] theory of mathematical communication gives it as: a source which sends a message via a transmitter using a channel, which could be subject to interference or 'noise', to a receiver used at the destination.[11] This model has limitations – it tells us nothing about meaning and understanding of a message in terms of the dynamic interaction between the participants. However, as health professionals, we should take note of their concept of 'noise' because it can interfere with message transmission and we should strive to reduce anything that may interfere with our interactions with role players. Apart from noise, there are other factors that act as barriers in communication, such as the tendency to evaluate and judge another person's statement or failing to listen to what is being said.[65]

We will now return to what is involved in the decoding and encoding of messages in order to understand their meaning. Several steps are involved in human communication between a sender and receiver: a sender decodes signs by using at least a one code system to send a message to someone else, who, in turn, encodes the message and ascribes meaning to it. There is no guarantee that the intended meaning is interpreted correctly but usually, there should be shared meaning if the communicating parties share the used code systems. It should be noted that not all messages are understood by all members of a shared social or cultural group, even though they share common backgrounds,[56] since each person has personal meanings for signs. We all have different life experiences based on denotative and connotative meanings. Meaning needs to be contextualised and thus, health professionals use specific signs (jargon)[66] in the medical code to share and exchange information. This jargon can effectively exclude non-professionals from understanding the information. Participants attach 'denotative' and 'connotative' meanings to the signs used. A dictionary contains denotative meanings as there is an unambiguous and very conventional relationship between a sign and its referent.[54] Connotative meanings, such as feelings, implications and associations arise from the denotative meaning.[54] Each participant attributes denotative and connotative meanings to messages based on life experiences. Let us consider a possible connotative meaning of the word 'exposure'. To a practitioner, an 'exposure' might be an X-ray emission, while to the public, an 'exposure' might imply that someone has experienced freezing cold, germs or hazardous substances.

Two other popular models are TA (transactional analysis) and NLP (neurolinguistic programming) but neither model is evidenced across all training and development literature in radiography. TA was originally developed in the 1960s[67] and has been related directly to, and advocated in radiography by Booth[68] as a model which could be used to enhance communication skills. TA refers to styles of interpersonal communication and focuses on a process, rather than a structural model of communication. The familiar three ego state model is used as a basis (parent, adult, child); each ego state having a discreet function (parent – controlling and nurturing; adult – logic and reasoning; and child – free/fun and adapted/conforming).[68]

Practitioners require training in TA along with showing individual effort to apply that learning in practice to increase their self-awareness of the three ego states and their potential contribution to any situation. This is most likely to be useful in a reflective manner, following any difficult interaction, rather than being used in the moment, at least until the practitioner has become an expert in TA.

The aims of the NLP communication model are to assist practitioners to become self-empowered and take responsibility for their contribution to each interaction.[69] The model focuses on how individual practitioners communicate with themselves; how that determines behaviours in practice, as well as how to communicate effectively with others. This model is a functional and process-orientated model, exploring the internal processing of information and explaining how each individual has a unique representation of any 'reality'. It explains how no two people will share completely a description of the external event being considered. It also describes the link from communication processes to how we feel, and our physiology, highlighting the dynamic, holistic, interactive nature of internal communication. It explores deeper aspects of values and beliefs and a range of individual filters, which determine behaviour and outcome, offering a powerful mechanism to reflect on, understand and change behaviour, if practitioners are honest and open with themselves about what is actually happening.

KEY POINTS

- Communication is a complex and dynamic process, hence researchers have used different models in their studies to explore and explain its process
- Looking at the range of models and the scope of using all five senses to communicate, and the individual nature of each person within any interaction – and within a health context the complexity and importance of the interactions – it is not surprising that sometimes when we reflect on outcomes, we may find areas where we could have been more effective
- As healthcare practitioners, with a passion to centre on and improve patient care, it is an on-going, continual process to develop and grow in the area of communication
- As healthcare professionals, we have the added responsibility of using our communication in a context where patients are vulnerable and in need of extra care

Chapter | 2 |

Communication with specific patient groups

Pauline J. Reeves

INTRODUCTION

The patient centred model of care in radiography (Fig. 2.1) was derived from research with practitioners and represents a philosophy of care which places the patient at the centre of the examination, allowing the patient's needs to dictate the process.[1] Both medical imaging examination times and radiotherapy treatments are relatively short, making good communication skills imperative; nowhere is this need more apparent than when we are working with young, elderly or otherwise vulnerable patients, such as cancer patients or those suffering from multiple injuries.

Radiotherapy practitioners are likely to see their patients over an extended period, such as 5 weeks while treatment is carried out, but medical imaging practitioners often will never see their patients again. There is, therefore, no opportunity to rebuild the relationship if the imaging encounter goes badly. This is especially crucial with children, whose bad memories of their X-ray examination are likely to affect their next meeting with a practitioner. Medical imaging practitioners also have to work hard to keep the patient, rather than the image, at the centre of their practice. Similarly, radiotherapy practitioners may become more focussed on getting their treatment parameters set up

than centring their attention on the patient who is being treated; in both cases, this distancing from the patient may act as an emotional safeguard for the practitioner, but can mean that the patient may perceive their care as less than optimal.

This chapter will use the concepts of patient assessment, care and communication from the patient centred model outlined in Figure 2.1 to examine how best we might place any one of these patients at the centre of the examination process. Patient assessment is about initial contact with the individual whereby the practitioner assesses things such as clinical information, signs and symptoms, but also the ability of the patient to cooperate with the examination and/or to take in information.[1] It is this assessment stage that reinforces the need for the practitioner to have excellent communication skills. Other health professionals such as doctors and nurses may take up to 45 minutes to assess their patients, whereas the majority of radiographic encounters in total are of a much shorter length than this. The practitioner typically has 2–3 minutes to assess their patient and gain their cooperation and only about 7–10 minutes to complete the whole examination in most cases. Patient care and communication are linked concepts – one cannot provide good patient care in radiography without the communication skills already referred to. We will look at how these three concepts apply in the cases of particular groups of patients.

CHANGED EMOTIONAL STATUS – THE CANCER PATIENT

Several studies have examined the needs and experiences of cancer patients, especially women with breast cancer[2-4] (see Chapter 22, Mammography). Practitioners themselves have written about how being recalled for additional

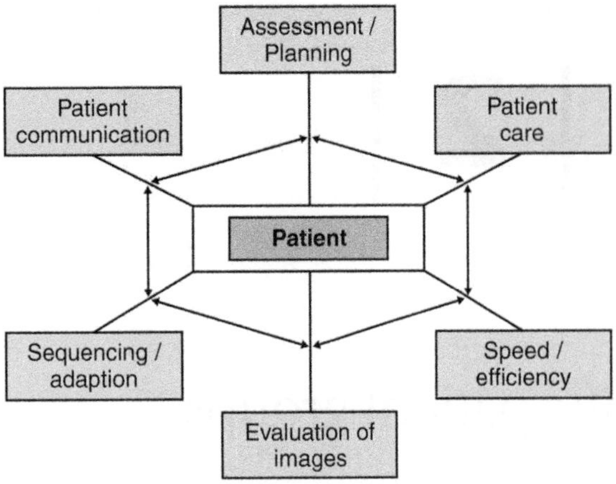

Figure 2.1 Patient centred model of radiography.[1] *(From; Reeves PJ. (1999) Models of Care for Diagnostic Radiography and Their Use in the Education of Undergraduate and Postgraduate Students. PhD thesis. Bangor: University of Wales).*

mammographic views after a screening appointment can be a shattering experience.[5-6] The individual's self-image as healthy is immediately threatened and one of the overwhelming feelings that patients report is one of loss of control.[5-7]

> ! The initial contact with the patient is crucial, whether attending for imaging or to begin a course of radiotherapy; in one study respondents stated that they wanted practitioners to introduce themselves, to explain their roles and to keep up a continuous flow of information during the procedure.[2]

While the patient may not take it in all at once, the provision of information helps the individual feel as if they are regaining some control over the situation.[7] Failure to respond to the patient's questions may be seen as deliberate withholding of information or dishonesty.[2] Initial assessment of the patient by the practitioner as to their emotional status may be difficult as patients with, or potentially awaiting, a cancer diagnosis go through a range of different emotions, including anxiety, grief, powerlessness and dread.[2-3] In these cases, patients may typically experience a sense of 'fear' about forthcoming radiotherapy treatment.[4]

Researchers also reported that the experiences of having radiotherapy and of being recalled for further mammographic screening, or additional views, reinforced the isolation of having a malignant disease. Even when treatment had been successful, there was always the fear of whether it would return.[2,4] In terms of patient care and communication, fear may manifest itself in a number of ways: the

patient may be very quiet and withdrawn or, in contrast, they may be snappy and even aggressive. As one patient stated, the practitioner 'should be prepared to receive whatever my response is. That is different for everybody'.[2]

> ! The radiotherapy practitioner needs to be mindful of the impact of the technology on those who start a course of radiotherapy. A linear accelerator is a huge piece of equipment, which most patients will never have come into contact with previously.[3]

In addition to this initial impact is the fact that the patient is left on their own during treatment. One patient described her experience as 'white knuckle riding' as she held tightly onto the equipment and 'counting the seconds' as the treatment took place.[4] Patients utilise different coping strategies to deal with the experience of radiotherapy but the practitioner needs to be alert to cues that suggest the ability to cope may be breaking down. Look out for patients who need emotional support; there may be signs of tearfulness or a patient who may linger at the end of a treatment and want to talk. A number of publications warn practitioners against becoming too concerned with the pressures of throughput and the potential for becoming too engrossed in the technology.[8] While we accept that technology is at the heart of what we do, for patients the environment can be very depersonalising, e.g. one patient talked about feeling 'like a piece of meat on a slab'.[3,8]

To summarise therefore, patients would like practitioners to give them as much information as possible, as this helps them feel in control of, what can be, a very scary situation. The practitioner should assess the patient at the start of the examination or treatment, watching for any signs that the patient may need emotional support and permitting them to express any concerns. It is important that the patient is made to feel that the practitioner understands what they are going through and is there to provide support where it is needed.

CHANGED PHYSICAL STATUS – THE TRAUMA PATIENT

A large part of the work of the medical imaging practitioner is undertaken with patients suffering from minor or major trauma. It is critical that the practitioner assesses the patient before commencing the examination because it is, unfortunately, the case that many patients from the A&E department may be intoxicated and/or may have taken drugs. In either case, this could well affect the patient's ability to cooperate with the examination. The actual behaviour manifested by the patient is subject to considerable variation and the practitioner needs to be alert to the potential for bizarre and even violent behaviour.[9] Such behaviours may include any or all of the following:

* Unexplained change in personality or attitude
* Sudden mood swings, irritability or angry outbursts
* Periods of unusual hyperactivity, agitation or giddiness
* Lack of motivation; appears lethargic or 'spaced out'
* Appears fearful, anxious or paranoid[10]

It is this variation in potential reactions that demonstrates the need for patient centred care; the practitioners must take their cues from the patient as to how to proceed with the examination and should not be afraid, if all else fails, to send the patient back to A&E with a request for them to be given time to sober up, when appropriate. Examinations, such as those of facial bones, are a waste of time if the patient cannot keep still during positioning.

Practitioners should get into the habit of asking trauma patients how the injury occurred. History-taking may point towards the need for particular views: 'punching a wall' (*aka* 'I've been in a fight'!) indicates a possible 'Boxer's fracture' of the 5th metacarpal, in which case a lateral projection of the hand should be undertaken in addition to postero-anterior (PA) and oblique projections of the hand.[11] The mechanism of injury is also very useful information for the practitioner or radiologist who is doing the definitive report, as they are unlikely to have seen the patient themselves and therefore must be noted on the picture archiving and communication system (PACS).

> **!** The simple act of enquiring how the injury took place also indicates to the patient an interest in what happened to them. Research has shown that it is the attitude of staff (including interpersonal skills and provision of information) rather than the actual task of treating the patient, which engenders a perception of high quality care.[12]

There are three types of communication used in the trauma situation:[13]

1. Formal communication: used to convey information about the course of events. In a radiographic context, this might include information about the projections to be undertaken and the positions which the patient needs to adopt.
2. Diverting communication: while still connected to the examination, this type of communication was described as 'free and easy'. It is used to take the patient's mind off what is happening and may include enquiries about the patient's family or other information such as what they do for a living or how the accident happened.
3. Humoristic communication: the use of humour tends to be used after the main examination has taken place and may be initiated by the practitioner or the patient. Humour can be very powerful in putting the patient at ease, but needs to be used with care to avoid offence.[13]

Table 2.1 Levels of consciousness[15]

Level of consciousness	Signs
Fully conscious	Aware of surroundings Able to reply to questions Engages in conversation
Drowsy	Answers direct questions Obeys commands Responds vaguely when addressed
Stupor	Responds to pain stimulus Appears unaware of surroundings Makes no response when addressed
Coma (complete unconsciousness)	Makes no response, even to painful stimuli

In another study of nurses working in acute trauma, researchers identified that the nurses used a specific speech style or tone of voice, which they termed 'comfort talk', which was used in response to expressions of pain, fear or lack of understanding by the patient and served four main functions:[14]

1. To help patients 'hold on' or bear the pain
2. To get information from the patient
3. To explain procedures
4. To communicate a sense of caring to the patient.[14]

Examples of the types of phrases used included: 'You're doing great'; 'Hang in there'; 'Where does it hurt?'; 'Can you sit up for me?' etc. Such phrases are also utilised in medical imaging and radiotherapy departments; it is said that these short, often rhythmical phrases are easy for the patient to perceive and are used with all ages. Comfort talk may be used to distract children during procedures. The voice intonation may also be slower and louder than in normal conversation, with clearly marked pauses.[14]

With all trauma patients, the practitioner needs to be alert to a change in the patient's level of consciousness (Table 2.1) and should be ready to initiate resuscitation procedures if required.

Changes in levels of consciousness should be reported to staff in the A&E Department when the patient is returned. The practitioner should continue to talk to the patient, even if they appear to be fully unconscious, as research has shown that hearing is the last sense to go.[16] This also applies when undertaking mobile radiography of patients in the Intensive Care Unit (ICU) as studies have shown that this environment may cause significant psychological distress.[17]

CHANGED AGE STATUS – CHILDREN AND ADOLESCENTS

The intellectual development of children was first outlined by Piaget and is divided into four broad stages:[18-20]

0–24 months

Over this period, the child moves from simple reflex actions to a discovery of consequences through repetition and devising new ways to achieve the same ends. From the age of approximately 6 months, the child will experience 'separation anxiety' when removed from the proximity of its parents and will demonstrate this by crying or screaming.

2–7 years

The child begins to use verbal and symbolic representation. Speech evolves from the egocentric, i.e. when the child identifies himself as separate from the mother, to the social, i.e. when the child sees the actions of other children and adults. During these stages, the child begins to form crude concepts with a rapidly expanding vocabulary. By the age of 3, the child begins to lose separation anxiety as they recognise that the parent will return, however their judgement is dominated by their perceptions and 'magical' thinking may prevail. The child's independence gradually develops over this period. By the time they are 7, children can draw with meaning and detail and begin to understand rules and respond to reasoning. They can tell jokes and enjoy relatively fluent conversation.

7–12 years

The child begins to use concrete problem-solving and logic. Their confidence and sense of morality develops, as does their curiosity about the workings of their environment. By the time they are 12, they enjoy being given responsibility and have good coordination skills, including balance and relatively fine manipulation. They are able to express preferences for different subjects.

12 years onwards

Thought processes become more abstract and multiple processes may occur concurrently. They become more globally aware and questioning of the world around them. They become concerned about what people think of them and self-esteem and peer-pressure may become an issue. By the time they are 16, they will have developed their own tastes and may have high levels of skill in one or more areas.[18-20]

> **!** For the practitioner, communication with children includes the need for effective communication with parents, especially where the child is very young. Studies have indicated that, as with adult patients, the provision of information is important to both children and their families.[21]

In the case of imaging, the family may not necessarily know what examination they have been referred for and the procedure needs to be explained to both the child and their parents. Communication, which is tailored specifically to the needs of the child, can increase the chances of completing an imaging examination successfully and without distress or the need for undue restraint. For very young children the use of distraction techniques (such as pictures on the wall, for them to look at while the exposure is taken) is likely to be very helpful.[20] Toddlers tend to be suspicious of strange people[21] however, and as the examination progresses, they are likely to respond to the 'comfort talk' described above.[14] However, children of school age or older may well perceive this as being talked down to. Older children are likely to respond to the use of their name, together with the establishment of eye contact and adoption of an open posture. Explanations that they can understand are really important, together with demonstrations of what will happen, e.g. giving the child a ride on a moving table or a practise using the child's favourite toy.[20] Using drawings and interviews to determine children's perceptions of their X-ray examinations can also be effective.[22] Children often have fears about the equipment, including the worry that the tube would come down and crush them. Therefore, time spent explaining and demonstrating what will happen is time well spent.[22]

A good practice recommendation is that all radiology departments, where there is regular imaging of children, should have a lead practitioner who is a paediatric specialist.[23] Such posts have also been established in the majority of radiotherapy departments.[24] In both cases, such individuals can act as 'Children's Champions' in helping to ensure the provision of suitable child-centred services. Departments should also make use of play specialists who are now available in the majority of hospitals and whose skills can reduce children's fears of both routine and more complex procedures.[25] In the case of radiotherapy, fear of the technology is compounded for young children by the need for separation from the parent, albeit for short periods.[24] It has been proven that the use of play specialists can reduce the number of children who require either general

> **!** Spending time establishing a relationship with the patient and family, with lots of praise and reassurance, will help make the sequence of treatments much easier.

Box 2.1 **Paediatric special interest groups**

Both radiography professions have established paediatric special interest groups to promote best practice in the examination and treatment of children and adolescents.

The Association of Paediatric Radiographers (APR) is the medical imaging group. The APR committee consists of a maximum of 10 elected members from throughout the UK and a Council representative from the Society of Radiographers. Study days are arranged, usually twice a year in the Spring and Autumn, at venues throughout the UK. Any practitioner with an interest in paediatric radiography can apply to join and the study days are open to all. They also publish newsletters and guidance documents, which are available on the Society of Radiographers' website. This group has been in existence for over 30 years.

In 2008, the Specialist Paediatric Radiotherapy Radiographers Interest Group (SPRRIG) was formed. As of 2011, this group has a membership of approximately 18 practitioners, some of whom are specialist radiotherapy practitioners who have dedicated time allotted to paediatric radiotherapy; others are radiotherapy practitioners with an interest in paediatrics. The Group tries to get together twice a year.

Both groups have very similar aims; to act as sources of expert knowledge and to provide advice, support and professional development to those working with children with a view to driving best practice and developing standards for the examination and treatment of children.

(All information correct at the time of writing.)

Box 2.2 **Example of an adolescent cancer unit[27]**

The Young Oncology Unit (YOU) at Christie Hospital in south Manchester is just one of 16 units partly funded by the Teenage Cancer Trust. YOU provides care for patients from 16 to 24 years of age, suffering from cancer and related illnesses. Opened in 1998, it is a 13-bed ward with facilities which include a games room, relaxation lounge and therapy room. The unit provides a range of activities, trips and events through a dedicated activities coordinator. The Teenage Cancer Trust is in the process of developing a further 15 units at hospitals across the UK. The units provide the opportunity for patients to support each other, surrounded by a team of medical specialists who have an interest and expertise in teenage cancer. It is believed that the concentration of medical expertise within these units can improve chances of recovery among adolescents by over 15%.

(All information correct at the time of writing.)

! Adolescents want factual information without the use of medical jargon and to be told in advance what to expect from any examination or treatment; equally they want healthcare professionals to really listen to what they have to say and to give them the opportunity to ask questions and have them properly answered. They want healthcare professionals to appear warm and caring and to reassure them, make them feel safe and try to make their visit to hospital fun[26] (see Box 2.2).

anaesthetics or sedation for their radiotherapy treatment. Some departments have various models and toys to simulate scans, masks and treatment and many centres work closely with nearby specialist children's hospitals. (See Box 2.1 for Paediatric special interest groups.)

The special case of adolescents

It is only recently that Trusts have recognised that adolescents need special consideration when attending for examination or treatment.[7] Not really an adult and no longer a child, a diagnosis of illness, particularly cancer, can have a negative effect on teenagers who are struggling with emotions, self-esteem and relationships. This age group requires special consideration in communication, as their perceptions of healthcare may differ from those of their families.[26] The importance of information as a means of imparting a sense of control cannot be over-emphasised[7] and it is imperative to involve adolescents in the decision-making process regarding their care.[26] While they did not wish to be treated like children, many adolescents typically feel that their questions were not always answered in an understandable way.

In addition, the relationship with their parents needs sensitive handling, so that they do not feel excluded at times when the adolescent asserts their need for independence and confidentiality, e.g. the young person should be given the choice as to whether they wish to have a parent or guardian in the room with them for their X-ray examination. It has also been recognised that parents have an important role in ensuring compliance with treatment regimes such as skin care and such things as examination preparation, e.g. taking laxatives before scanning or barium appointments, as this is an age at which the adolescent is inclined to test boundaries.[20-26]

DIFFERING AGE STATUS – THE ELDERLY PATIENT

Recent media reports have pointed out that the proportions of elderly people in the population, both in the UK and worldwide, are increasing.[28-31] This is attributed both to the falling birth rate and greater life expectancy. Since the 1970s, the adult life expectancy in the UK has risen from 72 to 80 years.[32] This has been associated with better healthcare and nutrition, however older people tend to be automatically assumed to have greater levels of illness and poor health. It needs to be remembered that ageing is a natural process[28] and not an automatic predictor of poor health.[30] Recent newspaper reports have highlighted the fact that older people do not necessarily receive acceptable treatment when in hospital.[28,30] In a recent study of practitioners in Norway, respondents reported negative attitudes towards patients suffering from dementia[34] (see Chapter 3, Communication with patients with disabilities and additional needs). Practitioners generally highlight issues of time pressures which have to be weighed against the lack of physical mobility of elderly patients and their perceived desire for prolonged conversations resulting from isolation and loneliness.[31] Interestingly, good guidance publications have highlighted the need for specialist paediatric imaging practice, however there has been no such mention with regard to geriatrics.[28-30]

As the patient ages, there are physical changes to vision (especially perception of depth), hearing, balance and coordination; all of which may make the person more predisposed to falls. Individuals often experience postural hypotension, whereby they feel dizzy when changing position from lying down to sitting up or from sitting to standing. The skin becomes thinner and can be broken, e.g. when subjected to shearing forces from being moved about on an X-ray table. This may act as a trigger for the formation of pressure sores in more elderly patients.

> **!** The body's ability to regulate temperature also decreases and older patients should be protected from the cold and draughts.[30] This requires special consideration and understanding from the practitioner.

The patient may also experience some degree of psychological change, particularly functions such as short-term memory. This does not necessarily imply that the patient has dementia. The incidence of dementia is highest in those over 80 but, unfortunately, is not confined to that age group. Patients with dementia may show resistance to being treated or examined, often accompanied by confused, agitated and even aggressive behaviour.[34] The stress of being in unfamiliar surroundings may exacerbate these symptoms. It is important to realise that the patient has no control over this and under no circumstances should they be chastised. It is important that you stay calm and in control, remembering that the patient is not really angry at you; their reactions arise out of fear and frustration.[38] Distraction techniques may work, such as asking the patient questions about themselves. Other recommended techniques include listening carefully to what is being said and proposing alternative solutions where possible, e.g. erect instead of supine positioning.[38] Impairment of memory processes in dementia raises issues for the radiotherapy practitioner with regard to patient consent, both initially and as the series of treatments progress. When communicating with dementia patients, in whatever context, it is recommended that the practitioner should speak slowly and distinctly, asking only one question at a time and waiting for the answer.[39] Face the patient at the same level as they are and use eye contact. At all times be courteous, calm and reassuring (see Chapter 3, Communication with patients with disabilities and additional needs.)

In order to be perceived as providing quality of care to any group of patients, practitioners must reorient themselves away from solely being concentrated on the task of imaging or treatment, to really placing the individual patient at the centre of the process and caring for their psychological needs[28] as well as just providing physical care.

KEY POINTS

- Holistic care means attending to the psychological needs of our patients not just the task at hand
- All groups of patients expect practitioners to give them information about what is about to happen
- This makes them feel in control of an otherwise difficult and potentially frightening experience
- Patients attribute the perception of 'quality' to examinations where the practitioner appears interested in them and projects a warm demeanour
- Non-verbal communication, such as eye contact and use of an open stance, is also important
- Attitudes to groups of patients such as children and the elderly are improved by specific knowledge and experience

ACKNOWLEDGEMENTS

Acknowledgements go to radiotherapy colleagues at the Society of Radiographers and in centres nationwide who were kind enough to e-mail the author details of their practice with children.

Chapter | 3 |

Communication with patients with disabilities and additional needs

Hilary Bungay

INTRODUCTION

There are over 10 million people in the UK living with a limiting long-term illness, impairment or disability.[1] This represents approximately one-sixth of the population and means that it is highly probable that practitioners working in medical imaging and radiotherapy departments will be caring for people with a disability regularly in the course of their everyday practice. A disabled person is defined[2] as someone who has:

> ... *a physical or mental impairment that has a substantial and long-term adverse effect on their ability to carry out normal day to day activities. The term impairment covers long-term medical conditions such as asthma and diabetes and mental impairment, and also includes mental health conditions such as bipolar disorders, learning difficulties, learning disabilities and autism*

These definitions are medical definitions and represent an approach to disability, which attributes disability to an individual's health condition or impairment. This medical model of disability is a deficit model and highlights what is missing or has been lost; it places disability in the person and regards them as suffering a tragedy and being in need of pity.[3] In contrast, the social model of disability focuses on what the person can do rather on what they cannot.[4] In this model, disability is created by the barriers in society such as inaccessible buildings, people's attitudes, resulting in stereotyping, prejudice and discrimination and organisations which have inflexible policies and practices in place. Recognising the existence of these barriers within radiography and applying the principles of effective communication should help to overcome communication difficulties with people with a disability.

Radiotherapy practitioners see patients over a number of days and weeks and during this time they are able to establish a relationship with the person and become familiar with their communication skills and needs. Medical imaging practitioners on the other hand, generally spend less time with each patient and it has been suggested that rather than considering the individual needs of the patient, the interactions with patients tend to be task-focused and goal-orientated towards producing a medical image.[5] As a consequence, patients are in fact, often referred to as the 'chest in the bed' or the 'stroke on a trolley' and this emphasis on a person's condition focuses on the person's deficits rather than on their abilities. It is important to find out what and how the person is able to communicate and adjust the practice accordingly. Practitioners in the course of their work may also have to communicate about a person with a disability to other professionals or members of the public and in these circumstances, it is important to use the appropriate language, e.g. today the word 'handicapped' is no longer used because of the belief it is derived from begging 'cap in hand'.

> **!** In person centred care,[6] the term now preferred is 'disabled people' or 'people with disabilities' but not 'the disabled', as using 'the disabled' categorises people as a group rather than considering individuals in their own right.[7] Phrases which imply misfortune such as 'afflicted by' or 'suffers from' or 'victim of' should also be avoided.

In person centred care, the person should always come before the disability. Therefore, when referring to people with a hearing impairment, avoid using the terms 'deaf mute'; instead use 'deaf', 'user of British Sign Language' (BSL) or 'person with hearing impairment'. Similarly, avoid using the terms 'the blind'; instead use 'people with visual impairment'; 'blind people'; a 'blind or partially sighted person'. It is also the case that having a disability is *not* the same as having an illness and that disabled people are not patients or invalids *because* of their disability, they may be ill just as a non-disabled person has an illness and in that context, they are a 'patient'.

COMMUNICATING WITH PEOPLE WITH COMMUNICATION DIFFICULTIES

The ability to communicate may be compromised by disability and people with communication difficulties are at risk of not being able to communicate their symptoms or worries with healthcare professionals and this may adversely affect both their health, and their access to healthcare. Hospital environments can be particularly challenging for people with communication difficulties because not only are they anxious about their appointments, they may also be very unwell and their ability to communicate may be further affected by their condition. Furthermore, the surroundings are unfamiliar and they may be interacting with staff who do not know how best to communicate with them. Every disabled person has different communication needs; communication disabilities may be due to a physical disability, congenital conditions which resulted in hearing impairment or deafness, partial sightedness or blindness, or cognitive impairment such as a learning disability. However, communications disabilities may also be acquired as a result of trauma, a stroke or due to a degenerative illness. Medical treatments such as chemotherapy, surgery or ventilation may also affect peoples' ability to communicate in the short or long term.

> **!** Whether the disability is congenital or acquired may influence the communication skills of the individual and different techniques and strategies may be required to facilitate communication and understanding.

Communicating with people with communication difficulties requires us to consider individual needs and The Department of Health have produced: *The Essence of Care: Patient-focused benchmarking for health care practitioners*.[8] One of the 12 benchmarks of best practice for effective patient centred care *Respect and Dignity* requires that communication between staff and patients takes place in a manner that respects their individuality.[9]

Respect for the individual is also a key element of The Equality Act (2010) which replaced the Disability Discrimination Act (1995 and 2005).[10,11] Under the terms of the Equality Act, reasonable adjustment must be made to ensure that patients with a disability do not experience any barriers to accessing information. The Act explicitly recognises that disabled peoples' needs may be different to those of non-disabled people, however the Act does not require that all people should be treated the same, rather it requires that peoples' different needs and how they may be met is considered.

However, not only are we required by law to provide information to people with a disability in an accessible manner, we are also governed by our Code of Conduct and Ethics[12] (see Chapter 29, Ethical and legal considerations in professional practice). This requires us to ensure equality of care with no discrimination, and to identify individuals with communication difficulties and make adjustments to accommodate their particular problems. It is also necessary to be satisfied that appropriate informed consent has been gained prior to undertaking any examination or procedure, and this requires clear and effective communication. In earlier chapters, the authors outlined the principles of communication and applied the principles of effective communication with specific client groups. This chapter builds on these chapters and applies the basic principles of good communication in communicating with and about people with disabilities.

BARRIERS TO EFFECTIVE COMMUNICATION

There are a number of factors which create problems with communication for disabled people when attending medical imaging and radiotherapy departments, and these can be grouped using the social model of disability.

Staff attitudes

- Negative stereotyping of people, lack of knowledge or understanding of the nature of the disability and making assumptions about a person's abilities
- Staff under pressure and in a hurry, reluctant to spend time with the person ensuring they understand what will happen to them.

Organisational factors

- Lack of knowledge, or availability of resources to assist communication such as interpreters, induction loops, communication boards and specialist literature
- Rigid appointment times.

Environmental factors

- Noise levels can be a particular issue in imaging and radiotherapy departments because of noise from the equipment
- Practitioners are standing behind screens at a distance from the patient which can affect their ability to hear
- Low levels of lighting, common in imaging rooms, can make it difficult to see peoples' faces, facial expressions and lips
- Wearing face masks during some procedures.

- Can you identify other factors which form barriers to communication?
- Consider times when you had patients with communication difficulty in the department. How did you respond?
- How could you improve your communication with people in the future?

In the following sections, the communication difficulties faced by people with physical disabilities; sensory impairments, i.e. hearing and visual; and cognitive impairment are explored. Suggestions are made as to how to facilitate communication and it will be seen how applying the general principles of good practice in communication is central to communicating with people with disabilities.

PHYSICAL DISABILITIES

People with physical disabilities may arrive in the department in a wheelchair. It is important to realise that it is not correct to suggest or talk about a person as 'confined to a wheelchair' because in reality wheelchairs provide freedom for users.

> ! When speaking to someone in a wheelchair it is also important to speak to the person directly and not address the person accompanying them – the classic 'does she take sugar in her tea' is often quoted by disabled people to illustrate how they are ignored by others. If you are having a lengthy conversation with the person, it is good practice to position yourself at the same level as them, as standing over someone can be intimidating. Furthermore, rather than assuming that because someone is a wheelchair user that they will require assistance, ask them what assistance they require.

People who have a facial disfigurement due to congenital, trauma or tumour may find speech difficult. In Box 3.3 in the Stroke section below, there are some tips which may also be used to help communication with those who are unable to speak or find speech difficult.

HEARING IMPAIRED AND DEAF PEOPLE

According to Action on Hearing Loss (formerly the Royal National Institute for the Deaf, RNID), there are approximately 10 million people with hearing loss in the UK and over 800 000 people who are severely or profoundly deaf [13] and, as the population ages, these numbers are likely to increase. There are different levels of deafness, ranging from: mild hearing loss, where the person may experience some difficulty following speech in noisy environments; moderate hearing loss, where the person has difficulty following speech without a hearing aid; and severe hearing loss, where the person relies on lip reading with a hearing aid, and British Sign Language (BSL) may be their first or preferred language. Deaf people with profound hearing loss do not benefit from hearing aids and communicate using BSL as their first or preferred language. BSL is not just English translated into BSL, it is recognised as a language in its own right, and is a distinct language with its own grammar; it is a visual and spatial language, using sign and gesture. Most people who use sign language are pre-lingually deaf, that is they were born with little or no hearing or lost their hearing before speech was learnt, and for many people who use BSL, spoken or written English is their second or third language. [14] As a result of the absence of verbal communication in their early years, people who are pre-lingually deaf may also have a low level of literacy, [15] and this means that written information on patient information sheets or appointment letters may also be difficult for them to understand. Sometimes, healthcare professionals may write down instructions to supplement communication with deaf people but for this to be successful, it is important to make sure handwriting is legible and also that appropriate words are chosen.[15]

Few healthcare professionals are able to understand sign language and when deaf or hearing impaired people attend for appointments, they may experience difficulty in communicating with staff. Indeed, it was found that 42% of deaf and hard of hearing people who had visited hospital as a non-emergency reported difficulty with communication, and this increased to 72% among BSL users.[16] There is also a potential cost to the NHS when communication fails or breaks down, e.g. it is estimated that it costs the NHS £20 million per annum through appointments being missed because people do not hear their name being called, or through appointments needing to be re-booked with a BSL interpreter.[16] People who use BSL require a BSL interpreter to be present when they attend hospital appointments, and most hospitals have a register of interpreters that include BSL interpreters. Professional interpreters use simultaneous interpretation and therefore, when using an interpreter, it is necessary to give small amounts of information at a time. There is potential for issues around confidentiality and privacy as the interpreter may be well known in the local deaf community, and it may be appropriate to ask the patient if they have any objections to the interpreter being present during certain examinations or investigations.[14] If the patient does object, then it is necessary to ensure that as much information is provided as possible before the examination starts. With the availability of videophones, it is possible for the interpreter to continue to interpret without being physically present. Some deaf people can lip read but not all are able to and even those who can are not able to distinguish all the spoken sounds. The nature of mouth movements can make it difficult to distinguish many words from one another, and typically only 30–40% of speech can be understood through lip reading alone.[15]

! People of any age may be affected by hearing problems and it is important not to make assumptions about who may be affected.

The normal ageing process can lead to hearing difficulties but not in all older people; it is therefore important not to stereotype people and speak loudly or shout at all older people. People who develop hearing loss in later life will tend to use spoken English or whichever is their first language as their preferred language for communication, and use hearing aids. It is important to be patient with people with hearing loss, and people with hearing loss, unlike deaf people may like you to raise your voice and to speak loudly and clearly; this may cause issues with

---

Box 3.1 Communicating with people with a hearing impairment

- Even if someone is wearing a hearing aid, it does not mean that they can hear you; ask if they need to lip read
- If using an interpreter, talk directly to the person you are communicating with and not to the interpreter
- It is important to ensure that the person you are talking to can see your face
- Make sure you have the listener's attention before you start speaking. To do this, you can use waving, tapping on the shoulder or hand signs mimicking lights being switched on and off
- It is important not to speak too quickly or to speak over another person. Speak clearly but not too slowly and do not exaggerate your lip movements
- Use natural facial expressions and gestures
- If talking to a hearing person and a deaf person, do not just focus on the hearing person, as this excludes the deaf person from the discussion and decision-making
- Do not shout – it is uncomfortable for a hearing aid user, and those around you, and looks aggressive
- If someone doesn't understand what you have said, don't just keep repeating the same words, think of an alternative way to say it
- Find a suitable place to talk, with good lighting away from noise and distractions. You will need to also consider the person's privacy and issues of confidentiality
- Check that the person you are talking to can follow what you are saying
- Be patient and take time to communicate properly
- Use plain language, avoid jargon and unfamiliar abbreviations.

---

confidentiality and privacy. It is important to take this into account.

Box 3.1 contains a list of points which may help you when communicating with people with a hearing impairment.

According to research, 93% of communication is non-verbal; 38% involves vocal tones and 55% is attributed to body language. Therefore, for the hearing impaired person, although they lose 45% of communication through not being able to hear words (7%) or tone of voice (38%), there remains a large element of communication that they can pick up from the practitioner in the form of facial expressions, gestures, eye contact, personal space and touch – these can convey empathy and understanding and conversely impatience and irritation.

Within medical imaging and radiotherapy departments, there may be resources available to facilitate communication with hearing impaired people. For example, some departments have portable induction hearing loops in reception areas to enable people with hearing aids to hear when their name is called. Some manufacturers fit a loudspeaker device to chest stands and erect Buckys to assist communication with patients with hearing loss.

> **!** Although CT and MRI scanners, linear accelerators and simulators have integral speakers it is important that practitioners alert patients to the fact that they will be speaking to them through the speakers and ascertain whether the patients are able to hear through the system. If patients use a hearing aid which needs to be removed for the procedure, it is important to inform the patient about the procedure before the hearing aid is removed, and establish an alternative method of communication, e.g. hand signals to alert patients as and when they need to keep still or hold their breath if required.

VISUAL IMPAIRED AND BLIND PEOPLE

Only a small proportion of people with visual impairment are completely blind. Although most do have some sight, there is a considerable amount of variation in the level of vision people have and this can also be influenced by the available light. Visual impairment in adults may be the result of childhood blindness, cataracts, glaucoma or age-related conditions, and women are at more risk than men. People with visual impairment who attend medical imaging or radiotherapy departments have additional needs. Any information about procedures or investigations need to be provided in a format that is accessible, and accessibility is dependent on the level of impairment. If the person is unable to read, then any information that is usually provided in a written format may be translated into Braille or an audio recording could be made available. If the person is partially sighted, then the written information should be formatted to follow the recommendations of the Office of Disability Issues,[7] e.g. the font size should be a minimum of 16 points; the paper needs to be of good quality so there is no reflection or shine through of light; the text should be justified on the left side only; and italics and capitals should be avoided.

Once a visually impaired person arrives in the department, it is important to speak as you approach them, ask the person what assistance they need and if they request that you take them to the waiting room or treatment room, offer them your arm so that you can guide them rather than leading the way. Once in the X-ray or treatment room, the same principles apply as with any other patient and you need to ensure they understand what they are there for; have followed any preparation that was required and tell them what is going to happen to them.

> **!** If you need to touch them to position them, tell them when and where you will be touching them; you also need to tell them who else is present in the room. If you leave the room or move away from them, tell them that you are going and how long it will be before you return. You also need to describe any noises that they will hear. People who are visually impaired may be unable to see body language such as facial expressions and eye contact, but they will be aware of touch and personal space and these can be used to show empathy and warmth.

COGNITIVE IMPAIRMENT

Cognitive impairment may be present at birth due to a range of factors: genetic abnormalities, hypothyroidism or complications due to prematurity; it can also develop throughout childhood due to trauma, metabolic conditions or as a result of medical interventions such as chemotherapy. As people age, conditions such as dementia, stroke, brain tumours and brain trauma may affect their ability to communicate and people undergoing chemotherapy may experience a temporary or permanent cognitive impairment. There are different levels of cognitive impairment: at the lowest level, the person may experience forgetfulness and confusion; at higher levels, there may be decreased intelligence and a reduction in mental functioning. Communication with people with dementia, stroke and learning disabilities will now be explored.

DEMENTIA

There are currently approximately 820 000 people in the UK diagnosed with dementia.[17] Dementia can cause memory loss and communication difficulties. There are signs which may indicate that a person has dementia, one of which is confusion. Patients may repeat themselves, and may appear not to be paying attention or following the conversation. When a person with dementia attends for an appointment, it is possible that the practitioner will not initially be aware that the person has dementia, unless it is specified on the request form or if the person attends with a carer. It is possible that the person with dementia may have forgotten why they are at the hospital and who the people around them are. It may be necessary therefore to repeat information a number of times.

> **!** Dementia patients may have difficulty expressing themselves and use incorrect words or mix words up to refer to items or people and they may become frustrated and anxious as a result. It is not only verbal communication that can be an issue, as reading and understanding written text can also be a problem.

Box 3.2 **How to communicate with people with dementia**

1. Approach the person from the front so that they can see your face and when speaking to them give a 'cue' to show that you are talking to them, for instance through making eye contact, using their name, or touching their hand or arm
2. If possible, try and ensure that the environment is quiet and free from distractions; this can be difficult in a busy department but after a preliminary greeting, more complex information should be given in a quiet space
3. Speak to the person as an adult and not as a child. Speaking calmly and clearly, use short sentences, with simple language, making one point at a time. Avoid questions that require complex answers
4. Give the person time to process the information and respond; do not hurry them and try and avoid being too quick to try and guess what the person is trying to express or pressure them to respond
5. Be aware of your own body language, use touch if appropriate, listen carefully to them and look at their body language
6. Do not correct, contradict or argue with the person
7. Do not patronise the person or speak down to them and do not speak to others who are present, as though they are not there.

Box 3.3 **Strategies that you can use to communicate with people who have had a stroke[18]**

1. Establish communication: can the person use yes or no, or thumbs up/down accurately? If so, ensure you ask questions which require a yes or no answer
2. Do not rush: give the person time to take in what you say and respond, and do not interrupt them
3. Adjust communication to the right level: use a normal tone but speak slower and use shorter sentences
4. Use visual aids to reinforce verbal messages: use facial expressions, gestures and communication charts, if available
5. Do not pretend to understand a person who has aphasia: be honest and ask them to start again
6. Be positive and encouraging
7. Remember that the person has not become less intelligent
8. Stand or sit where you can be heard clearly and where there are no distractions.

The Alzheimer's Society[17] has produced a series of 'top tips' for nurses caring for people with dementia. One of these, on communication, aims to promote effective communication with the person who has dementia. The list in Box 3.2 has been adapted from the Alzheimer's Society guidance as they apply equally to practitioners and all healthcare professionals interacting with people with dementia.

COMMUNICATION DIFFICULTIES DUE TO STROKE

Approximately 150 000 people per year have a stroke. One-third are left disabled in some form, and there are about a quarter of a million people living in the UK who have a disability as a result of having a stroke.[18] One of the most common effects of strokes are communication problems. These may be due to either physical or cognitive impairment or a combination of both, resulting in the person losing their ability to speak or to understand the spoken word. In this case, reading and writing may also potentially be affected. When a person has a stroke they may lose their speech completely or what they say may not appear to make sense. Their intelligence however, is unaffected and it can be very frustrating for them as they may

believe that they are talking normally, but other people may not understand what they are saying. The words that come out of their mouths may not be the words they want to say. Some people may be affected by muscle weakness of the mouth; this may affect breath control and their speech may be slurred, nasal or have a jerky rhythm. Others may have dyspraxia, which is the inability to control and coordinate the movements required to speak normally or make deliberate sounds.

COMMUNICATING WITH PEOPLE WITH A LEARNING DISABILITY

There are around 1.2 million people in the UK with a learning disability, and approximately 210 000 have a profound learning disability. Learning disability is defined as: 'a significantly reduced ability to understand new or complex information to learn new skills (impaired intelligence); with a reduced ability to cope independently (impaired social functioning), which starts before adulthood with a lasting effect on development'.[19] Many people with a learning disability also have physical and/or sensory impairments, e.g. it is estimated that around 40% have hearing loss and 40% have visual impairment.[20]

People with a learning disability experience difficulty with communication. This may be in expressing themselves as they only have a few words or signs that they are able to use; some may have difficulty speaking clearly and are reliant on others to interpret for them. Their comprehension and level of understanding may be such that they only understand a few words and are unable to understand complex sentences. People with a learning disability have a broad range of abilities and needs and it is important in person- or patient-centred care to treat each person as an individual.

> **!** Practitioners are often working in pressured environments with large numbers of patients requiring medical imaging or radiotherapy. However, if time is not taken to understand how a person with a learning disability communicates and then be able to properly communicate with that person, this can lead to distress and the examination or treatment having to be abandoned. This places further pressure on department workloads and may also result in the person's treatment being delayed.

There are signs that you can look out for when communicating with a person with a learning disability, to assess whether they understand what you are saying.[21] These include:

- Loss of concentration
- Loss of eye contact
- Changing the subject
- Agreeing with everything you say
- Repeating the last word you say
- Fidgeting
- Becoming nervous or anxious
- Answering inappropriately or inaccurately.

If the patient with a learning disability is accompanied by a carer, then this person may be able to advise as to how best to communicate with the patient. There are a number of strategies which may help with communication[20] and in Box 3.4 these have been adapted for practitioners.

There are a number of resources which can aid communication with people with learning disability. Some Trusts have produced 'Easy Read' leaflets, which explain hospital procedures using pictures and simple language with a large font size. Macmillan Cancer Support have produced a series of books for people with learning disabilities and their carers. The books cover health screening and diagnosis and treatment of cancer. The series is available free of charge from their website. The NHS Screening Programme also produces literature for women with learning disabilities about cervical and breast screening. It is important that people with learning disabilities understand what examinations and treatment they are having so that they are able to consent. Under the Mental Capacity Act (2005),[22] every adult should be assumed to have capacity to make

---

> **Box 3.4 Communicating with people with learning disabilities**
>
> 1. Make sure the person can see and hear to the best of their ability – that is they have their glasses and hearing aids if used
> 2. Ensure the person is comfortable and the environment is not too noisy
> 3. Gain their attention before you start communicating by using their name or by touching their arm
> 4. Use simple language making one point at a time
> 5. Use the environment to support what you are saying, e.g. by demonstrating the equipment
> 6. Use a variety of methods to communicate such as: signs (Makaton or Rebus are two sign languages used with people with learning disabilities); gestures; pictures; the Hospital Communication Book or Easy Read information leaflets
> 7. Give people time to respond and be aware of all their communication signals
> 8. Check that they have understood your information and you have understood theirs, ask them to tell you what they think is going to happen, and ask their carer whether your interpretation of what the person is trying to communicate matches theirs.

a particular decision unless it is shown that they lack the capacity to do so. To support the decision-making process, every effort should be made to present the information in an accessible way. People with a learning disability often agree and say 'Yes' to everything that is suggested. Using the guidance provided in Box 3.4 may help to ensure understanding so that consent is genuinely given.

KEY POINTS

Although there are some strategies which are specific to certain disabled people, such as BSL and Braille, there are a number of communication strategies which may be effective with all people with disabilities. These include:

- Facing the person with whom you are communicating
- Addressing the patient and not the carer
- Ensuring there are no distractions
- Being aware of body language
- Speaking clearly and slowly
- Do not patronise the person
- Give the person time to respond and do not hurry them

Chapter | 4 |

Interprofessional communication

Leonie Munro, Suzanne M. Henwood

CHAPTER OUTLINE

This chapter will consider the following aspects of interprofessional communication (IPC) in practice:

- Requirements to enhance IPC among persons in a health organisation
- Methods of IPC
- Barriers that impinge on IPC within a healthcare organisation context
- Communication within a healthcare organisation

INTRODUCTION

The aim of this chapter is to explore and address some reasons why interprofessional communication (IPC) is important for healthcare professionals and others in health organisations. Over the past decades the expansion of subject content, as well as the increasing complexity of patient care, have resulted in further specialisation in all the healthcare professions.[1] Despite some moves towards 'multi-skilling', no single healthcare professional can meet all the complex needs of a patient.[1] In other words, an integrated team approach is essential for effective patient care. Service delivery to patients does not occur in isolation and necessitates communication between different groups of health professionals.[2]

It is generally agreed that good teamwork and effective communication underpin quality service delivery in any successful organisation. Healthcare organisations are no different.[3] We believe that interprofessional communication is an essential element of that communication in a multidisciplinary healthcare setting.

UNRAVELLING INTERPROFESSIONAL COMMUNICATION

Embedding effective interprofessional communication (IPC) in health organisations is vital to quality service delivery, preventing breakdowns in communication between the role-players.[4-5] IPC takes place when members of different professions interact to exchange information verbally, non-verbally, in writing or through information technology.[6] Factors that impact on effective IPC have been extensively researched in order to improve healthcare service to patients.[4,7,8] Specific examples of improving IPC in healthcare include: the use of checklists in operating rooms;[4] cooperative documentation system usage;[9] joint compilation of organisational policies[10] and openness, respect and trust.[7,10]

The need for IPC is not new. Each profession frequently uses specialised vocabulary and language, such as abbreviations, esoteric signs and symbols, resulting in message failure in IPC.[11] The use and interpretation of clinical terminology often leads to comprehensibility problems between doctors and nurses, e.g. the former would use 'febrile' and the latter 'pyrexial' when discussing a feverish patient.[12] Members of different professional groups learn to think, speak and act in the specific patterns which their profession has developed, often creating obstacles in IPC.[11] Professionals should work together in a coherent and purposive combination of highly specialised professionals within a multidisciplinary team, accepting each individual's knowledge and skills by allowing professional autonomy. Fear of loss of professional autonomy is one of many barriers that impact on IPC.[13] Another barrier relates to fear of losing a sense of professional identity. One analogy is that wishing to retain the sense of having a 'fruit salad', instead of creating a 'smoothie', where each individual component loses something of its unique identity. The challenge is to retain professional identity, yet benefit from all that the integrated working of teams offers.

It is not surprising that there is a unique professional identity. Values, attitudes, behaviour and customs[1] form each profession's culture, which impacts on how health professionals interact with patients and other professionals. Professional cultures may contribute to a 'silo' approach to patient care and interprofessional learning early in professional education programmes can help to build bridges.[1] However, this must be supported by appropriate professional socialisation in clinical practice if these changes are to be embedded in reality. Otherwise the interprofessional focus remains an academic or theoretical perspective, not replicated in the clinical arena.

There is consensus in the literature that, over time, effective teamwork and effective IPC improve patient satisfaction; reduce service delivery costs; improve job satisfaction; and enhance the image of the health organisation.[1,5,7,10,11,13,14]

So against this background, our objectives are to highlight: IPC education; different methods of IPC; the role of non-healthcare professions (such as human resource management, administrative personnel, information technology and support personnel) who contribute (and have contributed over time) to service delivery in health organisations.[10,11] A respectful and partnership approach to care is, we argue, the way forward. This may challenge some professional groups and some individual staff, who wish to cling to the old hierarchical approaches and more autocratic styles of communication and teamwork.

TEAMWORK: INTERPROFESSIONAL COMMUNICATION AND PROFESSIONAL COLLABORATION

Many researchers[1,4,5] link poor communication, or a lack of communication, to their studies of poor health outcomes, high mortality rates and medical errors. High staff turnover, lack of job satisfaction, and low professional esteem, are also attributed to lack of teamwork and poor IPC.[5,7,14] Some practitioners have expressed difficulty communicating with nurses and believe that other health professions are neither familiar with the scope of radiographic practice, nor respectful of the radiographic profession. On the other hand, practitioners have indicated that from their perspective, they both respect and understand other healthcare disciplines. It would be interesting to see if other professional disciplines had a similar view of understanding others, while feeling they were not completely understood.

It would seem that at least some health professionals think that they respect and communicate well with members of their own profession[7,12,15] but experience problems with other professions, especially in a hierarchical structure. Doctors are usually perceived by nurses as having the

most power and authority.[7] Doctors and nurses may have discrepant attitudes: doctors being satisfied with their collaboration with nurses in the team, whereas nurses' ratings were the opposite, showing dissatisfaction. This shows a communication or understanding gap, which may lead to issues between professionals in practice. It has been argued that effective IPC requires equal status[1] for each health profession, since the focus is on quality service delivery to patients. With the advent of more extended clinical roles in nursing and allied health, it will be interesting to see if this perceived hierarchical gap reduces.

Briefings at the beginning of a shift;[5] precise unambiguous face-to-face communication handovers, namely the transfer of roles and responsibilities from one person to another[8] and interdisciplinary morning meetings[16] have been shown to enhance effective teamwork and quality healthcare, minimising the 'blame game' when things go wrong. Dysfunctional conflict in a team does not serve the interests of any of the role-players, and thus collaboration should be embedded in horizontal and vertical communication in an organisation.[3] For example, multidisciplinary meetings enhance both teamwork and management of patients with breast cancer.[17] It is the cross-professional meeting and working which can break down previous barriers and ensure better continuity and quality of care. This has successfully been introduced in some system-based, or pathology-related, disciplines and perhaps now is the time for a more general introduction of such styles of working to form truly integrated teams which are patient focused.

Interestingly, according to some authors, interprofessional collaboration in healthcare is based on voluntary participation and negotiation.[18] According to them, very limited empirical research has been done on the determinants of interprofessional collaboration. Several elements may impact on collaboration in healthcare organisations, namely:

- Systemic determinants, such as educational and professional systems
- Social factors, such as the power that exists between health team professionals
- The philosophy and structure of an organisation
- Team resources
- Administrative support
- Coordination and communication mechanisms
- Interactional determinants that address mutual trust, respect and communication
- The willingness to collaborate.

Collaboration may depend in part on professional education.[19] It has been recommended that IPC education should be included in all health training programmes at qualification level[1] to bring about a change in professional cultures that seem to act as barriers to effective IPC. In some institutions, this has been taken further to ensure interprofessional learning at qualification level: learning together

– working together, setting up an expectation of collaboration at all levels, right from day one.

INTERPROFESSIONAL COMMUNICATION EDUCATION

Past educational systems, in many instances, may have become multiple silos leading to a fragmentation[1] of academic knowledge as well as limited, or no opportunities, for healthcare professionals to interact with other disciplines and professions. There is a modern desire to introduce initiatives from the beginning of professional socialisation, yet this also raises questions about how you then integrate that change of practice into an existing clinical culture, where interprofessional working and an integrated team approach may not be evident.[20]

It may take time to change the culture of professionals in clinical practice, but there are already a number of significant moves in that direction, which can only help to improve the focus on holistic and integrated patient care; improve service delivery and increase staff satisfaction by ensuring that their desire to make a real difference in patient care is being realised.

ORGANISATIONAL COMMUNICATION

Organisations have existing structures[3] that indicate designations of personnel, usually in terms of fields of specialisation and departments. Figure 4.1 is an example of a healthcare organisation that is broadly divided into administrative services and direct health provision services. The overall responsibility of the organisation in this example resides with the chief executive officer (CEO). The medical manager's (med man) span of control includes medical specialties, such as surgery and radiology; pharmacy; and allied health professionals, such as medical imaging practitioners and radiotherapists; occupational therapists and physiotherapists. Communication can be

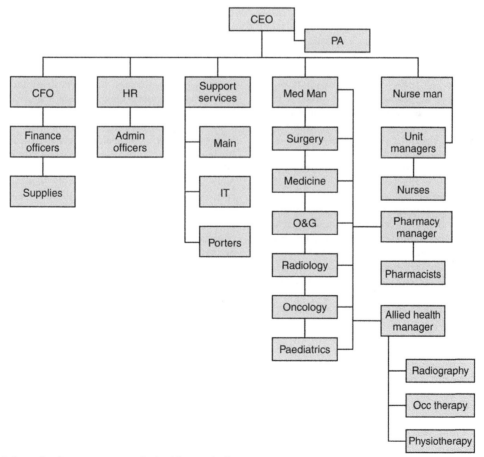

Figure 4.1 Example of an organogram of a health organisation.

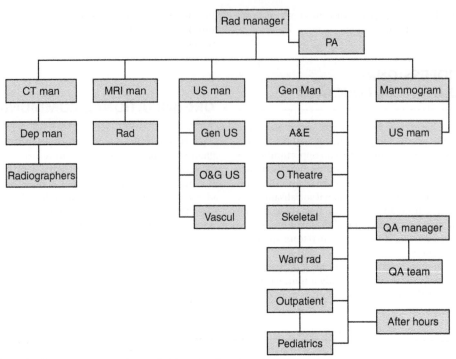

Figure 4.2 Example of an organogram of a medical imaging department.

vertical – both up and down – as well as lateral. If we consider a radiography department then the structure could resemble Figure 4.2, which indicates additional levels of service delivery within the department. Communication, in our example in Figure 4.2, would involve communication between all members of the radiography department. Such communication would be lateral and vertical.

Interestingly, there is reportedly a move away from the traditional hierarchical structures to a more 'web' approach, or flatter structure.[21] This raises some interesting questions in healthcare about how cross-disciplinary teams can be managed differently to enhance interprofessional working and how new advanced and consultant practitioner roles can be introduced without adding additional layers to existing structures. The new roles may even create confusion or conflict between managerial and clinical positions in relation to organisational structure and need to be carefully introduced to avoid introducing new silos of activity or conflict with existing roles.

An example of how changes to service delivery have to be reflected in organisation structures is the introduction of film-less imaging services. If we return to Figure 4.1, then communication between the radiography department and the IT (information technology) department would be even more important, since the latter's expertise is essential for provision of a film-less imaging service. New connections and new ways of working need to be explored to keep pace with the technological changes occurring in practice and the wider distribution of electronic images across a range of departments. This cannot be achieved without effective IPC.

There are predominantly two communication networks in organisations:[3] informal (the grapevine) and formal. It cannot be overemphasised that when communication takes place in a health service setting, relevant legislation pertaining to patient confidentiality[22,23] and professional ethics[24] should be adhered to. It would be unacceptable for example, for any health professional to discuss a patient's medical history with staff who lack a specific role or patient care responsibility that would require them to be party to that history. But alongside this need to contain information, there is also a need to share information between clinical departments to ensure continuity of care. Clear dissemination processes and policies are required to handle information exchange appropriately.

The informal or grapevine network of information is also an issue within staff groups. Miscommunication, or inaccurate interpretation of information, can lead to occupational stress and job dissatisfaction.[3] High level formal communication should be frequent[3] and detailed in order to ensure that accurate information is passed to all departments. Departments then need to explore how best to disseminate and apply that information to individual staff to ensure accurate and timely communication. This is especially important if staff begin to work across teams and hear information from a variety of sources. There needs to be accuracy and consistency in how that information is passed on. While traditional forms of communications, e.g. meetings, notice boards, etc. are still valuable, consideration should also be given to how technology can be used to keep staff informed. Examples of this may include effective use of e-mail or local hospital intranet sites.

Each communication channel has advantages and disadvantages in terms of their ability to convey messages in an organisation.[3] For example, since face-to-face communication includes verbal and non-verbal messages, it provides the maximum of information. During interactions, verbal and non-verbal communication underscores mutual influences.[26] However, when face-to-face communication is compared with electronic communication,[27] face-to-face is often limited in organisational communication in that status differences in group members may determine participation, with higher status members participating more. Electronic communication[3,27,28] allows rapid transmission of information in both internal and external communication, but its use should be underpinned by appropriate e-mailing ethics and etiquette,[29] particularly when used in IPC. The use of e-mailing should also include professional ethics and standards. In addition, it is important to ensure that the system is secure to minimise any risks of breach of confidentiality.[29] This is of special importance in IPC where patients' rights should be safe-guarded.[24] Video-conferencing can also be used in IPC and professional collaboration, as it includes all the benefits of face-to-face communication, yet takes into consideration potential geographic or cost constraints of meeting face-to-face in person.[31] The use of telemedicine in IPC is another system of electronic communication.[32-33]

To summarise, there are many communication options in IPC and professional collaboration, including: hard-copy text; face-to-face communication; telephonic; e-communication; videoconferencing; telemedicine.

Any one aspect of health service delivery cannot be viewed in isolation as the inputs and expertise of a range of other professionals should be included.[10-11] No health service problem has a uni-dimensional solution[11] and it is important to involve other professions in order to obtain a range of opinions before arriving at a decision. As healthcare becomes increasingly complex and inter-related, requiring rapid information flow and immediate responses, there is an ever greater need for interprofessional communication.

The need for a move to greater interprofessional working and therefore the need for further improvements in interprofessional communication is no longer something to discuss or debate. It is already here. Now, our task is to ensure it is effectively implemented throughout all healthcare provision to ensure the best possible outcome for patients and staff alike.

KEY POINTS

- Communication in a healthcare organisation is said to be a 'core component of professionalism'[23]
- Communication has to be interprofessional to ensure that a quality service is provided in modern healthcare settings. It is no longer an optional component to explore, but an essential set of skills and a cultural approach which we must all learn to adopt to enhance practice
- From the first entry to qualification level training in healthcare, through post-qualification and postgraduate education routes, IPC should be central to healthcare development and practice
- Through continuing professional development, existing cultures should be challenged where they have not yet begun to make the shift to more integrated and interprofessional communication and care, to break down the gap between newly qualified staff ready to work interprofessionally and existing cultures maintaining a uni-professional approach
- Role boundaries are changing and there is a need to be fully patient-focused in order to care for the patient holistically
- Staff need to be truly respectful and inclusive of all professions and all support staff, respecting and valuing difference, while recognising the unique role of each individual professional group
- Each person in the team has a valuable role to play and full inclusivity and interprofessional working can only increase patient care and staff satisfaction

Section | 2 |

Psychosocial aspects of patient care

Chapter 5

Cultural and social diversity issues in patient care

Segun S. Adeyemi

CHAPTER OUTLINE

This chapter will focus on the following psychological principles of interaction:

- Personality
- Behaviour
- Attitude
- Culture
- Social class

INTRODUCTION

The global world community is multicultural with different countries becoming multicultural societies. Differences in cultures may be due to nationality, ethnicity, customs, religious beliefs, language, political orientation, physical features, beliefs and experiences.[1] Culture helps develop the values, norms and behaviour of the people who identify with that particular culture. The culture of any particular group of people has been developed over centuries and forms the basis of their traditions. Because of this, it is often difficult for such groups of people to disengage themselves from their time-tested values. Meanwhile, living in a different country through emigration or work means that the culture of their native land is transferred to their new country of abode. This results in those people having to live within two cultures. The mixing of the two cultures is called 'multiculturalisation' and this process can cause behavioural change among such groups of people.

The healthcare environment consists of diverse cultures. This diversity is a result of the variety of patients with individual personal characteristics and representing different age groups, sex, race and religion (see Box 5.1). In addition, the wider healthcare team who care for the patients may have cultures which are different from those of their patients. However, both the practitioners and patients have to interact to enable the successful management of the patients' medical imaging examination or radiotherapy treatment.

It is essential that practitioners have knowledge of these psychological principles, since each individual is different. It will also serve as the building block that ensures that practitioners understand the factors which might affect patients' interactions with them during imaging for diagnosis or radiotherapy treatment. Based on this knowledge, practitioners will be able to manage their interaction with patients and thus establish methods of coping.

PSYCHOLOGICAL PRINCIPLES OF INTERACTIONS WITHIN HEALTHCARE

Caring for patients in the radiography and radiotherapy departments involves complex psychological and social factors. Psychological factors of personality such as who you are, the values and attitudes an individual has, and the situation of the environment, affect the behaviour of both patients and practitioners. This in turn determines the type of interaction that takes place during such an encounter.

Principles affecting behaviour have been developed over the centuries through the study of psychology or the science of behaviour. There are five principles or approaches: (1) behaviourist; (2) psychodynamic; (3) cognitive; (4) humanistic and (5) social constructivist.

The behaviourist approach

The proponents of this approach believe that environmental factors such as culture have a big influence on how people behave. The concept is on the role of learning either

Box 5.1 **Definitions**

Culture: refers to that complex whole which includes knowledge, belief, morals, law, customs and any other capabilities and habits acquired by man as a member of society.[2]
- It is also learned, shared and transmitted values, beliefs, norms and ways of a specific individual or group that guide their thinking, decisions, actions and patterned ways of living.[3]
- Culture is a framework of beliefs, expressive symbols and values, in terms of which individuals define their world, express their feelings and make judgements.[4]

Diversity: refers to the divergence among people rooted in age, culture, ethnicity, experience, gender, sexual orientation and various combinations of these traits.

Gender: refers to the socially constructed roles, behaviors, activities and attributes that a given society considers appropriate for men and women.[5]

Sex: is the biological and physiological characteristics that are used to define men and women.[5]

Ethnic: relates to large groups of people classified according to common traits or customs.

Ethnicity: relates to the sense of identity an individual has based on common ancestry and national, religious, tribal, linguistic or cultural origins.[2]

Race: refers to a group of people united or classified together on the basis of common history, nationality or geographical distribution.

Religion: is a set of beliefs based on the idea of a sacred being.

Language: refers to a body of words and the systems common to a group of people who are of the same community or nation, the same geographical area or the same cultural location.

Values: permanent and important beliefs which can influence thought and behaviour.

Attitudes: readiness to respond in a certain way to a person, object or situation.

through conditioning or associative learning, also known as stimulus or response psychology. The response approach considers the influence of environmental stimuli on the responses produced in relation to the reward or punishment that follows. Innate or inherited factors have no relevance in peoples' behaviour, i.e. the individual's subjective experiences do not count. This means that an individual's behaviour can be used to determine how that person perceives and feels about things or events around them. This theory assumes that people will behave in certain ways to obtain some desirable consequences, while avoiding those that will not. For example, if a patient had a bad experience in imaging or radiotherapy, this will affect his interaction with practitioners the next time he visits the imaging or radiotherapy department for examination or treatment.

> **!** In medical imaging or radiotherapy, how the practitioner greets the patient and explains the procedure forms the basis of the patient's impression within the first few minutes. If a negative impression is formed during this encounter, it will be difficult to erase and the subsequent practitioner and patient interaction will be affected.

The psychodynamic approach

This approach emphasises that people's behaviours are affected by the forces within the individual. An individual's behaviour is determined by unconscious thoughts and memories, which can either be partly inaccessible, i.e. preconscious; or totally inaccessible, i.e. unconscious. These unconscious thoughts can be made conscious through dreams and interpretations. In this case, the role of behaviour has not been considered.

Both the behaviourist and psychodynamic approaches are deterministic, since people are driven by forces beyond their control, either within or without, through reinforcements. For example, patients' concerns about their illness differ according to the stage of their disease. This is due to the 'fear of the unknown' of what might be discovered during imaging or fear of complications from radiotherapy treatment. All these will affect the patients' behaviour towards practitioners.

Cognitive approach

This theory proposes that an individual's thoughts, i.e. cognitive processes, enable reasoning and decision-making to take place. An individual can either learn the information from other individuals or can acquire it through experience.[6] This can then be communicated to others using speech. How this happens has been explained as selective interpretation of perceptual data organised into new pattern of thoughts and relationships.

> **!** Individual's feelings, motives, attitudes, memory and cognition have an effect on the individual's behaviour. For example, if the practitioner focuses on biases such as culture, race, ethnicity, etc., this will result in the stereotyping of patients, which will affect the interaction between the practitioner and those patients.

Humanistic approach

The humanist's perspective emphasises the positive aspects of human behaviour in terms of the possibility of growth and achievement. This means that an individual's behaviour is dependent on that person's experience. They stress that each individual has a unique perception of the world and it is this perception that shapes how that person behaves. The humanists argue that no two people will behave in the same way under the same conditions. In clinical practice, each patient comes as a unique individual person and consequently, the way the individual interacts with the practitioner will be unique to that person at that point in time. This essentially determines the personality of the individual. For example, the way a patient perceives the practitioner's attitudes in terms of empathy, verbal and non-verbal communication will determine how the patient will react and consequently behave towards the practitioner during the procedure.

Social constructivist approach

Social constructionist psychology emphasises that knowledge is culturally created. This means that social learning comes before development. Learning between people comes before individual learning. What this indicates is that people understand their social world through images and social representations shared by members of a social group. This is indicative of people learning through imitation of a role model. Children copy what their parents do and internalise these, which then forms the basis of their behaviour in the future. Therefore, people's attitudes are shaped by the environment and the commonalities shared by groups of people. These in turn determine their behaviour and interaction with members of the healthcare team. In this area, religious beliefs about illness can determine the way patients behave during imaging or radiotherapy treatment. In addition, cultural differences affect the interaction between the practitioner and the patient due to the differences in expectations from both parties.

So, what can we learn from these psychological principles, and how do they affect the practitioner patient interaction in medical imaging and radiotherapy? It is noted that the way patients access healthcare is determined by their beliefs and previous experience within the radiology or radiotherapy department. Another factor which influences a patient's decision as to whether to use healthcare services or not, is their symptoms, since the influence of a given symptom varies for different people.

In addition, it is important to consider an individual's health-related behaviour, such as the effects of diet, exercise and smoking; and the demographic characteristics of age, gender and ethnicity. On the other hand, socioeconomic standards and group values are paramount players in affecting behaviour towards accessing healthcare. While the list is not exhaustive, an issue worth mentioning is compliance/non-compliance, with instructions given for a particular examination or treatment. This aspect will be revisited below.

HUMAN CHARACTERISTICS OF INTERACTION

The quality of care provided for patients in the radiology and radiotherapy departments should be optimum, irrespective of their personal dispensation, gender, age, race, religion and language. Providing suboptimal care goes against the professional's duty of care and professional standards[7,8] (see Chapter 29, Ethical and legal considerations in professional practice). It is important for practitioners to understand the perspectives of the patients they care for because the practitioners' perspectives may differ from those of their clients, especially if they are from different cultures. The practitioner is therefore required to be culturally sensitive, in other words, required to consider the patient's cultural needs.

Personal characteristics

Individuals are different in the way they perceive things. They tend to perceive what they want, need and expect. This creates a form of diversity in addition to the characteristics of gender, race, religion, culture, language and age. Perception is further affected by the physical, mental and emotional status of the individual, the time of the day and the nature of the environment. Also, the person's beliefs, values, attitudes and expectations will influence such perception. In the medical environment, the perception is two-fold: that from the patient and that from the practitioner. This brings with it certain expectations from both parties and if not handled properly by the practitioner, will result in a bad experience for the patient.

The variety of patients, i.e. children, adults and the elderly, who attend both the imaging and radiotherapy departments require specific care.

> **!** Children should not be managed in the same way as adults and it is essential that appropriate language is used for this group of patients

However, special considerations need to be given to patients who present with a form of disability. The elderly population is increasing in the UK and according to statistics, elderly people will form over 23% of the population by 2025.[9] The elderly pose other challenges for practitioners, since some may have a form of disease or condition, e.g. dementia, which makes coordination and remembering difficult.

Another problem with patients with dementia is that they may also like to communicate in their native language, which the practitioner may not understand. The problem becomes more critical, especially if the elderly patient's culture is different from that of the practitioner. Hearing and language problems may affect their understanding of the instructions given by the practitioner. For those patients with impaired hearing, the practitioner should avoid shouting at them. Additionally, the practitioner may use sign language to communicate or use the services of an interpreter who is able to speak the same language as the patient. (See Chapters 2 and 3 for Communication with specific patient groups and Communication with patients with disabilities and additional needs, respectively.)

Interacting with this group of people during examination or treatment requires the practitioner to be sensitive to their needs and to adopt strategies aimed at ensuring the provision of adequate care. These patients should not be treated differently from other patients, as this represents a form of discrimination, which is against the law. In the UK, the government passed the Equality Act in 2010,[10] which states that an individual should not be discriminated against based on his or her race, gender, religion or disability. In Western culture, respect for the elderly is far less than in Chinese, Asian and Middle Eastern countries, where old people enjoy a great level of respect and the family structure is well bonded.

Gender

The gender of the patient affects the interaction with the practitioner. What is considered normal and accepted varies within different cultures. For example in Western culture, patients of either sex can be attended to by practitioners of either sex. The preference for a same sex practitioner is more dominant in Middle Eastern countries and most especially, the Arab community. This is due mainly to the influence of the Islamic religion on culture. In order for a female patient to be examined or treated by a male practitioner, the use of a chaperone is required. It is also not unusual for the husband to insist on being in the examination or treatment room with his wife. In cases when a chaperone is present, practitioners should always ensure that the person is protected from the radiation exposure. It has been found in women of Canadian-European descent and Canadian South-Asian descent that the women prefer a same gender family physician for gynaecological examinations.[11] The women's choice has been based on physicians' behaviours, attitudes, communication style, age and the stereotyping of physicians, while their cultural beliefs, norms and values influence their decision.

In Saudi Arabia, the basic beliefs about male/female relationships are influenced by religion. For example a female cannot be alone with a male unless he is a close relative, although exceptions do exist. Segregation of sexes is the norm in all areas of the society, whereby boys and girls are taught separately from elementary school up to University level. Hospital treatment and wedding ceremonies also follow the cultural tradition.

It is also forbidden for females to expose parts of their body, including their hair, in Middle Eastern culture, while this is acceptable in Western societies. If the practitioner requests a female patient from a Middle Eastern culture to expose a part of her body, this could lead to embarrassment and anxiety. For example, giving instructions to change into a gown for an examination, the practitioner must be aware that there may be issues concerning certain items of clothing such as the Hijab worn by Muslim women, especially if her male chaperone is not her husband. Also, certain items worn on the body by East-Asian women represent cultural artefacts, therefore the practitioner should be cautious in telling the patient to remove them, as the patient may be reluctant to do so. The practitioner must be able to explain why the patient has to remove the artefact. In addition, family members often accompany patients to the hospital and often stay with them during the exposure. The presence of family members in the examination or treatment room can become problematic due to the use of radiation, so the practitioner needs to be able to explain what is required of the family member during the procedure.

Another important factor in diversity is the use of personal space or proximity. This is the distance or closeness that two people talking to each other maintain. In Arab countries, individuals tend to stand close to each other. This is also true in some European cultures such as the Italians and the Spaniards, who tend to maintain close personal space while talking, unlike people from Great Britain who prefer more personal space. Practitioners have to be culturally sensitive on this issue when interacting with patients.

The use of touch as a form of communication means different things in different cultures. While it is acceptable in Western culture for people to touch each other, it is unacceptable in other cultures. For example, the Spanish speaking countries use 'touch' a lot during conversation, while in Western countries, the handshake is used only for greetings. However, in some cultures, touching patients by a same gender healthcare professional may require permission. In most Islamic countries, touching is uncommon and is forbidden between the opposite sexes. In carrying out an examination, the practitioner needs to position the patient, which means having to touch certain bony landmarks on the patient's body, as well as moving the patient. In this instance, the practitioner should explain clearly what he intends to do and why, in order to avoid any misunderstanding and to be able to carry out a successful examination.

Different gender or sexual orientation affects the approach healthcare providers should take when dealing with same sex patients such as homosexual 'gays' and 'lesbians'. In the Western world, prominence has been given to such relationships through the Equality Act, recognising same sex relationships and marriages.[10] Practitioners dealing with these groups of people must accord them the appropriate duty of care, even if they do not agree with such relationships.

Race

The race or ethnic background to which an individual belongs determines the culture that influences the individual's values, attitudes, perceptions about health and consequently their behaviour. The British and Chinese have long established traditions about health issues. They regard looking after their health as extremely important, which means that practitioners interacting with people from either of these nations must be aware of that culture relating to healthcare. In some cultures, the decision to access healthcare services is often taken by a senior member of the family. This translates into 'the family comes first' and practitioners should have the skill to deal with such patients. South-Asians and South-East Asians have strong family values which include obedience and thus they will not discuss family issues or conflicts with strangers.[12]

Religion

There are various religions throughout the world, including Christianity, which comprises various faiths and denominations, Islam, Buddhism, Hinduism. Religion plays a vital role in many cultures. Often the word 'religion' is used synonymously with culture. This is because some religious practices have become part of the culture. For example in the Christian religion, some denominations fast for 40 days, starting from Ash Wednesday until Easter; Muslims abstain from food and drink during daylight in the Holy month of Ramadan. Scheduling an examination or treatment during this period for patients from both religions can be problematic, especially if the examination or treatment means that those patients will not to be able to carry out their religious duties. For example, in Arab and Muslim countries, the culture is influenced by the Islamic code, which stipulates the need to pray five times a day, and a dress code. (Dressing has been covered in an earlier section under gender.) Therefore, if a patient from that culture presents for examination or treatment, the practitioner needs to be conversant with the prevailing cultures of their patients at that time. The practitioners should respect the patient's belief system and should not attempt to incorporate their own culture into the patient's culture.

Communication and language

In a hospital setting, effective patient centred care depends on effective communication between practitioners and their patients. Poor communication skills would affect the practitioner–patient interaction and the provision of quality patient care. Communication is a process in which two individuals attempt to exchange their ideas and meanings. When two individuals from different cultures try to exchange a set of meanings, this process results in intercultural communication.[13] They may not share the same views about certain aspects or they may have different ways of thinking, so communication between practitioners and patients is complicated because of cultural differences.

Language is the most obvious cultural difference. In any communication, language plays an important role. If the practitioner and the patient are from different cultures, then there may be linguistic problems.[14] So what is language? Language is a medium through which messages are passed between individuals. The messages may not necessarily result in a better understanding because of obstacles in the medium such as cultural and linguistic barriers, which could distort these messages and cause misunderstandings between the practitioner and patient.

There may be instances when the patient becomes difficult simply due to misunderstanding the practitioner's instructions or due to cultural differences, which may hide certain feelings. For example, a patient may not be convinced about the necessity of some technical aspects, such as taking a deep breath for a chest or abdominal X-ray examination or filling the bladder for an abdominal ultrasound, and may not understand why this is required. Practitioners should minimise the use of acronyms, technical jargon and phrases, as in many cultures, word equivalents may not exist or the same word may have different connotations.

Verbal communication is important while giving instructions but at the same time, the non-verbal aspects such as body language, gestures, spatial awareness and eye contact should not be ignored, as they play a vital role in intercultural communication. Verbal communication becomes more difficult when an interaction involves people who speak different languages. This type of communication is directly affected by language, as the client needs to listen to what the practitioner or the healthcare provider says. When verbal communication is used effectively, it enables the practitioner to develop an immediate rapport with the patient. Where the issue of language barrier exists, this can be minimised through the use of interpreters who can either be trained hospital staff or a family member accompanying the patient.

Initially, verbal communication can also be influenced by cultural values. The busy practitioner may wish to complete the examination as quickly as possible in order to devote time to other patients. However, some patients, e.g. the elderly, may want some explanation about their examination, while others may like to talk to the practitioner, e.g. because they are lonely. If the practitioner ignores this and proceeds with examination instructions, the patient may become offended. This would also be contrary, e.g. to the culture in Saudi Arabia, where it is important to follow social courtesies before business or personal work is carried out.[15]

It is normal in the UK to call patients by their first name and then family name (surname). This may be an issue in some cultures, such as in Asian cultures, where people are addressed by their family name followed by the first name. In this instance, the patient may feel that the practitioner is disrespectful and this may result in the patient not cooperating fully with the practitioner. This aspect can also affect the practitioner who has come from another culture, where calling either the elderly or someone of a higher hierarchy by their first name is not the norm.

Non-verbal communication is also culture dependent. What is considered normal and accepted varies with different cultures. For example, in Indian culture, shaking the head from side to side means 'yes', while shaking the head up and down means 'no'. Therefore in a multicultural environment, the practitioner's body language such as posture, facial expressions, gestures and eye contact can make the patient feel uncomfortable, which may lead to an uncooperative attitude. The practitioner must also assess the patient's body language for signs of understanding. For example, maintaining eye contact when speaking to a patient is seen as a sign of sincerity, politeness and respectfulness in Western and Middle Eastern culture. On the other hand, West Indians and East-Asians avoid direct eye contact, since it can be considered as being rude and defiant or an indication of sexual overtones, especially if both parties are of different sexes.[16]

One aspect of verbal communication which can prevent successful interaction between the practitioner and the patient is the issue of 'accent' or dialect. When a practitioner giving instructions to a patient has an accent, and the patient listening is a native speaker, then the possibility is that the patient's attention might concentrate on listening to the accent instead of what the practitioner is saying. Checking the patient's comprehension is important to ensure that the instructions given have been understood.

Finally, the use of written communication should not be ignored but whatever information is provided, it should be written in clear and simple language and one which the patient will understand. (Further information on communication can be found in Chapters 1–4.)

KEY POINTS

- The principles of personality, gender, race/ethnicity, religion and communication/language form the key elements of human interaction
- It can be seen that culture pervades all psychological processes
- Effective care requires an understanding of the varying cultural and social backgrounds of patients and how this may impact on their experiences
- There needs to be an appreciation of the intra- and inter-psychological processes that may affect both the patients' and healthcare professionals' behaviour within the healthcare environment
- Professionals need to be culturally sensitive and avoid stereotyping patients by using their own standards for comparison

Chapter | 6 |

Psychological aspects of patient care

Terri Gilleece

WHY DO PRACTITIONERS NEED AN UNDERSTANDING OF PSYCHOLOGY?

Radiography is a profession where we must develop a wide range of skills. The need for technical competence is obvious since we utilise technology in order to produce images or treat patients. However, we cannot function as health professionals without demonstrating the humanistic caring qualities that must be the focus of patient centred care.

It is easy to become task-centred rather than patient-centred. Time pressures and staffing issues can result in a 'busyness' that gives patients the impression that we are in too much of a hurry to take time to focus on them as a person; that we are not interested in them. To avoid this we must view the patient holistically, paying attention to their psychological, spiritual and physical needs. These conflicting requirements can undoubtedly cause tension for the practitioner resulting in anxiety and lack of confidence, especially for newly qualified practitioners.

In gaining an understanding of the psychology of patient care, we also gain a more in-depth understanding of ourselves as individuals and as healthcare providers. This can help us to deal with difficult and stressful interactions with patients, colleagues and with our own thoughts, feelings and reactions to these encounters.

THEORIES OF PSYCHOLOGY

Research has indicated that healthcare professionals who are aware of theoretical psychological approaches have more successful interactions with patients than those without such knowledge.[1]

There is general agreement that there are three main schools of thought in the field of psychology that apply to the healthcare setting:

- Psychodynamic
- Behavioural
- Humanistic

Psychodynamic approach

Based largely on the work of Freud, this embraces the concept of unconscious motivation and behaviour. Freud postulated that every event experienced by an individual throughout their life, or even before birth, shape how a person behaves and may determine decision-making in later life. Freud's model of the human mind has three levels: the *id*, the *ego* and the *superego*. The id is the infant personality that requires us to satisfy basic desires. As we grow, we become aware of the world around us and develop a more realistic view and an understanding that we cannot fulfil every desire. The ego allows us to consider our actions; it can be thought of as the reasoning part of our personality. The superego is the part of our personality that develops as we cultivate our morality or values. It has a governing function on our behaviour.

Table 6.1 Coping mechanisms

Mechanism	Description and function
Rationalisation	Making excuses or finding acceptable reasons for things we really know to be wrong. Allows continuation of bad behaviour, e.g. a person who is overweight and continues to eat a poor diet blames his genes and metabolism for weight gain
Suppression	Consciously excluding thoughts or feelings that are painful or unpleasant, sometimes called 'motivated forgetting'. A person who has a fear of attending the dentist may 'forget' that it is time to book a dental check-up
Sublimation	Transformation of socially unacceptable or aggressive behaviours into socially acceptable pursuits. Participation in sports can reduce aggressive behaviour and is an acceptable way of releasing tension
Repression	Unconsciously eliminating a painful or traumatic event from memory. (This is different from suppression, which is a conscious mechanism.) The purpose of this mechanism is to protect the individual from emotional overload
Reaction formation	Unconsciously avoiding the urge to do or say something by doing the exact opposite. It is a way of protecting the individual from rejection or instigated as a barrier against being hurt, e.g. when a teacher tries to explain a concept and the student insists they understand, even though they know they have not come close to comprehension
Regression	Reverting to a less mature state – a temporary denial of adult responsibility. Serves to reduce tension and allow abdication of certain responsibilities, e.g. patients who assume a very dependent role or who become very demanding
Displacement	Redirects the source of frustration from objects felt to be dangerous or unacceptable to an object felt to be safe or acceptable. It reduces anxiety by transferring emotions such as guilt or anger, e.g. a teenager who has had a disagreement with a parent may displace their anger by slamming doors or chastising a sibling
Denial	A person is faced with a fact that is too uncomfortable to accept and rejects it instead, insisting that it is not true, despite evidence to the contrary. This prevents acceptance of the unacceptable, e.g. some alcoholics refuse to accept that their patterns and quantity of alcohol consumption are any different from that of the normal population

In terms of healthcare, important aspects of this theory are the mental defence mechanisms (also called ego defence mechanisms or coping mechanisms). These processes allow us to cope with rising levels of anxiety. With the exception of rationalisation and suppression, which are conscious mechanisms, the others are unconscious processes (Table 6.1).

Behavioural approach

This approach focuses on repetitive or 'learned' behaviour that the individual develops in response to reward or reinforcement. The champions of this approach hypothesise that such principles determine all or most of human behaviour. These ideas began with the work of Pavlov[2] who described 'classical conditioning'. Pavlov fed his dogs at 1.00p.m. every day; at that time a bell was rung in a nearby building. He noticed that if he was late feeding his dogs they salivated when they heard the bell; they had developed a conditioned reflex. Other researchers went on to refine classical conditioning and demonstrate that it was possible to encourage behaviour outside of the normal range associated with a specific animal;[3] 'operant conditioning'. This is also achieved through regular reinforcement or the use of rewards. A clear example of this is the training of dogs to assist those with various disabilities.

! The conditioning approach can often be observed in paediatric patients who have had previous hospital encounters. If they have had a negative experience with injections, surgery or imaging procedures, they view the hospital environment as ominous.

Frequently in these situations, the child is in a state of distress before they arrive in the imaging or radiotherapy department. Conversely, a child who has had positive experiences in the hospital environment can view a visit to hospital as a place where they will be given 'stickers', or a time when parents will reward cooperation with sweets, a new toy or a visit to a fast food chain.

Humanistic approach

This approach emphasises the importance of how the person functions in the present. It is a result of the individual's strengths, aspirations and conscious free will. It is of importance within the healthcare sector because it is concerned with understanding interpersonal interaction, asserting that each individual can fulfil personal ambitions and reach their full potential. It embraces the concept of unconditional positive reward – demonstrating that some behaviours are unacceptable but still treating the individual with respect, empathy, openness and trust.[4,5,6] This could equally be described as professionalism within the clinical setting.

Theoretical versus practical application

The approaches discussed above each have their merits and limitations. Indeed, many other approaches have been developed to define human behaviour, but are beyond the scope of this text. Frequently, behaviour may be best understood by employing an 'eclectic approach', a combination of the theories, to appreciate a person's actions and reactions. We must be mindful that critical evaluation of our own behaviour as healthcare staff, through reflection, can be the most useful starting point for understanding the behaviour of others.

The following sections contain definitions of some of the behavioural states that affect the patients we are likely to encounter in the healthcare environment. By recognising these in patients, we should be better able to offer personalised care, appropriate to the needs of that individual.

STRESS, ANXIETY AND DEPRESSION

In everyday life, the terms 'stress', 'anxiety' and 'depression' are often used interchangeably. We all experience stress during our daily lives. The signs of stress can vary: increased heart rate, muscle tension, lack of concentration and fatigue can all be attributed to stress. Stress can come from any situation if we perceive that we do not have the ability to cope with the events or the likely outcomes of the event. Stress is a very individual experience and what may be a stressor to one person may not seem significant to another, possibly because of better/different coping mechanisms or social support.

During times of stress, adrenaline is released causing a rise in blood pressure and other negative changes and effects. One of the negative effects is anxiety. With anxiety, fear overcomes all emotions, accompanied by worry and apprehension. Some people describe feelings of impending doom. Other symptoms are chest pains, dizziness and shortness of breath and panic attacks, constant aches and pains, palpitations, chronic fatigue, crying, over or undereating, frequent infections and loss of libido.

Since stress leads to anxiety, it can be difficult to differentiate the two, but symptoms of anxiety persist independently of stressors. According to the *Diagnostic and Statistical Manual*, 4th edn. (DSM IV), anxiety is:

> *a clinically significant behavioural or psychological syndrome or pattern that occurs in an individual and that is associated with present distress or disability or with significantly increased risk of suffering, death, pain, or disability, or an important loss of freedom.*

Stress is regarded as a normal reaction and is usually short-lived. The DSM IV states that for anxiety to be diagnosed, the condition should have persisted for at least 6 months.[7]

There are varying definitions of depression. It is generally agreed that the symptoms are similar to that of stress or anxiety but much more intense and often accompanied by thoughts of self-harm or suicide. There is also disagreement among mental health professionals about how long symptoms have to be present for the diagnosis of depression to apply.

> **!** Depression is common within the general population but the diagnosis of a life-limiting disease can certainly increase the individual's susceptibility to depression. However, not all patients with serious conditions such as cancer develop depression.

For the purposes of this text, it is sufficient to note that psychologists and general practitioners regard stress, anxiety and depression as unique entities but the effects that they may have on our patients are the same.

The feelings associated with any of these three conditions can be generated by: new situations,[8] the presence of strangers, concerns about personal appearance or being asked to do things in public that would normally be viewed as socially inappropriate. If we look at the hospital setting from a patient's perspective, we can see multiple opportunities for the generation of stress and anxiety: patients may not have been in an imaging or radiotherapy department before, the staff are unfamiliar to them, they may have surgical scars or a disfiguring injury and we may require them to remove clothing and follow instructions. In addition they are, in most cases, in hospital to have a condition diagnosed or treated, so they are already anxious about the implications of their illness.

Patients often find themselves irritable, tense and restless; they may exhibit anger or hostility. Where the illness is on-going, the patient may cope with feelings of anxiety by employing denial as a mechanism to reduce the impact of disruptive situations. This can be useful in the short term, however, it can have adverse effects if continued for longer periods and can even lead to non-compliance with medical treatment.

ANGER AND AGGRESSION

While aggression in the hospital setting is frequently associated with the A&E department (where alcohol and drugs are commonly a factor), with mental health or learning disabilities, every practitioner is likely to experience interactions with angry and aggressive patients because behaviour is altered in the hospital setting. The main reasons for patients behaving aggressively are:

- Lack of information
- Cognition clouded by pain, medication or psychotic illness
- Perception of intentional, avoidable or malevolent events.

According to research, people do not become aggressive because they have a desire to hurt another person; rather their aggression is a way for them to channel their emotions so that they can rebalance their social status or restore a negative self-esteem.[9] For example, an attempt to impress their peers by attacking an innocent victim because it will raise their 'status' within that peer group; to achieve a feeling of power and control by making others feel inferior, sometimes by demonstrating physical superiority; or as a way of removing stressors by hiding feelings of embarrassment or fear.

Illness or trauma can result in feelings of emotional weakness, vulnerability and personal inadequacies. As it is impossible for patients to avoid or escape from the situation in which they find themselves, the remaining 'primitive' instinct is to regain control through aggression.

Anger is generally viewed as a negative and undesirable emotion. By allowing patients the opportunity to dissipate their anger – simply by providing a listening ear, we can sometimes circumvent the frustrations that build-up and lead to aggression. Similarly, providing information to the patient can reduce their sense of powerlessness.

Imagine if you were on your way to take an exam. You are on a train that has stopped. You don't know why it has stopped. The exam is due to start in 30 minutes and you are still 10 minutes from the university. The train has been stationary for 15 minutes and there is no explanation as to why you are not moving.

The lack of information means you cannot make an assessment of how much longer you are likely to be delayed or what effect the delay will have on your ability to take the exam or perhaps progress to the following semester. If an announcement is made that there is a minor fault that has now been rectified and the train will get underway again in a matter of minutes, you are likely to feel as though frustration has been eradicated.

> **!** It is important that practitioners do not respond to patient aggression with anger. We should aim to:
> - Enhance self-esteem
> - Give back the patient's sense of control
> - Provide an outlet for anger
>
> Allowing the patients time and space to 'air their views' can be of enormous assistance in achieving all three of these goals.

MAKING CHOICES DURING TIMES OF STRESS, ANXIETY AND ILLNESS

As stated above, depression, anxiety and stress can be common responses to illness and hospitalisation. This is not surprising given that the basic elements that underlie these conditions are fostered in such circumstances:

- Patients are in an unfamiliar environment
- They are required to relinquish control to health professionals
- They are separated from family and friends
- Normal 'distractions' such as social activities, pets and coping mechanisms are denied to them.

In addition to the difficulties listed above, there is likely to be: anxiety over the physical pain of the presenting condition; worry about pain associated with investigations or treatments; recovery time; prognosis; loss of income; and placing additional burdens on loved ones.

High levels of anxiety can have an impact on how we process information and make decisions. Psychologists have suggested that we have 'cold' and 'hot' cognitive states. The former is associated with logical decision-making, largely devoid of emotion, while the latter is associated with irrational, emotionally-charged decisions,[10] and is often the state that our patients experience. When anxiety levels are heightened the ability to process, store and recall information is distorted.[11] As a result, patients are likely to behave in an emotional rather than logical manner. They can panic and accept the first available solution. They may deny the gravity of the situation and behave in an abnormally 'normal' manner, giving an outward appearance of having understood, digested and accepted the situation.

They may employ diversion mechanisms to shift responsibility for the situation to others or divert attention to other things, e.g. booking a holiday or getting a new kitchen.

While it is impossible to predict the outcomes of investigations prior to attendance at hospital – and it would be irresponsible and unethical in most circumstances to take the patient through all possible outcomes and scenarios prior to having investigations completed – it is necessary to provide the patient with as much information as possible *prior* to them making important decisions.

> ⚠ It is good practice to make information available to the patients in a variety of formats. An explanation of the situation, in simple terms, with an opportunity for questions, should be supplemented with written information for the patient to keep and later discuss with loved ones.

Ideally, a second discussion should ensue before decisions are finalised so that the patient has had the opportunity to assimilate the information, form questions after quiet reflection and possibly search the internet for further information. On the latter point, patients and families will frequently find inappropriate or even factually incorrect information from electronic sources – patients do not always wish to disclose that they have been surfing for information and may keep this worry to themselves – it can be a good idea to ask if they have looked up their condition and then have a discussion about what they have found and perhaps guide them to reliable sites.

COMPLIANCE

Compliance or rather non-compliance with advice and instructions in the medical imaging and radiotherapy department can be of particular importance because of the fact that we are frequently using ionising radiations, have long waiting lists and have budgetary restraints. For example, if a patient has not adhered to instructions for bowel preparation prior to gastrointestinal imaging, the examination may have to be repeated. This becomes a financial cost to the department, increases waiting times for other patients and means an additional radiation dose for the patient. In the radiotherapy department, non-compliance can have long-term repercussions for the patient, e.g. failure to adhere to bladder filling protocols for those with prostate cancers can result in geographical miss of the target organ and bladder necrosis.

It is therefore important to understand why patients do not comply with the information they are asked to follow. It is also important to examine staff attitudes to those patients who are obviously contravening medical advice. Most of the literature available in this area deals with non-compliance in treatment regimes for chronic disorders but as our interest lies in understanding the reasons underlying non-compliance, it should be logical to attribute the same reasoning to our patient set. We should also bear in mind that some of the patients we deal with could be with us because they have not been taking prescribed medications or implementing changes in lifestyle that have been recommended.

- Complexity of treatment regime
  - Taking one set of medication may be easy to maintain or taking a few tablets for preparation may be possible but if there are multiple drugs to be taken at different times on different days, this can cause patients to opt out of all treatments. Patients lose track and simply give up on the treatment or they see their lives as being controlled by the treatment regime
- Protracted treatments
  - Patients having prophylactic treatments and those with chronic disorders spanning many years are among the groups that are least likely to comply with treatment. Patients will cite reasons such as, 'How do I know if I still need the drugs if I don't stop taking them?' Sometimes patients on long-term treatments will stop medication as way of regaining control that they feel has been removed from them
- Adverse reactions
  - It may seem obvious that in such circumstances, the patient would return to the prescriber/pharmacy and explain the problem, but not all patients have the ability to do this. Some may also believe that because they have a poor reaction to one drug they will react in the same manner to all drugs for the condition
- Poor communication
  - If the patient was under severe stress when the treatment was explained, they simply might not understand the treatment process (see above), or may have had too much information given at one time – information overload.
- Lack of follow-up
  - If the patient does not have regular follow-up appointments with an appropriate healthcare professional, they can feel as though their condition is of little importance and therefore it doesn't matter whether they continue to take medication or not
- Success of the medication
  - Ironically, if the medication has had the desired effect, the patient may feel that they have recovered from their illness and no longer have need of the treatment
- Knowledge and understanding of the condition/treatment
  - If the patient has not been provided with enough information, in the correct manner and at a level

appropriate to their needs, then they can underestimate the long-term implications and side-effects of not complying with advice. The patient's knowledge of their condition has a greater effect on compliance than intelligence

- Mental impairment
  - The conditions for which the patients are receiving treatment or co-morbidities may cause mental impairments such as forgetfulness. It is also possible that some of the medications will have this effect on the patient
- Treatments involving lifestyle changes
  - Compliance for treatments involving lifestyle changes can be as low as 15%. Patients use *rationalisation* as a mechanism to justify the continuation of a behaviour they know to be detrimental to them, e.g. smoking after being diagnosed with cancer of the larynx – patients say they need the cigarettes to 'steady their nerves' and help them get through the radiotherapy treatment
- Denial
  - The patient has such difficulty dealing with their diagnosis/prognosis that they simply deny that there is a problem. Since they feel there is no problem, they feel they need not follow the medical advice.

It can be difficult for busy practitioners to deal in a caring manner with patients who present in their department due to non-compliance with prescribed drug regimes or medical advice, or who are having on-going treatment but flouting the advice provided. We can feel that we are wasting our time with such patients when others are more deserving. By reflecting on the possible reasons for non-compliance, we should be able to understand the patient and in some instances address their behaviour by offering solutions that will aid both the patient and ourselves. For example by encouraging the patient to set a target for only smoking half the number of cigarettes they normally would – they may find this less of a hurdle and be more willing to engage in it, if they believe they can be successful in reaching this target. We can reinforce the information relating to their illness – patients can forget the majority of what is said at consultation and while they retain the diagnosis, the instructions are often forgotten – although research has shown that we are more likely to retain information provided at the start and finish of a consultation. We can provide contact information for organisations that provide assistance for their particular condition.

Compliance and non-compliance in the medical imaging and radiotherapy departments

As stated previously, most of the research in the area of compliance centres around patients with long-term illnesses or on preventative medicine. Our daily encounters with patients tend to be more transient and subsequently, while the above list of reasons for non-compliance can be of use to us, we may find it most helpful to focus on 'poor communication' area that we should focus on and we should also consider phobias (see below).

Other patients may have difficulty in complying with our requests because of difficulty with communication. When anxious, it can be difficult for patients to process information and instructions. Again, taking time with the patient and being careful not to hurry them can achieve the required results. Demonstrating the task you want the patient to perform while repeating the instructions can be a considerable aid to compliance.

PAIN

According to the *Oxford English Dictionary*, pain is:

1 a strongly unpleasant bodily sensation caused, e.g. by illness or injury. 2 mental suffering.

In radiography practice, it is fair to say, that we give great consideration to the first definition, i.e. organic pain, but can overlook the second, i.e. psychogenic pain, although it is no less real or no less distressing for the patient. In actual fact, psychogenic pain can be more distressing for the patient because it can persist for longer periods of time and treatment options can be less acceptable to the patient because there can be a stigma attached to psychological interventions. It has been documented that negative mood states experienced by those with anxiety or depression can cause an individual to feel an increased level of organic pain,[12] which can be relieved through support and practical help.

Just as psychological states can have a negative effect on feelings of pain, they can have a positive effect too. We have all heard of the 'Placebo' effect. The placebo is of no therapeutic value whatsoever, but the administration of a placebo can reduce the intensity of pain. This is partly through the production of natural endorphins[13] that result from a conditioning reaction where the expectation is that medication will help. However, it will only help at the site at which we anticipate pain relief.[14] Empathy and consideration can produce similar effects to the placebo.

> **!** When patients are admitted to hospital, the feelings of fear and loss of control can intensify symptoms associated with physical pain. Other practical issues can affect pain levels too: being in a strange uncomfortable bed, not having their own pillows, lack of sleep, lack of privacy and forced daily routines associated with ward tasks.

With most patients we can communicate easily, assess levels of pain and take actions to alleviate it where possible – providing extra pillows on the imaging couch, altering the technique to make the patient more comfortable, etc. By asking the patient if there is anything that can be done to relieve their pain, we are offering them back some control and acknowledging their distress.

PHOBIAS

The *Oxford English Dictionary* defines the term 'Phobia' as a strong irrational fear. The main phobias that we encounter in our patients are 'belonephobia' or 'trypanophobia', i.e. specific fear of needles or fear of injections; and 'claustrophobia', which is fear of confined spaces. Other phobias such as 'agoraphobia', which is fear of having an anxiety attack in a situation from which it is difficult to escape, can prevent patients from attending appointments or put them in a state of high anxiety if they do manage to make it to the appointment. We may also encounter situations where the patient experiences the fear of being left alone in unfamiliar surroundings. This is known as 'isolophobia'.

Frequently, patients may recognise their phobias are irrational but because of the nature of phobias, logical thinking or persuasion will do little to counteract the very real feelings they are experiencing. Depending on the extent of the phobia, it may be possible to achieve success by taking time with the patient and demonstrating such things as a member of staff lying on the bed and going into the scanner – sometimes letting the patient use the controls of the couch may help. The important thing to note is that these patients require extra time, hurrying them certainly will not be of benefit. On occasion, medication can help reduce their anxiety levels and allow the procedure to be completed. It is useful to have prior knowledge of the patient's phobia in advance of booking a slot for these patients so that additional time can be allocated or so that prescribed medication can be made available.

CHILDREN, ADOLESCENTS AND OLDER ADULTS

So far in this chapter, there has been an assumption that in general, we are dealing with the adult patient. As this group spans the ages of 18–65, it represents the broadest section of patients and illnesses. In addition to a variety of conditions becoming prevalent in this age group, this is also the time in life at which major life changes are experienced along with the associated responsibilities and pressures; it can be described as the busiest time in life. It is during this time that personal relationships are developed and indeed dissolved in some cases. Financial responsibilities increase, people have children and for some individuals, the role of caring for elderly or sick parents adds to the other responsibilities. Illness during this time can increase stress and pressures, and indeed stress itself can become debilitating if it is allowed to progress to more serious levels. It can manifest in physical as well as mental ill health. Anger and aggression responses and coping mechanisms have been discussed in relation to this age group.

There are special considerations that must be applied to other age groups because the developmental process is incomplete and does not allow for rational thought and reasoned behaviour. Perhaps the obvious age groups are children and adolescents, but we have an ageing population in this country and this section of society can require some specific considerations also. (See also Chapter 2, Communication with specific patient groups.)

Stage development

'Stage' theories have been used in the literature to describe the transition from infant behaviour that requires us to satisfy our basic needs to socially acceptable, well-reasoned adult behaviour.[15,16] Each of the aforementioned theories assumes that development takes place in fixed stages within age bands. In recent years, there has been movement away from the traditional stage theories and there is now general agreement that children learn in incremental steps rather than fixed age bands. This reflects current thinking in healthcare that we should be focused on the individual as a unique entity, regardless of the age of the patient. However, it can be helpful to have a working understanding of stage theories such as Piaget's,[16] as his developmental framework is still widely used for the purpose of informing educational provision, health strategies and social care policies.

The developmental framework is of particular use to healthcare staff when dealing with those children who are unfamiliar with the hospital environment, e.g. trauma situations or initial investigations. Frequently, children and adolescents with health problems will have a deep understanding of their condition, medications and procedures. However, we should be careful not to assume this to be true of all patients, as it will depend greatly on the communication with practitioners, parents, interactions with their peers, particularly those with similar health problems, and to some extent, their level of intelligence.[17] For this reason, practitioners who are dealing with children and adolescents should ascertain the participant's level of knowledge and understanding before explaining procedures by asking if they have had the particular procedure/treatment before; asking what they remember/know about it; and giving the patient a chance to express worries or concerns. This allows practitioners to correct any misunderstandings and 'pitch' an explanation at the appropriate level.

Infants and children

We should not assume that very young children are incapable of appreciating what is happening to them, but it has been shown[18] that they respond best when we use familiar objects to explain procedures and events. In many hospitals, we can call on play therapists as part of the multidisciplinary team. On occasion, these specialist practitioners can work with the children before they enter the hospital environment. They can use toys and games to eliminate fears and anxieties.

Our actions and the behaviour of the parents and carers of the children can also be of great significance. At only 4 days old a baby can distinguish its mother's, or primary carer's, face from other faces. Children generally associate the presence of a parent with reassurance and comfort, and babies between 7 and 12 months can be very wary of strangers,[19] and become visibly and audibly upset at their close proximity. Parents are therefore encouraged to stay with the child at all times and it can be useful, particularly in this infant age group, to let the parent take on as much of the task as practicable to avoid anxiety for the child. Nevertheless, we should bear in mind that babies and children are capable of perceiving the feelings of those around them. Thus if children recognise stress and tension in parents or carers they can become fraught and upset. Therefore, practitioners must also be aware of the parents' needs, taking time to reassure and calm their anxieties when required.

If it is necessary to separate the child from the parent, special attention should be given to the information provided to the child and comforting the child throughout the procedure. Care is needed when choosing phrasing for explanations and common comments such as 'I'll pick you up in just a minute' – time can seem so much longer to children, and comments akin to this can lead to mistrust if the child feels as though staff have lied.

> **!** The child can also pick-up on the anxiety and stress of practitioners. Dealing with babies and children can be a daunting task for a variety of reasons, as diverse as difficulty relating to children because of lack of experience with paediatric patients; because of the severity of the diagnosis in such a young age group or because of difficulties in dealing with parents.

Response to parent interventions may be classed into four typical practitioner reactions,[20] as shown in Table 6.2.

Adolescents

Adolescence has been formally described as the period between puberty and adulthood. In real terms, it can be difficult to define and understand. Physical and biological changes make adolescence a problematic time but social and cultural pressure can intensify the complexities. Ill health during this time only serves to compound the situation. This is a time when this age group is learning to be independent, to reject parental constraints and values, and develop their own identity. When adults are faced with an illness, they usually rely on family support as a coping mechanism. It can be very confusing for adolescents who have just found some autonomy, to revert to seeking physical and emotional help from their parents. Some may however, regress to child-like behaviours as a result of overwhelming fear; others may become indifferent and employ denial as a coping strategy.[21]

Hospital procedures often require the removal of clothing. This can be embarrassing and distressing for any age group of patient but can be particularly difficult for adolescents who are more likely to be self-conscious about their body, particularly when encountering a member of the opposite sex.

Other difficulties can arise with practicalities such as where adolescents are placed in the hospital setting. Adolescence tends to be a time of less acute illness than early childhood or later adulthood, but traumatic events, accidents and death can be significant during this period. An adult ward or clinic may not be appropriate. Adolescents can view the other patients as elderly, even if they are not, and they can become withdrawn because of difficulties in communicating with the other patients because of lack of common interests. The older patients in the ward can have a worse prognosis than the adolescent and a poorer quality of life. Careful explanation of the adolescent's condition should also include an explanation that others in the ward are suffering from other types of illness and that each patient's prognosis and progression is different. Practical issues can arise due to lack of appropriate services in areas designed for adults, particularly if adolescents need access to tutoring services' parents live a long distance away and need to avail of parental accommodation and so forth. Adolescents can become angry at being treated in a paediatric setting where they perceive their maturity to be underestimated and again, can find little in common with younger children in the ward.

> **!** In legal terms, consent for procedures should be sought from parents but unless there is a mental impairment, adolescents should be included in the decision-making process. Failure to provide information and explanations can leave these patients feeling disenchanted and disempowered. Students and younger members of staff can be at an advantage when dealing with adolescents because they may relate better to those closer to their own age group and it may be easier for students and young staff to empathise with the adolescent patient.

Table 6.2 Practitioner reactions to parents

Reaction	Explanation
Facilitative	Recognition of the parents' role, giving support and removing barriers
Enforcement	Practitioners seek to take control over the actions of the parent and care of the child because they feel threatened by parental input. They try to enforce rules to help them maintain this control
Mutuality	Practitioners consider the parents to be the 'expert' in identifying the needs of their child and a relationship of trust is built between parents and practitioners
Avoidance	Practitioners use this protective but negative defence mechanism that can be displayed by practitioners if required to deal with demanding parents or those who express contradictory views to their own. Practitioners can develop feelings of hostility and anger, but recognise that this is not professional behaviour – denying that they have such feelings allow avoidance of the problems

Tolerance and understanding, particularly in response to frustration and anger, are key skills for dealing with the adolescent patient.

Older adults

As medicine and technology improve and our understandings of health protective behaviours increase, so too does the life span of the population. As with adolescence, it can be difficult to find a fixed definition for the beginning of this group. Simply applying a chronological age is not always appropriate as there are many unfit, unhealthy 60 year olds and many fit, healthy, independent 80 year olds. Our preconceptions of the older person do not always change in-line with the demographics of the older patient. Other similarities can be made with adolescence, as the 'older age' is a time of great transitions. However, instead of moving towards achieving respect and independence, this population can view themselves as experiencing loss; retirement can lead to loss of income and more importantly, feelings of loss of purpose and structure. For some, there is physical and/or mental decline that causes them to become more reliant on others and of course, there is loss associated with the death of family, friends and partners. Other individuals may embrace the transitions of older age in a more positive way; they see it as an opportunity to gain freedom from working life, to have financial independence and to develop new interests and hobbies.

> **!** Looking at a date of birth on a request form, it can be easy to assume the patient will be deaf or demented, because old age is often associated with negativity in our society. While it is inevitable that older people are more likely to experience illness and loss, it should not be assumed that they would respond to these issues differently from those who are younger.

Research has found that older people are just as satisfied with life and more positive about themselves[22] because they find it easier to adapt to changes in circumstances and modify their personal goals.

This does not mean that every older patient we come into contact with will be cheerful and happy to see us. They too will experience the fear and apprehension that can cause aggression and disagreeableness discussed earlier in this chapter. However, with this age group, practitioners are very often guilty of underestimating the intelligence and capabilities of the individual; infantilising the person, which intensifies the patient's feelings of anger and aggression.

Dementia

Alzheimer's disease and other forms of cognitive decline are becoming more frequent in society because people are living longer. In Europe, 1% of 60–64 year olds are estimated to have some form of dementia, while 25% of the 80+ age group are estimated to be affected by these disorders.[23] Dementias are often accompanied by depressive illness because of the physical changes in the brain structure but also because confusion and forgetfulness can cause stress and agitation. One of the main issues for dementia sufferers is depersonalisation.[24] This is of particular importance in imaging and radiotherapy departments because we do not get an opportunity to build up a relationship with the person; we do not get a chance to know the person and identify their capabilities. It can be very tempting, particularly in a busy department, to speak to the patient's carer and ignore the individual who should actually be the focus of our attention. This can lead to frustration, distress and agitation in the patient, making imaging or treatment impossible. To avoid this, attention must be focused on the patient, allowing extra time for that individual to absorb information and instructions. These should be given in a non-patronising manner, avoiding the use of child-like language and gestures. (See also Chapter 3, Communication with patients with disabilities and additional needs.)

DYING AND BEREAVEMENT

Bereavement is a characteristic response to the loss of someone or something that is of great importance to us. The emotions associated with bereavement, or the anticipation of such a loss, are the primary feelings of fear and anger. These primitive emotions are usually coupled with two others: guilt and sadness.

Fear is an emotion that has been mentioned many times in this chapter. There are a number of causes of fear in relation to death. For the practitioners, carers and family members, there can be fear that the event to be encountered will surpass their coping mechanisms, particularly if they have not had to deal with such an event before. For the patient, the fear of loss of control, both physical and mental aspects 12, can be more intimidating than associated pain. Because a lot of this pain is anticipatory, it can build for extended periods and it can be difficult to find appropriate coping mechanisms.

Anger too can be a destructive emotion, it can be directed towards loved ones or practitioners because of the frustration and injustice the patient feels at their diagnosis. However, anger can sometimes be a constructive emotion if it is directed at the disease, as it can give some patients the impetus they need to overcome physical difficulties, 'put up a fight' and give them an added quality to the time they have left with their loved ones.

Sadness is the emotion that most of us would attach to the bereavement process. The physical loss of someone who is an important part of our lives can leave us feeling a metaphorical void. These feelings can be so strong that the sense of emptiness can be described as having a physical quality.[8]

Guilt is the fourth emotion frequently related to the normal grief reactions. It arises from self-blame associated with bereavement and loss. We can apportion blame to ourselves out of a sense of not having acted sooner to persuade the individual to see a doctor; not having taken them seriously when they complained of symptoms; not having convinced them to give up smoking or change their lifestyle. These feelings of guilt should decrease as we accept the death.

It has long been accepted that there are stages of grieving. Among the most widely accepted is the Kubler–Ross model. It describes five stages: denial (protective mechanism, cushions the impact of reality); anger (feelings of injustice and frustration); bargaining (attempting to negate effect); depression (sense of helplessness with acknowledgement of loss) and acceptance (of the inevitability of the situation).

Regardless of which 'model' of bereavement we prefer, it is inarguable that death (or the anticipation of death) provokes strong emotions within the patient, their family and those responsible for the care of the patient. It is a traumatic event, but the emotions should be transient. Prolonged failure to move towards acceptance requires specific professional assistance. (See also Chapter 8, End-of-life care.)

Death and children

Dealing with a child who has a terminal illness is always an emotionally stressful situation. The death of a child can make practitioners feel powerless. It is a situation that has more significance for practitioners than the death of an adult, but there are more similarities than differences between the grief processes of the age groups. As adults, we know that it can be difficult to accept the concept of death, but for children the permanency of such an abstract concept can be impossible to grasp, most children are unable to accept the finality of death until around 9 years of age.[25] However, although they may not fully understand death, they are aware of death at a very early age.[21]

> **!** Some children seem to grasp the inevitability of their condition without an open discussion of their prognosis. Indeed, some children will even seek to protect their parents from this truth by acting as though they are well. Others see their illness as a punishment for something they have done in their past.

Parents too can blame themselves for the child's condition and seek answers. Medical imaging practitioners, who are not in a position to build an on-going care relationship with these children and families, can be spared some of this turmoil but they can face problems when the children or their parents ask direct questions. Practitioners should not be tempted to give trite reassurances, but responding with complete honesty can cause distress too. It is an area where non-verbal indicators are of importance; often the patient or relatives just want to have a listening ear. In other circumstances, referral to the specialist practitioner responsible for information and support is the best course of action, or if the department does not have this facility, referral to a counsellor or consultant may be the appropriate course of action.

KEY POINTS

- The psychology of behaviour is demonstrated by both patients and practitioners within the healthcare environment. By trying to view the situation from the patient's perspective and understanding the processes involved, we can hopefully be more tolerant to the behaviour that may be upsetting to us as healthcare practitioners

- The primitive reactions of 'fight or flight' can have an enormous impact on individuals and it can be difficult for some people to employ appropriate coping mechanisms to allow them to deal with situations in a way that is acceptable in the eyes of society
- Society is changing and behaviour that would not have been considered acceptable to the older generation is now, not just tolerable, but appropriate in the eyes of the public
- As society changes, the views and expectation of what the NHS is, what it should provide, and the public's rights to access services has also changed. In parallel with this, people's views of their own 'place' in society have changed. They tend to be more assertive and demanding; this undoubtedly affects the attitudes to staff delivering a service that is paid for by the public we treat
- Providing any form of public service can be difficult but with the added stresses, anxiety and concerns of pain, illness and prognoses this becomes even more so. Experience is a great master when it comes to working with and understanding others but a basic knowledge of psychology and reflective practice can provide a strong foundation regardless of age or background

Chapter | 7 |

Beyond a diagnosis of cancer

Elaine Parry-Jones, Samantha Glendinning, Kimberly Williamson

CHAPTER OUTLINE

This chapter will focus on:

- The potential psychosocial issues that may be experienced following a diagnosis of cancer
- The importance of the role of the practitioner in ensuring that all patients receive the appropriate treatment in a supportive patient centred environment and that caregivers are provided for
- The need to adapt practice to meet the ever increasing pressures of healthcare delivery using highly technical equipment while meeting government targets

INTRODUCTION

Latest figures (2012) state that over 2 million people are living with cancer in the UK alone; therefore the potential impact of this disease is huge. Alarmingly, the lifetime risk of receiving a diagnosis of cancer currently stands in excess of one in every three[1] individuals being directly affected; therefore, the indirect affect of those supporting a relative or family friend could be seen as virtually all-encompassing. Improved screening and associated treatment regimes have led to improved survival rates.[2,3] As the number of cancer survivors is expected to continue to rise at a significant rate, it is important that research and development is concentrated in this area to ensure holistic patient care is achieved and maintained for all.

Understandably, a diagnosis of any major illness can and does affect each and every individual in a different manner. Notably, this is not only applicable to the person in question but also to their family and friends, and this is imperative to adapting the approach used during discussions in order to meet their individual needs. An issue that is of key importance to one patient, e.g. removal of a breast due to a mastectomy, may be seen as relatively insignificant to another patient who is more concerned with the signs that cannot so easily be covered up, such as hair loss. This detail is of paramount importance when trying to ensure holistic patient care is achieved for all.

A personal statement by one patient explains, 'Cancer takes you to the threshold of life, from that point you are forced to consider the value of your life'.[4] However, others may not feel this at all.

For most patients, the initial issue which will impact on how they begin to come to terms with their diagnosis is likely to be influenced as a result of how they present with their disease. They may present as an emergency via the A&E department due to a brain haemorrhage, as a result of a primary brain tumour, or via routine screening, e.g. the national cervical screening programme. Alternatively, as a result of requesting a GP appointment having been aware of a lump for a number of weeks; but attributing it to a benign cause. If the latter is the case, there may be associated psychological issues of blame for a delay in their own diagnosis. With current lifestyle trends being so hectic – many people work full-time and often care for either children or other family members – it can prove difficult to fit in non-routine appointments and sometimes people are not seen as a priority, when they should be. Whether the person is alone or accompanied by a relative or friend will also have huge implications to hearing and taking on board the news of the cancer diagnosis.

In addition to the circumstances in which a person finds out about their diagnosis, the manner in which they are told is likely to remain with them forever; long after any treatment is completed and side-effects have subsided. It is therefore important to remember this when involved with all patients at any stage in their cancer journey. Equally, it is worth acknowledging that a whole range of responses may be experienced; those involved should be reassured that any reaction to the news is normal.

Several patients strive for something called 'normality'; and then there is the question of what is normal? It can probably be described as a period of time without any massive significant happenings; it is what you are used to. Some patients state they can cope for so long and with so much and then they reach burn-out; it is important that they have access to the appropriate healthcare professionals at that stage.

One of the many traumatic stages is that of waiting for results or being sent for further tests to establish the extent of the disease; some report this as being more horrific than the initial diagnosis. Patients themselves may make assumptions about why they are now being sent for an additional MRI scan. Ensuring that an appointment is made with the counselling service or specialist nurse is important at this time.

> **!** Patients experience all kinds of emotions, including a momentary change of character; some patients feel anger towards those that appear to be carrying on as normal and whom they perceive as not having a care in the world.

Patients may question the unfairness as to why they have been the unlucky one, when they followed a strict healthy lifestyle, taking necessary precautions and yet other people appear to drink and smoke excessively and go on to lead normal healthy lives. This leads to the question 'why me?' This unfortunately is often left unanswered by the medical staff; potentially causing frustration and a lack of confidence in their ability.

Patients may feel abandoned and anxiety will be increased, especially while they wait for treatment to begin; particularly in the knowledge that they have a cancer growing inside them. While for the majority of patients this cancer will either be surgically removed or ablated with radiotherapy and chemotherapy; it is worth paying further attention to those patients for whom the cancer is inoperable or who are given a 'watch and wait policy'. The emotional implications for this on the patient and everyone involved can be catastrophic.

It is important throughout the entire patient journey that a patient centred approach is utilised and this is of paramount importance when it comes to the decision-making stage. Some patients experience difficulties in taking on board the information and having to make decisions; questions arise such as, 'Am I making the right choice?' Others may feel that they do not have any say in their treatment. Therefore, the level of information needs to be specifically tailored to meet the patient's needs; for some this will be simply wanting to be told of the absolute minimum, while others will thrive on gaining knowledge; completing a crash course in breast cancer in order to achieve some control and be in a position to make an informed decision. Either way, patients need to feel involved. Some patients find using visualisation techniques beneficial. 'Charlie Cavernoma' does become easier to talk about with others than the alternative. Research has shown that the provision of adequate information and support to individuals affected by cancer is an important role in facilitating better adjustment and coping.[6] In particular, the benefits include a better understanding of the illness and treatment options available, better sense of control, reduced fear, reduced anxiety and depression. In addition to this, there is improved communication with the health professionals and the family members. People use different coping methods. Some will count the days in-between treatments and visits to the hospital and consider that as 'free' time; so any disruption should be kept to a minimum. If an injection can be delivered at home avoiding a hospital visit, this could improve quality of life issues.

Is there life after a diagnosis of cancer or is it a case of continuing with life regardless of a cancer diagnosis? For some, the chapter in their life can be closed and they can move on, while for others, the impact is much longer term. Particularly for those who have a physical change, e.g. a colostomy bag to deal with. Interestingly, it is worth considering whether the diagnosis of cancer will lead to a change in lifestyle; possibly becoming healthier or making the decision to have a positive change in their direction in life.

> **!** A comment from one patient states, 'Whilst cancer takes away part of your life it gives you the opportunity to choose the life to continue to lead rather than the one it interrupted'. The question that everyone needs to ask is: 'Have I treated just the cancer or have I treated the person?'[4] Ultimately, for many patients, they will simply want to return to what they used to do.

BEYOND A DIAGNOSIS OF CANCER: THE EFFECT ON FAMILY AND FRIENDS

Just like a pebble thrown into a pond and the concentric circles rippling out from where the pebble hits the water, the diagnosis of cancer causes an effect on many people and not just the patient alone. Family members and friends will be there to help and support in many ways; understanding treatment options, managing side-effects, informing others of the patient's illness, as well as the emotional support with help to deal with the psychological stress that a diagnosis may bring. Depending on the relationship to the patient, i.e. spouse, parent, child, sibling, friend, etc. will depend on the effect this diagnosis will have, and although many of the feelings experienced by these people are categorised under similar headings, the experience for each will be different due to their individual perspective. The conflicting emotions which may be experienced include disbelief, fear, feeling a sense of guilt, being angry, feeling neglected, lonely or potentially embarrassed, to name but a few.

Telling loved ones – parents, children, partners and friends – can also be extremely taxing and worrying for the individual concerned. For some patients, this can be the hardest aspect to deal with. A common fear among patients is, 'How do I tell the children?' A parent may struggle with the explanations of cancer and what the diagnosis could mean for themselves and the family. There can be concern that what they say will upset the child and therefore in trying to protect the child, there is a decline in sharing the details or perhaps just not knowing the words to use to explain in a simplified manner for the child to understand. There are many references for doctors about communicating with patients and disclosing the diagnosis of cancer, however, a study identified an issue in that parents do not have any of these guidelines and are left to disclose their diagnosis to their families alone.[5] Dealing with the reactions of others to the news can often be problematic, as there can be reactions of disbelief, shock and not knowing what to say.

> ! Patients report feeling lost, lonely, numb, frightened and disempowered, as though they are an outsider looking in. This could be attributed to the loss of control. This feeling of loss of control continues throughout treatment; appointments are often given with an assumption that the individual will do everything that is asked of them, irrelevant of the impact this may have on their life outside of the hospital.

Treatment side-effects are another feature that is often seen as beyond the patient's control and yet a constant reminder of what they are dealing with (see Chapter 13, Radiotherapy-related treatment reactions).

Many patients diagnosed with cancer will require the support from a family caregiver or friend. Caregivers play an important role in the management of cancer in all manner of support tasks, including physical, psychological, spiritual and emotional domains. They can also act as an intermediary between family and friends; monitoring phone calls and providing respite from well-intentioned callers. However, the caregiver will have their own emotional responses to the diagnosis and prognoses and will therefore require their own support systems too. Caregiving can have a considerable impact on the caregiver's life. Family caregivers experience increased levels of anxiety, depression and psychosomatic symptoms. There are also restrictions on their normal roles and activities, strain in marital relationships and diminished physical health. As the spouse of the patient, the burdens include employment issues, physical, social, time and financial concerns.

Often, the family caregiver is the one most responsible for managing the side-effects of treatment and the symptoms of disease at home, as the patient's condition deteriorates. The more time the caregiver spends doing the tasks for the patient, the more the caregiver's schedule is altered and the more the caregiver experiences emotional distress and suffering. The caregiver role will be affected by the patient's prognosis, stage of illness and goals of care. When a patient is undergoing treatment for curative intent, the side-effects from treatment from chemotherapy or radiotherapy may need management in a hospital setting and therefore the burden to the caregiver is more emotional support, whereas when the intent is palliative, the emphasis is on symptom management and supportive care, which tends to be undertaken in the home setting. This will ultimately depend on the caregiver being available and there will be increasing emphasis in the amount of caregiving tasks. If there is a presence of pain in a cancer patient, this can adversely affect the mood of the caregiver, particularly the level of depression and anxiety. This is particularly increased if the patient is younger. Gender of the caregiver is also an influential factor; psychological distress is generally higher in female spouses when their husbands are distressed. This may be to do with the society roles that men and women undertake, e.g. women are taught to nurture and attend to the needs of their nearest and dearest. In contrast, the experience of male spouses is often dependent on how well adjusted their wife is, e.g. if the wife is stable emotionally, then the husband suffers less from her physical condition.

For some couples, the diagnosis of cancer can strengthen their relationship. Fear of losing a partner can remind couples how much they love each other. This can also be said of any family or friend relationship. It can help them to re-evaluate their priorities and of the importance of the relationship. For others, including those with significant problems before the diagnosis, the stress of cancer may highlight the need for change. Changes in responsibilities and roles can lead to feelings of frustration, resentment and guilt; these changes may include physical tasks such as who cooks or who pays the bills. Alternatively, these changes could be emotional, for instance, a spouse becoming overprotective or taking on a parental role. Physical intimacy may become difficult with the effects of treatment, but also changes in body image may affect a person psychologically and may lower libido and lead a partner to feel unloved or neglected.

> **!** When a child finds out their parent has cancer, there will be the feelings of being scared, e.g. afraid that their parent might die; afraid that someone else in the family might catch the disease; or possibly afraid that something might happen to the parent at home and they won't know what to do in that situation. A child in this sense is not just a young person but it crosses all age groups, as we are all somebody's child.

Many young children and teenagers think that they need to protect their parents by not making them worry. They often feel that they have to be perfect and not cause trouble because one of their parents is ill. This can often lead to feelings of guilt, as it is difficult to maintain the facade of being perfect all the time. Children will need space to feel sad or to vent their anger and frustrations. It may be when they are laughing and having fun that they suddenly feel guilty for having a good time. With so much to deal with in the patient's life a young child/teenager may at times experience feelings of neglect. This may be due to the reduction in the time a parent has to spend with them or that the parent is not sharing and communicating in the way they had done in the past.

It is becoming clear that children's levels of anxiety are related to whether they are told about the illness and to the quality of the communication with their parents. Evidence suggests that where children are told the diagnosis by their parents, their anxiety levels are lower. This is based on the level of knowledge the child has about the illness and where anxiety is higher it is related to the inability to discuss the illness with their parents and therefore a more limited knowledge of the subject. Young children may become overly clingy, impulsive or want to stay home all the time. Older children or teenagers may be angry or distant and withdraw from family activities.

Some children may at times feel embarrassed to be out in public with their sick parent, particularly when there are physical reminders of the patient's disease such as loss of hair from chemotherapy or disfiguring facial surgery. Alternatively, it could be because they don't know how to answer people's questions about their parents' illness.

As an adult coping with the diagnosis of a parent with cancer, there are different connotations. The society that we live in today means that many people do not live in the same town or area that they grew up in, therefore, the family becomes widespread around the country or even the world. Communication with parents is consequently often via the telephone. As an adult, there are many responsibilities that must be managed; that of being a provider for your own immediate family unit, work pressures and financial commitments, etc. and therefore it is difficult to drop all these responsibilities at home to go and be with the parent, however much they feel they ought to be there. Often, a feeling of obligation is incurred by the child in assisting the parent, particularly when the parent has been widowed or separated, as they don't want their parent to be dealing with the situation on their own. With so many personal responsibilities, the priorities of individuals may vary. In an act of balancing these responsibilities, a dilemma for the child is at what stage should they go back to their parent's home; immediately following the diagnosis; while they are on treatment or thereafter? This could be in an emotional support capacity or as a caregiver following the side-effects of treatment. Alternatively, do they wait for the time that the parent may require help due to a physical requirement, when a lot of care tasks are involved as the patient becomes more palliative?

As a friend of someone with cancer, they may not know what to say or how to act. Some may avoid talking about cancer for fear of upsetting the patient. This could cause people to distance themselves from the patient or vice versa. For some, helping others makes them feel good and will benefit both patient and friend in an act of altruism. For some, they may perceive an increased risk of the disease where a lack of knowledge has led to a belief that they can catch the disease. This may lead to them distancing themselves, which may ultimately affect the relationship.

PRACTITIONER RECOGNITION AND RESPONSE

It goes without saying that living with cancer is a frightening, traumatic and life-changing experience associated with a host of physical and psychosocial implications. As stated, a diagnosis of any cancer can bring acute emotional distress and individuals and their families struggle with the concept about why the disease struck, the significance and the implications of the diagnosis for their future and the changes that may follow. It is imperative that practitioners involved with these patients are mindful of these concerns, so they can offer the appropriate advice and support, offering to listen to how the patient proposes to tell their loved ones; establishing what their specific concerns are; using examples of how they may discus their situation.

> **!** it is vital for practitioners to ensure that all those who are affected are treated within a patient centred, holistic environment throughout the continuum of their cancer journey.

! To be an efficient practitioner, teamwork and excellent communication skills are vital. This teamwork, the fact that routine practice is fraught with technical challenges and difficulties, along with the constant use of professional vocabulary has had a great impact upon patient experience. This has led to the perception that radiography can sometimes be seen as an 'uncaring profession'.

This can add stress and anxiety to patients at an already potentially intense emotional and psychological time. This is not helped by the inconsistency in the manner in which practitioners deal with individual patients, as witnessed in many departments across the country. If different members of staff are dealing with patients on a daily basis, leading to the possibility for discussions and information not being handed over, this results in a lack of rapport with the patient and the potential for psychological problems to be missed. As healthcare professionals, we should strive to establish a patient centred and patient focused environment. Excellent patient care and communication should be on par with technical skills within daily radiography practice. This is reinforced by legal, ethical and professional responsibilities tied into duty of care and Standards of Proficiency. (See also Chapter 29, Ethical and legal considerations in professional practice.)

Practitioners can play an important role in not only recognising psychological issues in patients and their families but also in responding appropriately to them. A key skill that practitioners possess is the ability to reassure. The question often arises as to what is 'normal'? To confirm to a patient that their reaction is normal and how to deal with it, is often received with great relief. As a result of this, it is highly important that all those involved are skilled and experienced within this area in order to ensure that the patient in question receives the ultimate level of care.

To offer constant reassurance throughout the patients' cancer journey can have a huge impact upon how they cope. Taking time and reassuring claustrophobic patients during an MRI appointment will make their next visit easier and less frightening than if their fear was ignored.

! Patients should feel that their concern is listened to and valued and will be addressed with empathy. Although they may be experiencing common issues seen daily by the healthcare professionals it will be new to the patient.

The abilities to empathise and to offer sympathy are key skills that should be held by practitioners. Patients can be intimidated by the machinery and radiography equipment is often referred to as being like 'something from Star Trek'. Patients who are receiving a course of radiotherapy can often find it very difficult to explain to loved ones what the treatment entails, especially those who require a mask or immobilisation device. Allowing their loved ones into the treatment room to observe the set-up or even taking pictures for the patient can explain what a thousand words could not. This can help reduce the sense of isolation and the feeling that no-one understands what they are going through.

Language used should be appropriate to a patient's level of understanding. In-depth use of medical terminology may not be suitable; therefore it is paramount to judge the patient's individual level of understanding. Good use of open body language should be used to convey openness in communication. Interactions and communication with patients can be adjusted on an individual basis, which should take into account disability and age. Patients that are hard of hearing will need to be taken away from a noisy waiting room or the background drone of a CT scanner so information can be passed on with clarity and ease. Care should also be taken to respect patients' religious and cultural beliefs. This is especially apparent when it comes to patients undressing. Again, this needs to be established on an individual patient basis. Some patients may want a gown; others will prefer to change in the treatment room. Some female patients may feel uncomfortable undressing in front of male practitioners, especially apparent perhaps after a total mastectomy. Alternatively, male patients may feel just as uncomfortable undressing in front of females, in particular for those procedures where the pelvis area needs to be accessed. Maintaining and respecting patients' dignity should be at the forefront of daily practice.

The adjustment of appointment times to fit around the patients' lifestyle can be extremely beneficial. This helps not only the patient in giving them a sense of control but enables them to continue with their normal activities, for instance, parents may wish to continue with the school run, but it also helps their friends and family; disruption to the children will be lessened if their routine is unbroken. Friends and family may be helping with travel or childcare provision and this will lessen the impact on their lives too.

One of the recurring comments from patients regarding radiotherapy treatment is, 'it is just like a conveyor belt here'. Work load within radiotherapy and radiology departments are high, with the average patient given a 10 minute appointment slot. This produces huge time pressures on staff. With government-led targets in place, this is unlikely to change. To improve the patient experience, consideration of the environment should be taken into account. Communication and information should be delivered away from other patients and the hustle and bustle of the department. Private clinic rooms should be utilised so the patient feels like they have had one-on-one time with the appropriate member of staff. These issues, along with the advent of advanced and consultant practice, have led to many radiotherapy departments training and employing clinic review practitioners. Not only can these staff members offer more in-depth advice on side-effects and management but they have longer, uninterrupted, one-on-one time with the patient. If seen regularly throughout treatment, they can build a strong rapport with the patient and with a strong rapport in place, psychological issues and concerns should be more easily diagnosed and addressed as patients are more likely to open up and discuss their issues. All staff should be consistent in the information they provide and there should be uniformity across a department.

! Patients often want to hear a certain answer and will ask several staff members the same question. Parity is vital to instil confidence. Assumptions should not be made about how much knowledge the patient has, or indeed, how much they want to have.

If a psychosocial issue is suspected, it is important to elicit the correct information from the patient. This is not always easy as patients are often reluctant to bring up their distress, leading to the fact that many patients with anxiety go undetected. Untreated distress has been shown to result in poorer physical functioning and greater pain, resulting in longer hospital stays and thus higher medical costs, adding a burden on to the patient, their family and the healthcare system.[6] Consequently, it is important for psychological issues not to be ignored. (See also Chapter 6, Psychological aspects of patient care.)

Once it has been recognised that an issue with a patient is apparent, then practitioners can play an important role in the referral of the patient to the appropriate service. Holistic care can play a vital role in reducing stress and anxiety in cancer patients. Referrals can be made to services available within the appropriate area. Complementary and alternative therapies have proven useful in reducing anxiety in patients. Referring to a hairdresser or a wig provider can be greatly beneficial for patients who are struggling with hair loss and the associated body image issues. Just as importantly, a referral to a financial advisor can be as advantageous to a patient who may have had to give up work as a result of their disease.

Health-related quality of life is the level of function and wellbeing a patient has in regard to their physical, psychological and social domains. A useful tool in addressing quality of life issues is the distress thermometer, as it is used to highlight increased anxiety levels. The distress thermometer is 'a one-item self-reporting screening tool for measuring psychological distress in cancer patients'.[7] Quality of life tools are not currently used routinely within radiography practice but it is important for practitioners to be aware of such tools. Screening tools can prove especially useful for those patients who have been coping up to a point, then reach 'burnout', which may be the case at some point in the duration of a long radiotherapy course.

With the increasing rate of cancer survivors, and the ever changing dimensions of radiography practice, it is imperative for practitioners to stay at the forefront of current research and latest advances to ensure holistic patient care is achieved and maintained by all. You cannot advise or guide a patient if you are not aware of the information yourself. Ensuring that the patient is fully aware of all the support and help available is paramount. For example, making patients aware of information prescriptions can help to reduce the feeling of isolation as they can be used as a source of key information on conditions, and can let people know where to get advice, where to get support and where to network with others with a similar condition. Additionally, ensure patients are aware of 'pastoral prescriptions' they can get from their GPs for those who are seeking non-medical and holistic ways to help enhance their treatment.[8,9] Assumptions that someone else has dealt with these psychosocial issues should never be made.

KEY POINTS

- A diagnosis of cancer is associated with not only acute but also chronic psychological and emotional implications that can require adjustments to daily routines
- The reactions and responses related with a diagnosis are not limited to only the patient, as family and close friends can be equally affected
- An individual's reaction to a cancer diagnosis; be it for themselves or a loved one, is unique and no two given situations will be dealt with and managed in the same way
- Practitioners can play a role in not only recognising distress in those living with cancer but also by reacting appropriately to it and ensuring that all are treated within a patient centred, holistic environment throughout the continuum of their cancer journey

Chapter | 8 |

End-of-life care

Terri Gilleece, Murray Schofield

'How people die remains in the memory of those who live on'

(Dame Cicely Saunders, 1918–2005)

CHAPTER OUTLINE

This chapter will focus on:

- Palliative and end-of-life care considerations for terminally ill patients

INTRODUCTION

At some point during their career radiographers may come into contact with patients who have terminal and life-limiting illnesses. Some radiographers work in positions where they may encounter sudden death at first hand and others, for example therapeutic radiographers, may experience the unexpected passing of patients before the completion of a planned course of palliative radiotherapy. The practitioner's approach to the patients and their family members can have a significant impact on those for whom they are providing care. Likewise the experience of dealing with a patient's death can have a major and significant impact on the radiographer.

The contact and relationship radiographers have with their patients can vary immensely according to their roles. Medical Imaging practitioners tend to have short bursts of contact with patients, but can get to know patients who have repeated imaging for chronic conditions over a long period of time. Those in the radiotherapy setting have the opportunity to build a stronger bond with their patients as they see them daily throughout a course of treatment. These repeated encounters with the patients can mean that their passing becomes more personalised and more difficult to deal with, but some radiographers find such situations easier to cope with because the death is foreseen and not unexpected. The terminally ill patient and their family have the opportunity to have discussions, make choices and accept that death is a natural process.

Sudden or unexpected death situations can arise at any time during student training or throughout a radiographer's professional career. Not all patients will have the opportunity to 'plan' their passing. This can be much more traumatic for all concerned. Cognisance should be afforded to staff who have been exposed to situations with outcomes that result in death, and opportunities to access counselling services should be provided.

Not all deaths that affect staff will happen while the patient is in the department, on occasions staff will learn of the demise of a patient after their treatment has ended. The effects can be felt just as acutely by those who have known the patient.

Everyone working in the healthcare environment, whether training, recently qualified or vastly experienced can find themselves having to manage and cope with end of life situations. It is important therefore that the concepts of Palliative and End of Life Care are introduced early to afford all of those who come in contact with terminally ill patients the knowledge, understanding and compassion to best deal with the experience.

PALLIATIVE AND END-OF-LIFE CARE

The terms 'palliative care' and 'end-of-life care' (EoLC) are often used interchangeably; however, there is a distinction to be made between the two terms:

Palliative care has been defined by the National Institute for Clinical Excellence (NICE) as follows:

> ... *the active holistic care of patients with advanced progressive illness. Management of pain and other symptoms and provision of psychological, social and spiritual support is paramount. The goal of palliative care is achievement of the best quality of life for patients and their families.*[1]

End-of-life care has been defined as:

> *Care that ... enables the supportive and palliative care needs of both the patient and family to be identified and met throughout the last phase of life and into bereavement.*[2]

While both palliative and EoLC offer support to the patient and their family members, palliative care places the emphasis on helping the patient to live with the highest possible quality of life for the limited time they have, while EoLC helps to ease their passing and offer bereavement support to the family after death. Palliative care can last for an extended period, and will form part of the EoLC pathway.

> **!** The philosophy of palliative care is that we should encourage the view that dying is a 'normal' process, but at the same time offer support for people to live as actively as possible, for as long as they are capable of doing so.

We should provide relief from pain and other distressing symptoms but view the person's psychological, social and spiritual needs with the same consideration as we give to their physical requirements. The purpose of palliative care is not to change the time frame of the person's death by shortening or prolonging life, but to make the person more comfortable in moving towards death.

The symptoms that most often cause distress are pain, anorexia, nausea, vomiting, constipation and lassitude. It is essential that the family are offered the same level of support as the person who is in the last stages of life. If the family are distressed, this distress can transfer to the patient. If the family are supported, they can in turn offer comfort and support to the patient.

The *Oxford Text of Palliative Medicine* captures the philosophy of palliative care with the statement:

> *Palliative care rehabilitation at its best is the transformation of the dying into the living ... The restoration of a patient to a person.*

EDUCATION

In its response to the End of Life Care Strategy 2008, The Society and College of Radiographers identified that this ideal is not always achieved. In an effort to rectify this problem, recommendations suggest that:

> *Providers of Higher Education need to consider if educational programmes deliver the required learning outcomes for end of life care.*

It can be advocated that education for practitioners falls into two broad streams. One being the academic experience that provides the underpinning theoretical knowledge; and the second being the clinical placement, that allows the student to gain the practical and technical skills required. The former should arguably provide the theoretical basis for end-of-life practical skills.

Unarguable, more work is required to prepare the practitioner who is about to enter the workforce and interact with the public. The integration of this knowledge and the accompanying skills will take place as current Higher Education Institutes redesign courses and implement modes of delivery.

What is the experience of the practitioner out in the department; what practical help can be given to them to both help themselves and the patient? Table 8.1 suggests a number of areas where a practitioner might be able to gain useful insights that could help them. Much of this is discussed in detail in the following paragraphs.

Self-knowledge

In simple terms, this is an awareness of one's own strengths and weaknesses built up over time, from experience. This may come from a formal learning process or be experiential. However, whatever the source, there is the possibility that this can be linked into more formal models of reflection, which may then highlight areas of learning and understanding.

It would appear safe to assert that practitioners of all disciplines will come from a variety of backgrounds with differing personal and professional experiences. Many may unfortunately have gained such experience initially through the loss of a family member or in caring for a family member who has had a terminal illness. In the current climate, others, such as those serving in the armed forces, may be exposed to the extremes of injury and death on a day-to-day basis.

A legacy of this may well be the development of coping mechanisms that allow an individual to function. In whatever context the experience has been gained through, this idea of self-knowledge can be augmented by a supportive environment within a department.

Table 8.1 Possible requirements for practitioners	
Possible requirements	
Self-knowledge	Gained from life and professional experience
Professional knowledge	Knowledge of what is required professionally of the individual in a given situation – Care plans – Not for resuscitation, Crash procedures, CPR
Holistic approach to patient care	An awareness of the psychological and physical wellbeing of the patient
End of Life Care Strategy	Does the hospital recognise this and act accordingly?

PROFESSIONAL KNOWLEDGE AND HOLISTIC APPROACH

For practical purposes, these two particular facets can be combined. This is about an individual in a department having the professional knowledge to deal with a given situation. But it is also about recognising a bigger picture of the patient's journey.

For example, any practitioner trained in cannulation for the administration of contrast media should also be trained to recognise any signs or symptoms of allergic reaction. We must make ourselves aware, from the patient's care plan, that a particular individual has requested that they do not wish to be resuscitated.

The onus is on the individual treating a patient to have this knowledge; however, it can be argued that it is equally important that a department provide support to the member of staff. In a practical sense, this is about making the department a comfortable environment in which to learn and having the relevant information readily available.

There are many practical skills such as good communication and good planning that will make the patient's journey less stressful as they approach the latter phases of their life. It is an everyday situation and part of the professional role for a medical imaging practitioner to query the justification for an X-ray examination request.

This can require tact and good communication skills but may also allow a patient to be left in peace and relative comfort, rather than have an unnecessary radiograph. In effect, the practitioner is acting as an advocate for the patient (see Chapter 29, Ethical and legal considerations in professional practice).

Continuing Professional Development is recognised by the Health Professions Council as:

> ... a range of learning activities through which health professionals maintain and develop throughout their career to ensure that they retain their capacity to practice safely, effectively and legally within their evolving scope of practice.

! Part of this responsibility can be very simple but important: factors such as knowing how and when to transfer a patient from their bed to a couch or treatment table or what kind of personal protective clothing is required, if any, for a patient who is suffering from MRSA. It can be emotionally upsetting for a patient to be approached by staff in such clothing, especially if their condition has not been properly explained to them.

CARING FOR THE DYING

Often palliative care is associated with a cancer diagnosis, but it should be noted that a large proportion of people suffering from non-malignant life-threatening or life-limiting diseases, and their families, require specialist palliative care. Dementia care, cardiology, respiratory disease and neurology, are all areas where patients frequently require palliative and EoLC, but this list is by no means exhaustive and anyone with a serious illness of any kind may find themselves in need of such services.

Previous research has found that patients with non-malignant disorders experience debilitating symptoms of the same magnitude as those with malignant diagnoses, but were not offered the same level of relief. There have been noticeable differences[3] between provision of palliative services for patients with non-malignant disorders in the UK and USA. This distinction developed partly because of the way in which palliative care is financed in the UK; for many years, the majority of funding for palliative care in the UK has been through charitable organisations. This has made it difficult to devise national strategies and set standards. The development of the National Council for Palliative Care[4] (NCPC), an overarching charity for all those involved in the provision, commissioning and use of palliative care throughout the UK, has sought to promote the standard and availability of palliative services throughout the country. Other strategies and policies have been developed as a result of appreciation of the problems in this sector. In 2004, the Health Select Committee of House of Commons[4] noted that:

> *Lack of palliative care for non-cancer sufferers … is the greatest inequality of all in palliative services.*

The recognition of the severe lack of coordination of services and the shortfall in service provision in this sector has led to a number of changes at government level. The National End of Life Care Programme (NEoLCP) was implemented in response to the department of health report, 'Building on the Best: Choice, Responsiveness and Equality in the NHS'.[6] The objectives of the NEoLC Programme are three-fold:

- Greater choice for patients, irrespective of their diagnosis, with regard to where they wish to live and die
- A decrease in the numbers of emergency admissions of patients to hospitals when they have expressly wished to die at home
- A decrease in the number of patients transferred from a care home to a hospital in the last week of life.

These aspirations resulted in the development of the End of Life Care Strategy in 2008.[2]

A clearly defined care pathway comprising 6 steps is now in place to help healthcare staff ensure that those in need receive well-planned, coordinated, high quality, patient centred care that is tailored to the needs of the specific individual. Training in the principles of palliative care for general staff across the healthcare sector is available through the website of the EoLC programme.[7]

The pathway outlined in Figure 8.1 has been developed for adult patients in England. The other parts of the UK have developed equivalent strategies for their devolved regions, but all aspire to the same quality and standard and seek to rectify previous disparities in availability of specialist palliative care. (Links for regional initiatives are provided at the end of this book.)

NEONATES, CHILDREN AND YOUNG PEOPLE

While the care pathway and other initiatives outlined above consider the needs of adult patients and their families, it takes no account of the specific needs of children and young people who are diagnosed with an incurable health condition. It is estimated that over 23 500 children (0–19 years) fall into this category each year,[8] while the number of neonates requiring access to specialist palliative care service annually is estimated at 1473. Figures also show that 10 400 young adults (20–30 years old) who have had a diagnosis of life-limiting or life-threatening condition in childhood, die each year.[9]

These children and young people have different care needs from adults. Despite their medical conditions, the children and young people still need to be given the

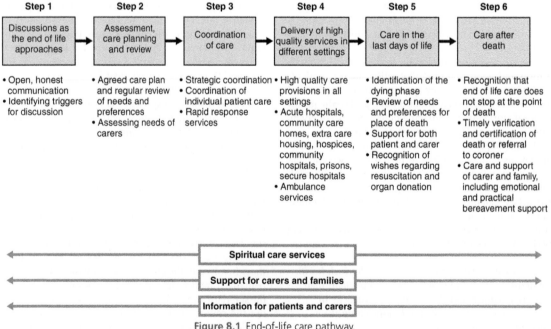

Figure 8.1 End-of-life care pathway.

opportunity to develop physically, emotionally and cognitively throughout their illness, which may continue over a considerable period of time. Frequently, the parents of these children want to take on the majority of the care but doing so can have serious implications for families both emotionally and financially, especially if one parent has to give up work. Parents will need breaks and access to respite facilities to ensure continued care for other children in the family and to have the opportunity to simply take some time out for themselves and their partners. The need for specialist palliative care for this group of people is further complicated by the fact that many will have co-existing disabilities. A distinction needs to be made between palliative and disabled children's care and the correct level of physical, psychological and emotional support offered to the children and their families. For those suffering from familial conditions, the parents, or indeed the children themselves, may have had to witness siblings with progressive diseases moving along the same end-of-life pathway.

Particular problems can arise during the transition phase from the paediatric to adult care services. With improvements in medical technology and drug development, more children with life-limiting and life-threatening diagnoses are now reaching adulthood. The Association for Children's Palliative Care[8] (ACT) has highlighted the potential problems faced by these individuals and developed a dedicated transition care pathway to empower the young people to take control of their own decisions. The considerations required in respect to this have been included in some of the regional palliative care recommendations.

OLDER PEOPLE

It is a well-accepted fact that as a nation, we are living longer. Improvements in healthcare, nutrition and health education mean that the death rate has fallen over the last four decades. But with an ageing population, it is now predicted that the death rate of the older population will begin to rise,[10] putting pressure on hospitals, hospices and social care, not simply because of the increase in numbers but because of the period of increased ill health at the end-of-life.[2]

Two-thirds of those who die every year in the UK are aged over 75. As people age, they are more likely to have multiple health problems. It is estimated that 29% of people over the age of 85 with cancer, circulatory and respiratory problems also have dementia. Organising a structured approach to their end-of-life care can be very difficult because of the number of different medical teams involved.

According to the End of Life Care Strategy, 70% of people want to die at home but in reality, few have their wishes fulfilled and 60% of people die in hospital. It is estimated that 40% of EoLC patients who do die in hospitals have no medical necessity for acute hospital care.[11]

These figures reflect the difficulty in providing palliative and EoLC for this older age group within their own homes. Often, family members are unable to provide round the clock care for their relatives because of work and commitments to their own children. The complicated nature of multiple illnesses and/or dementia also means that home care becomes impracticable.

END-OF-LIFE CHOICES

The EoLC pathway affords people a chance to record their wishes so that there can be no ambiguity as to their preferred place of care (PPC), resuscitation, organ donation and when they wish treatment to cease. Early consideration of the EoLC plan should be encouraged, as illness or even medication can sometimes have a detrimental effect on mental faculties. The Mental Capacity Act, 2005 states that: Although those involved in the patient's care will seek

> **!** 'Every adult has the right to make his/her own decision and must be assumed to have capacity to do so unless it is proven otherwise'

> **!** Even if the patient has difficulty in articulating their views, every effort should be made to offer them the chance to make decisions regarding their care.

to accommodate their wishes, fulfilment cannot always be guaranteed for a number of reasons. Providing care at home for a terminally ill relative can be extremely demanding. Despite wishing to remain at home, there may be insufficient support for the required 24-hour care that is necessary. There may be physical barriers to providing care in the home if appropriate adjustments cannot be made because the patient lives in a rented property or multiple dwelling such as an apartment block. Even in circumstances where families do make adjustments and initiate home care, they may find themselves unable to cope as circumstances change or the disease progresses, despite the support of the palliative care team. If subsequently, the patient has to be cared for in another environment, family can be left with feelings of defeat and guilt at not accommodating the patient's wishes.

Some patients prefer to be in a hospice setting because they feel that they are no longer a 'burden' on family. Hospices have the specialised staff and facilities to offer excellent EoLC. The high staff to patient ratio and tranquil environment means that patients can have a higher level of care than in an acute hospital, and staff can take more time with each patient to listen or just offer a physical presence. Psychologically, the move to a place of terminal care can be difficult for some patients to embrace.

Every effort should be made to avoid terminally ill patients being admitted for 'crisis' care to a general hospital. It is hoped that the number of patients dying in this type of environment can be reduced by the introduction of the EoLC register. Each person listed on the register has an identified care coordinator who links across all services to ensure effective discharge planning from the acute setting to a more suitable care location in a timely manner and the coordinator can also arrange access to fast track additional services where necessary.[12]

ENDING TREATMENT

Each person has the right to cease treatment at any time. As healthcare professionals, we have to respect that right, even if their decision does not fall into line with our own views. In promoting the patient's quality of life, we seek to maintain the patient's dignity, hope and control. We can do this best by respecting their views. Under the Mental Capacity Act (2005):

> *Individuals must retain the right to make what might be seen as eccentric or unwise decisions.*

We must, however, ensure that people make such decisions in the full knowledge of the pertinent information relating to their particular situation. Some patients will decide to cease treatment because they feel they cannot cope with the side-effects of treatment; they have been told that there is no hope of recovery; they feel as though they are a burden on their family or they have lost their trust in the medical profession. It is important to understand the patient's reasoning behind the decision to end treatment so that we can be sure it is an informed choice for the appropriate reasons.

ALTERNATIVE MEDICINE AND COMPLEMENTARY THERAPIES

The terms 'alternative' and 'complementary' medicine are often used together and indeed frequently shortened to CAM (complementary and alternative medicine). For the purposes of this text, the two forms of treatment will be separated out and defined to avoid confusion.

Alternative medicine can be defined as treatments that have either not gone through the process of rigorous scientific testing, or have been tested and found to be ineffective. They are used in an effort to elicit a cure for the condition or at the very least, to lessen symptoms and prolong life. They include a wide spectrum of treatments such as homeopathy, green tea polyphenols, selenium and shark cartilage, to name just a few.

Complementary therapies are more about integrating conventional treatments and therapies that will help to improve the patient's quality of life but not add to the cura-

> **!** Patients, for whom conventional treatments fail, may find that the use of alternative remedies and regimes reinstates a sense of control and empowerment that was previously surrendered to the healthcare team. Other patients use these modes of treatment as a form of denial that hope of a cure is futile.

tive properties of the treatments prescribed by physicians. Complementary therapies such as art therapy, reflexology, massage and music therapies can reinstate the same sense of control as alternative therapies for patients without offering false hope. They are often provided free of charge for terminally ill patients, unlike the alternative treatments which can be financially draining to patients and their families. These complementary therapies can have the added benefit of helping patients to accept their prognosis.

KEY POINTS

- As has been noted, practitioners from both medical imaging and radiotherapy disciplines will, on a regular basis, encounter patients whose health is seriously compromised. Situations in which a patient may die can occur either after a chronic long-term illness or in a more acute situation such as trauma. This can happen at virtually any time in a practitioner's career

- It is recognised within the profession and at governmental level that there are deficiencies in the EoLC of patients. The End of Life Care Strategy is a key document in both assessing and addressing the issues raised

- Rather than focusing purely on how to prolong an individual's life, the key focus should be about recognising how they can be supported both physically and psychologically, and about inclusion and support of the family in both care and bereavement

- Palliative care is often associated with cancer-related illness, while in reality, many patients with non-malignant but life-threatening or life-limiting disease processes require similar levels of care. This has been recognised and is included in the EoLC Strategy 2008. This has led to the creation of a well-defined 6-step care pathway. A limitation of this pathway is that it does not specifically address the issues surrounding neonates, children and young people, who will have differing physical and emotional needs from their adult counterparts

- Up to two-thirds of those who die in the UK are aged 75 years or above and often will have had multifactorial illnesses, including dementia. This can make it difficult for patient choices enshrined under the EoLC to be met, as patient choice to be treated at home cannot always be fulfilled. Up to 40% of this group of patients who do die in hospitals have no medical necessity for acute hospital admission

- Each patient has the legal right to end treatment at any time, as long as the requirements of the Mental Capacity Act 2005 are met. Professionally, this can be very difficult for those practitioners involved. However, it is part of our professional duties to ensure that a patient is suitably informed of their choice and that their comfort and dignity is protected throughout.

Section | 3 |

Radiation hazards and safety

Chapter | 9 |

Ionising radiations

Segun S. Adeyemi

INTRODUCTION

In medicine, ionising radiation is widely used. Ionising radiations are capable of ejecting electrons from atoms and include X-rays, gamma rays, beta particles and alpha particles. Alpha particles are not used in medicine but are emitted by natural radiaoctive sources on Earth. The application of radiation carries a risk, as it is capable of causing harm to human tissue, especially when an individual has received either low doses of radiation over an extended period of time or a large dose of radiation at one time. Globally, there is an increase in the numbers of people receiving ionising radiation either for diagnosis or treatment. Public concern about the possible risks associated with the use of ionising radiation is escalating as a result of misconceptions contained within the wealth of information available on the internet, and possibly fuelled by media coverage, which seems to emphasise negative or sensational aspects of ionising radiation, rather than the positive benefits. Meanwhile, radiation incidents in nuclear power plants such as Fukushima, Japan in 2011 and Chernobyl, Ukraine in 1986, have contributed to the public's negative perceptions of ionising radiation. Therefore, limitation of radiation doses received by members of the public and the people engaged in the medical use of ionising radiations is a vital means of promoting public reassurance and safety.

SOURCES OF RADIATION DOSES TO HUMANS

Radiations are energies which move through space either as electromagnetic waves or particles. Electromagnetic waves contain both electric and magnetic properties and transfer their energy to matter such as human tissue, by absorption. There are numerous sources of radiation, some of which are well known to all of us, such as the sun. The X-ray tube, which can change electrical energy into radiation, is familiar to hospital patients.

Radiations are all around us and we cannot get away from them. All human beings are exposed to radiations from space (cosmic rays and the sun); from radioactive materials (gamma radiation from rocks and soil); from radioactive gases (radon) and from radionuclides in our bodies, which we ingest in food and drink. The radiation from these sources is called 'natural radiation' and the radiation dose we get from them is referred to as 'background' radiation. Background radiation is regarded as the main source of exposure for most people. However, the dose received will vary depending on the geology and altitude of the environment where people live. For instance, people who live in areas containing granite rocks (such as Cornwall or Dartmoor in the UK), will receive higher doses than those people who live in a non-granite environment. Air travel also contributes to the background dose, due to the higher altitude. In the UK, Europe and Australia, natural or background radiation to the population is estimated to comprise 85% of the total radiation dose.[1] The largest contribution to background radiation (50%) comes from radioactive radon gas, which is a decay by-product from radioactive uranium in the earth. Food and drink add another 11%, while soil and rocks produce over 13%. Only about 14% comes from medical uses of radiation and less than 1% from nuclear fallout or discharges (apart from exceptional incidents such as Chernobyl and Fukushima), as shown in Figure 9.1.

Additionally, we are all exposed to some degree, to man-made artificial sources of radiation. Artificial sources include medical exposures (medical imaging X-rays, nuclear medicine and radiotherapy); the nuclear power industry; nuclear weapons testing and luminous paints. In this chapter, we are concerned with the X- and gamma-radiation used for medical purposes.

X-rays were discovered accidentally in 1895 by Willhelm Conrad Roentgen. They are produced in X-ray tubes, a special type of glass tube containing two metal electrodes with an intervening vacuum. When a very high voltage is applied across the electrodes, electrons are pulled out of one electrode (the cathode) and bombard the other (the 'target'). On reaching the target, electrons lose their energy by braking and by collisions and give off the excess energy as X-rays. X-rays are invisible, have no mass and charge and have much higher energy, higher frequency and shorter wavelength than most other electromagnetic radiations (such as light, radiowaves and microwaves). X-ray imaging is known to be the highest man-made contributor of radiation dose to the public, especially in developed countries such as the UK.

Gamma rays are produced by radioactive materials (radioactive isotopes) found in the earth, through a process known as radioactivity. Radioactivity is the disintegration of an unstable atom resulting in the spontaneous emission of a charged particle and/or gamma ray. Incidentally, radioactivity was discovered in 1896, just 1 year after X-rays, by Henri Becquerel. Gamma rays can also be found in radionuclide imaging departments or radiotherapy departments in hospitals.

Therefore, each patient exposure to radiation contributes to the background dose received, thus increasing the probability of the hazard. In keeping with the practitioner's professional code of ethics, the 'duty of care' emphasises that in carrying out an X-ray examination or radiotherapy treatment we should ensure that the patient comes to no harm. It is thus imperative that practitioners should ensure that the radiation they apply to patients does not exceed that required to obtain good quality images or treat malignancies.

 Differences between X-rays and gamma rays:

- X-rays come from electrically powered X-ray tubes, while gamma rays come from radioactive atoms
- Although there is some overlap, the energy of X-rays is mostly less than that of gamma rays
- X-rays are only produced when the X-ray tube is on, while gamma rays are produced as long as the radioactive source is active.

EFFECTS OF IONISING RADIATIONS ON THE HUMAN BODY

X-rays, gamma rays, beta particles and ultraviolet light are capable of ionising atoms in body tissues by removing electrons from them. This occurs due to the high energy of the ionising radiations, which can be transferred to atoms. This ionisation can break chemical bonds. Sometimes DNA molecules are broken directly (direct effect), or sometimes the radiation ionises water molecules, which then break DNA (the indirect effect). The most significant biological effect is damage to this DNA within the nucleus of cells (often called DNA mutation). The damage may be repaired by the cell or possibly not as sometimes the DNA may be so damaged that the cell can no longer divide. This is termed reproductive cell death. It is death in the sense that the cell can no longer produce offspring because its genetic material is no longer viable. If a lot of cells can no longer reproduce, visible tissue damage will result. Examples of tissue damage include skin reddening (erythema) or cataract to the lens of the eye. It should be noted that large doses are needed for tissue damage to occur. This is the basis of radiotherapy for killing cancerous cells. In other instances, the cell may repair its DNA, but

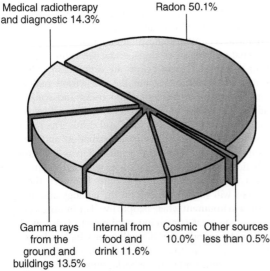

Medical radiotherapy and diagnostic 14.3%

Radon 50.1%

Gamma rays from the ground and buildings 13.5%

Internal from food and drink 11.6%

Cosmic 10.0%

Other sources less than 0.5%

Figure 9.1 Sources of radiation to the UK population. *(Reprinted courtesy of the National Physical Laboratory.)*

incorrectly. A gene mutation may be present, which can either be passed on to the cell's offspring, or can result in a cancer. These 'stable mutations', in which the cell is altered but still viable, can occur both at low and high doses. These are the most worrying possible side-effects of using medical imaging or radiotherapy X-rays. If sex cells (e.g. ova or sperm) in the ovary or testis are affected, a mutation can be passed on to a future child. Sometimes, however, the cell may simply repair itself with no visible damage to its DNA. It is important to note that cells which divide rapidly, such as in tumours, the lining of the gut, sex cells such as ova and sperm and the basal layer of the skin are more vulnerable to radiation than cells which divide slowly or not at all. Also some people may be genetically more susceptible than others, since some cancers (e.g. breast and bowel) have a genetic risk, with first-degree relatives of known sufferers being more likely to contract a cancer.

 Ionisation is the process of ejecting an electron from an atom which results in an ion pair consisting of a negative ion (ejected electron) and a positive ion (the residual atom).

Classification of ionising radiation effects

Radiation effects are categorised into two main areas: somatic and genetic. Somatic effects occur in the person who is exposed to ionising radiation. On the other hand, genetic effects occur in the offspring of the person irradiated and are also referred to as hereditary.

- **Somatic effects** concern the body of the person who is irradiated. The person can be an adult or child (after birth)
- **Genetic effects** concern damage to future as yet unconceived offspring due to damage to sperm or ova.

A further categorisation of radiation effects is into deterministic and stochastic categories, as explained below. Somatic effects can be either deterministic (tissue damage) or stochastic (cancer), while genetic effects are always stochastic.

Deterministic effects

Deterministic effects are often referred to as acute or nonstochastic. These effects cannot occur unless the radiation dose reaches a certain threshold, since the effect will not occur below that threshold. However, if the threshold value is exceeded, the severity of the effect increases with dose (i.e. the magnitude of the effect is determined by the amount of radiation exposure).

The damage due to these acute effects may manifest in tissues, e.g. skin reddening, cataract to the lens of the eye, vomiting and nausea, drop in blood count and sterility. These symptoms have been recorded in victims of the atom bomb blasts in Hiroshima and Nagasaki during the Second World War, and in people exposed to radiation at Chernobyl. Patients receiving radiotherapy for cancer may also experience some of these effects, while the sunburn people receive from too much exposure to ultraviolet light is also a deterministic effect. In diagnostic medical imaging, high radiation exposures from fluoroscopy procedures can cause similar effects. In nuclear medicine, although such effects may be caused by the ingestion of large quantities of radioisotopes, no occurrence has been reported up to the present time.

Stochastic effects

On the other hand, stochastic effects, which are sometimes called non-deterministic are random or 'chance effects'. The chance or likelihood of the effect occurring increases with dose and there is no dose so low that will give absolutely no risk of the effect. The effects may occur as a result of exposure to sources which are either external or internal to the body. However, the probability of the effects occurring increases with the dose and for conventional X-rays, such as chest X-rays, the risk is very low. Generally, the higher the dose, the higher the risk. All risks are additive, e.g. an individual having 100 chest X-rays is more at-risk than an individual having one chest X-ray.

In addition, if the sex glands (ovaries or testicles) are exposed to radiation, there is a small stochastic risk of inherited defects being passed to future children, via affected egg or sperm cells. It is important to guard against these risks by keeping all doses as low as reasonably achievable (ALARA principle). Stochastic effects include the 'induction' or commencement of a cancer and genetic damage. This tends to be the main fear of people receiving prolonged exposure to low doses of radiation for diagnosis or treatment. We are mainly concerned here with limiting the probability of stochastic effects in diagnostic medical procedures.

We need to be particularly concerned about damaging the human 'gene pool' when irradiating the body part containing sperm or ova. Incidents of hereditary defects will become magnified in successive generations as the effects of damaged genes are more likely to become manifest during gene mixing (i.e. one defective recessive gene from each parent results in an abnormality). It is clear that there is no such thing as a completely safe dose of radiation, although the risks are usually very small.

Bearing in mind that the risk from ionising radiation is a function of the dose received, the age of the individual, the size or area of the body receiving the radiation, type of radiation and state of pregnancy, it is necessary to know what the effect will be on the pregnant woman and the fetus, now discussed below.

- **Stochastic effects:** This is a chance effect whose probability of occurrence increases with dose, with no dose threshold, but the severity of the effect is not related to the dose received
- **Deterministic effects:** This is a dose threshold below which no effect will occur. But the severity of the effect will increase with a dose above the threshold.

Effects of radiation in pregnancy

Radiation effects on the unborn child *in utero* is referred to as 'teratogenesis', which is a type of deterministic effect and can include malformation. Irradiating a pregnant woman can produce serious effects, especially on the embryo in the first trimester, due to the high sensitivity of the embryo to radiation. The effects depend upon the stage of development, the radiation dose applied and the rate at which the dose is delivered. From the 9th day to the 60th day after conception, the developing embryo is very vulnerable to malformation damage, as the vital organs of the body are forming during this period. The effects produced depend on the body systems being developed at the time of exposure. The main effects are: growth retardation, congenital malformations, embryonic, neonatal or fetal death and possibly mental retardation or loss of IQ.[2,3] It is believed that a dose of about 100 mGy (milligrays) received by a developing embryo could be a threshold value for malformation. Although the fetus is less sensitive to malformation damage during the second and third trimesters, there is an increased risk of stochastic effects such as cancer induction.

Children and radiation effects

Doses received during childhood are known to greatly increase the risk of radiation-induced cancer. This is because at this early age, children are more sensitive to some forms of cancer such as the thyroid, which is estimated at 75%, breast cancer and leukaemia. Early exposure of the developing brain to radiation may result in impaired learning ability. Children are more susceptible to radiation-induced malignancy because their cells are more rapidly dividing and because they have a longer lifespan in which to develop that malignancy. Many tumours show a long latent or hidden period before malignancy. On account of these, stringent efforts should be made

by practitioners to reduce radiation doses to children. It is especially important to reduce children's exposure to computed tomography (CT), since this fast but high dose procedure is now by far the largest contributor to radiation dose from medical imaging.[4]

- A **latent period** refers to the gap or time delay that may occur between a dose of radiation being received and the effects becoming apparent
- **Teratogenic effects** concern the embryo or fetus in the womb. They may include mutation if the embryo is irradiated before or during organ development.

SAFEGUARDING PEOPLE FROM THE EFFECTS OF IONISING RADIATION

The somatic effects of ionising radiation were soon evident following the discovery and use of X-rays and radioactive materials some 100 years ago. Genetic effects caused by ionising radiation only became evident many years later. As a consequence of concern and awareness among professionals who use ionising radiation, some measures of safeguarding people was deemed necessary. This resulted in a body of experts being set-up in 1928 to provide measures of control, which later became known as the International Commission on Radiological Protection (ICRP).

Radiation protection practices in the UK fall within the larger framework of health and safety legislation. The Health and Safety at Work Act (1974) states that employers have a duty to 'ensure as far as is reasonably practicable, the health, safety and welfare at work of their employees',[5] while each employee's duty includes looking after their own and others' safety who might be affected by their actions or omissions at work. The Health and Safety Executive is responsible for enforcing radiation regulations. The UK ionising radiation regulations are influenced by the publications and guidance of the International Commission on Radiological Protection as well as the National Radiological Protection Board (NRPB), which is now part of the Health Protection Agency, as well as European Union Directives, which are concerned with protection of the worker, general public and patients in the field of radiation. There are two main UK regulations, the Ionising Radiations Regulations 1999, which cover workers and the general public, and the Ionising Radiation (Medical Exposure) Regulations 2000 for patients. Exposures involving the use of radiopharmaceuticals have additional regulations. These are Radioactive Substances Act 1993, Environmental Protection Act 1991 and Medicines (Administration of Radioactive Substances) Regulations 1978. In dental radiography, the 1994 Guidelines on Radiology Standards for the Primary Dental Care is followed.

The Ionising Radiations Regulations (1999)

These general regulations apply to all uses of ionising radiation, including teaching, research, industrial and medical. They set out basic safety standards which employers must satisfy in order to protect their workers and the general public against hazards arising from the occupational use of ionising radiation. The regulations specify the need for the employer to ensure that steps are taken to restrict, as far as reasonably practicable, the radiation exposure to employees and other persons. These include the provision of adequate protective equipment, setting up systems of work and the monitoring of employees' radiation doses. Protective equipment and measures for controlling ionising radiation require that the employer must mark out (designate) certain areas (controlled) where the likely radiation dose to personnel working in that area will exceed the recommended limit and also where access to the source of radiation or room is either controlled or restricted, and another area (supervised) where the dose is considerably lower than that specified for the controlled area and where members of the public have access (e.g. waiting area next to a X-ray room). The X-ray room, radiotherapy treatment room and the injection room in nuclear medicine are usually designated as controlled areas, while on the ward during mobile radiography, it is specified as an area corresponding to 2 metres around the X-ray tube and patient.

The regulations also require that employers appoint a radiation protection adviser, who is qualified to give professional advice on radiation protection issues, and a radiation protection supervisor, who is responsible for ensuring that radiation regulations and local rules are applied.

Annual dose limits are specified for different categories of employees such as classified workers (aged 18 years and over), for trainees, members of the public (excluding patients) and the fetus *in utero*. Dose constraints are also specified for comforters and carers. Female employees are required to declare their pregnancy so that risks to the developing child in utero can be minimised.

Furthermore, the regulations require the monitoring of employees to ensure that the doses received are below the set values for each category of employee. For this purpose, each employee is issued with a personal monitoring badge on a monthly basis or for a longer period, provided by an approved dosimetry service. Record of the doses are normally kept for a specified period of time.

Lastly, IRR 1999 specify that each employer should provide local rules which should take into consideration the prevailing circumstances in that particular area.[6] Local rules are simplified versions of the main regulations. According to Regulation 17(1), it is stated that:

For the purposes of enabling work with ionising radiation to be carried out in accordance with the requirements of these Regulations, every radiation employer shall, in respect of any controlled area, or where appropriate having regard to the nature of the work carried out there, any supervised area, make and set down in writing such rules as are appropriate to the radiation risk and the nature of the operations undertaken in that area.

Local rules are written and identify key working instructions intended to restrict exposure in controlled or supervised areas. They also emphasise the restriction of access to an controlled area, provide contingency plans in case of incidents or emergencies (see Fig. 9.2) and must specify the names of both the radiation protection adviser (RPA) and radiation protection supervisor (RPS) for the particular area where the rules are applicable.

The Ionising Radiation (Medical Exposure) Regulations [IR(ME)R] 2000

These regulations issued in 2000 and amended in 2006 are specific to the medical uses of radiation for diagnosis or treatment. They replaced the previous Ionising Regulations (1998) known as POPUMET (protection of patients undergoing medical examination or treatment). The key applications of IR(ME)R include exposure of patients as part of their medical diagnosis or treatment; individuals as part of their occupational health surveillance or as part of health screening programmes, or for medico-legal purposes and volunteers in research programmes.

The regulations identify four key roles: employer, referrer, practitioner and operator, who are assigned responsibilities for maintaining the principles of justification and optimisation of radiation exposure to individuals.[7]

IR(ME)R specify the duties of employers as providing a framework under which medical exposures may take place. These include written procedures and protocols for practical aspects of radiation exposure for every type of standard radiological practice and each standard type of equipment. The protocols must be complied with by the practitioner and operator. Other responsibilities include: providing referral criteria for medical exposures, including radiation doses; establishing 'dose reference levels' for typical examinations for groups of standard sized patients for broadly defined types of equipment and comparable with national reference levels. Also the employer must ensure that quality assurance for standard operating procedures is performed, and also certify that practitioners and employers are adequately trained in addition to receiving continuous professional development to enable them keep abreast of developments in their area of practice. The last part deals with the need to investigate radiation incidents.

Referrers are charged with the responsibility of providing sufficient information to a practitioner to enable justification of the procedure to be given. For example, a referrer

```
┌──────────────┐   ┌──────────────┐
│  Radiation   │   │  Radiation   │
│exposure starts│──│exposure fails│
│              │   │ to terminate │
└──────────────┘   └──────────────┘
                          │
                   ┌──────────────┐
                   │Switch off X-ray│
                   │ unit from mains │
                   │   isolator   │
                   └──────────────┘
                          │
                   ┌──────────────┐
                   │Stick a note on│
                   │unit to prevent│
                   │ further use  │
                   └──────────────┘
                          │
        ┌──────────────┐   ┌──────────────────┐
        │  Inform RPS  │───│RPA reports incident to│
        │   and RPA    │   │Healthcare Commission │
        └──────────────┘   └──────────────────┘
                │                    │
        ┌──────────────┐   ┌──────────────────┐
        │ Call service │   │Healthcare Commission│
        │   engineer   │   │investigates incident│
        └──────────────┘   └──────────────────┘
                │                    │
        ┌──────────────┐   ┌──────────────────┐
        │ RPS handover │   │Healthcare Commission│
        │ X-ray room to│   │makes recommendations│
        │service engineer│  │to prevent future accident│
        └──────────────┘   └──────────────────┘
                │
        ┌──────────────┐
        │Service engineer│
        │handover of X-ray│
        │ room to RPS  │
        └──────────────┘
```

Figure 9.2 Flowchart of the management of radiation accident for patient overexposure.

must provide adequate information on a request form for an X-ray or radiotherapy treatment, as the form constitutes a legal authorisation to allow subjecting a patient to procedures involving the use of ionising radiation. This document therefore confirms that the examination or treatment is purposeful and useful to the patient management.

Meanwhile, practitioners can only justify medical exposures after full consideration of risks and benefits and making the best use of the imaging modality available. A protocol which can be used for justification is the publication, *Making the best use of clinical radiology services*, by The Royal College of Radiologists.[8]

Finally, operators have the responsibility of carrying out the practical aspects of the radiation exposure through the selection of equipment and methods, to ensure that the dose is kept ALARA. In radiotherapy, the operator must ensure that exposure to the cancerous cells (target

volume) are individually planned and doses to non-target areas are kept ALARA, consistent with the radiotherapy purpose.

- **The Employer** must provide a framework under which medical exposure may take place
- **The Referrer** must provide adequate and relevant clinical information to enable the practitioner justify the exposure
- **The Practitioner** decides the appropriate imaging and justifies any exposure to radiation
- **The Operator** authorises and undertakes the exposure with regard to dose optimisation.

Radioactive Substances Act 1993

The Radioactive Substances Act 1993 is used together with the Environmental Protection Act 1991and is designed to protect the public and the environment. They require that users of radioactive materials are registered to keep such materials and are authorised to dispose of them using the best practicable means (BPM) through established disposal channels. This is to enable the achievement of a high standard of protection for the public and the environment.[9] Furthermore, they are authorised to accumulate radioactive waste and submit annual pollution inventories to the Environmental Agency. In addition, an exemption order for registration and authorisation is available for hospitals to enable them keep to certain levels of radioactive materials and waste. In order to ensure compliance with the regulations, the Environmental Agency conducts annual inspections of facilities which use radioactive materials.

The Medicines (Administration of Radioactive Substances) Regulations 1978

The Medicines (Administration of Radioactive Substances) Regulations 1978 (MARS) deal with patient protection. MARS is the UK legislation based on Article 5(a) of the European Union Directive 76/579/Euratom, which requires prior authorisation for the administration of radioactive substances to persons for the purposes of diagnosis, therapy and research. MARS is policed by the Health Protection Agency. According to Regulation 2 of MARS, doctors administering radioactive substances to humans must be trained and certified. The regulation also established a body called the Administration of Radioactive Substances Advisory Committee (ARSAC), whose responsibilities include the issuing of certificates for trained and qualified applicants. Each certificate is site-specific and procedure-specific or, in certain circumstances, for a particular patient. The certificate is renewable every 5 years. A revised ARSAC was produced in 2006 and it includes aspects of IRR 1999 and IR(ME)R 2000, Transport Regulations, training for clinicians undertaking positron emission tomography (PET) procedures and updated guidance on the handling of breast-feeding patients, which emphasises provision of written instructions to such patients and subsequent recording in the patients' medical notes.

> **!** **Best Practicable Means** is defined as 'that level of management and engineering control that minimises, as far as practicable, the release of radioactivity to the environment whilst taking account of a wide range of factors, including cost-effectiveness, technological status, operational safety, and social environmental factors'.

Guidelines on Radiology Standard for Primary Dental Care (1994)

Radiation protection in dental radiology follows the 1994 guidelines. These cover the education and training of personnel who use ionising radiation in dentistry, patient selection and clinical justification, diagnostic interpretation of the radiograph, equipment selection and quality assurance.

The various regulations and guidelines have shown a common theme, i.e. the minimisation of ionising radiation dose used in medical procedures. However, the practitioner's responsibility is to enable an improved outcome in the patient's condition through the application of ionising radiation. It is then pertinent to ask, will the patient come to harm as a result of the exposure or will there be a benefit from such radiation exposure? Therefore, no matter how small the radiation exposure is, there is a need to ensure that the application of ionising radiation does not cause harm to the patient.

At this point, it would be useful to consider various ways in which we can prevent the occurrence of deterministic effects while limiting the possibility of stochastic effects of ionising radiation to patients and staff from diagnostic and radiotherapy procedures to a level which is deemed acceptable by regulations. The use of such methods to prevent the effects associated with low doses of radiation will also provide protection against deterministic effects at high doses.

RADIATION SAFEGUARDING MEASURES

The aims of safeguarding people from radiation effects are:

- Producing and maintaining an environment where the level of ionising radiation is 'safe' for both workers and patients
- Assessing the level of risk and assigning the level of radiation considered safe
- Ensuring conformity with the hypothesis underlying the ALARA principle that all radiation exposures are to be kept 'As Low As Reasonably Achievable'.

Following from the above aims, the objectives of radiation protection are two-fold: preventing the occurrence of deterministic effects and limiting the chance of stochastic effects.

In practice, three principles for reducing dose in all radiological examinations have been recommended by the ICRP, a longstanding international and influential body responsible for setting radiation protection recommendations. In 1990, ICRP publication No. 60 recommended the 'triad' of justification, optimisation and limitation (JOL).[10] Justification and optimisation principles apply to patients, while limitation applies to staff.

Before any dose of radiation is given, we need to operate the principle of justification, i.e. deciding whether the procedure is needed and making sure that the likely benefits to the patient from the procedure exceed the likely risks. The risks are the stochastic and deterministic effects of radiation. But the risk of not having the examination (i.e. missed diagnosis and treatment) may far exceed the relatively small risks from radiation exposure. This needs to be weighed up carefully and the benefits may include more timely detection, enabling appropriate treatment and reducing death and illness. In this instance, we should be able to determine if the examinations requested are appropriate or unnecessary. According to the National Radiological Protection Board's 1990 publication, 20% of radiological examinations requested are not needed.[11] Alternatively, we can make use of other methods of imaging, which do not involve ionising radiation such as ultrasound and magnetic resonance imaging (MRI). Efforts should also be made to avoid repeating X-ray examinations without good reason, if one has already recently been performed.

Carrying out the examination brings into operation the second principle of optimisation, which is giving as low a dose as achievable if a diagnostic X-ray procedure is deemed to be necessary. Optimisation refers to methods of dose reduction. This is where the ALARA or ALARP (UK concept) principle comes into play. This includes the use of modern equipment which is known to reduce radiation doses, and good techniques by practitioners. In addition, unnecessary use of radiodiagnostic tests, which have been reported to be between 20% and 30% in the UK and Canada, are responsible for causing about 250 cancer deaths annually in the UK.[12] Also, reducing the number of routine projections performed for some examinations where certain projections will not provide additional information. For example, oblique projections of the spine are only carried out in special circumstances. The evidence for this has been provided by the Royal College of Radiologists. Dose optimisation techniques have to be considered in respect of digital radiography, which is reinforced in ICRP 2004, that all operators involved with digital radiography should receive appropriate training in aspects of dose management before using it clinically.

The third principle is limitation, i.e. restricting the dose as much as possible by limiting the amount to which people are exposed. This forms the basis of the dose limits set for people who work with radiation and members of the public who may be exposed to ionising radiation. The dose limits in the UK (and European legislation) are derived from the ICRP recommendations. Since patients have to receive radiation exposure for diagnosis or treatment, dose limits have not been set for them. However, there is a system of 'national reference levels' for radiation exposures resulting from common X-ray examinations and imaging departments are required to check their dose against this standard.

Radiation protection in nuclear medicine is significantly different from that in X-ray imaging. In radiographic X-ray examinations, protecting the patient is a priority and once the X-ray beam is turned off, no radiation remains in the patient or the environment. However, in nuclear medicine, after the administration of the radiopharmaceutical, the patient becomes a mobile source of radiation exposure. In the hospital, the hazard is to nuclear medicine staff, ward staff and visitors, while outside the hospital, it is to fellow travellers, colleagues at work and family members. In this case, such patients should be advised to limit contact with the people listed above during the course of the next 2 days. This is to allow the radiopharmaceutical adequate time to be eliminated from the body. Because of this, procedures which involve the use of radiopharmaceuticals are not recommended for pregnant women or those who are breast-feeding.

The second triad, which is commonly used in radiation dose reduction is time, distance and shielding (TDS). These three factors are basic effective methods of protection which help to keep the dose as low as reasonably achievable. From our knowledge of radiation effects, it is the duration an individual is exposed to radiation that determines the radiation dose received. Therefore, if the time of exposure is kept to a minimum, then the person (either patient or practitioner) will receive a reduced radiation dose. This appears to be the simplest and most important way of the reducing radiation dose. In actual fact, the practitioner should use the shortest time coupled with the appropriate tube current to reduce patient's motion, which will cause the image to be of no diagnostic value because of unsharpness. The resultant effect is a repeat examination and consequent increase in dose. This measure can also be applied during fluoroscopy through the use of intermittent fluoroscopy or selecting a low dose rate mode (pulsed mode) on the image intensifier. In radionuclide imaging the use of radiopharmaceutical with a short half-life is recommended and limiting the contact period the patient has with family members and carers after the procedure.

Distance is the second effective method of radiation dose reduction. The farther away an individual is from the radiation source, the less the amount of the exposure the person receives. This is based on the inverse square law, which specifies that the intensity of a beam of radiation from a point source is inversely proportional to the square of the distance from the source. This in effect means that when the distance is increased, the intensity of the radiation field becomes greatly reduced. Hence, by doubling the distance between the patient and the X-ray source, it reduces the radiation dose by a factor of 4. During fluoroscopy, the distance between the X-ray tube and the patient should be maximised (30 cm minimum recommended), while keeping the patient's anatomy as close as possible to the image intensifier. Staff should keep the maximum possible distance from the patient (at least 2 metres) to reduce the dose due to scattered radiation and should not expose themselves directly to the radiation beam.

Shielding assists in keeping the radiation beam to the area where it is needed. Many forms of shielding are available for protecting both patients and staff. Shielding in respect of X-ray room or treatment unit will be covered below. Gonad shields should be employed when examinations of areas containing highly radiosensitive organs such as sperm and ova are being carried out. The use of gonad shields for women and men including boys and girls is recommended provided their use will not obscure the area of interest, thus making diagnosis impossible. Wherever possible, patients should be given lead aprons, e.g. during chest and/or extremity examination. Comforters or carers should not be present with a patient during an X-ray examination unless it is absolutely necessary. If this is the case, such persons should be provided with lead aprons and they should not be within the useful X-ray beam.

The use of collimation to reduce the area of irradiation helps in limiting the patient's dose. In addition, it assists in improving the quality of the image due to reduction in the amount of scattered radiation produced either from radiation interaction with the patient or with the X-ray table. Most X-ray units and orthovoltage therapy beam units have collimators and light beam diaphragms which are used to keep the radiation field to the area of interest, apart from providing a visual indication of the radiation field.

The protective measures discussed above are applicable to different groups of patients, including children, pregnant women and practitioners and will be discussed further below.

Safeguarding children

The radiographic examination of children and neonates differs from that of adults in several important ways. The considerably greater radiosensitivity of the organs and bone marrow in children indicates that serious measures and strict rules should be applied to ensure that the radiation doses used are as low as reasonably achievable.

One of the problems in paediatric radiography is the common inability of children to cooperate during the exposure. Since they are unable to understand and follow instructions which require them to remain stationary during the course of the examinations, practitioners therefore need to ensure they are capable of reducing movement in order to obtain good quality images. This will eliminate repeat exposures, thereby reducing radiation dose. Various methods to reduce the radiation dose include the manipulation of technical factors of kilovoltage (kV), milliamperes (mA), time and distance. Others are collimation, shielding and the use of non-ionising radiation techniques.

The selection of optimum exposure factors of kV, mA and time should be used to produce diagnostic quality radiographic images while using the lowest radiation dose. It must be borne in mind that the use of a 'one size fits all' X-ray exposure approach in conventional radiography should be avoided, as children's sizes show wide variation

and use of a standard exposure value will often result in unnecessary over-irradiation. The use of the shortest exposure time possible is recommended, to eliminate movement unsharpness and reduce repeats.

In addition, restricting the child's movement through the use of immobilisation devices is recommended. Various apparatus for immobilising paediatric patients are available. Simple methods include the sandbags, foam pads or restraining devices, while others are specialised harnesses or devices. In some departments, dedicated and equipped paediatric rooms are available. These rooms have features which children are familiar with and thus provide a less intimidating environment.

Collimation is used to restrict the area of the volume of tissue irradiated and also minimise the amount of scattered radiation produced. This helps to contribute to improvement in image quality. Collimation of the radiation beam is performed by using the light beam diaphragm to limit the radiation field to the size of the patient, rather than to the image receptor or cassette. Obtaining diagnostic quality images requires the practitioner to be conversant with the techniques for paediatric examinations.

Gonad shields help to reduce the dose to the more susceptible regions in paediatric patients. The application of gonad shields depends on the area being radiographed and it is important that they are placed in the correct positions for males and females for whom the position of the ovaries vary. Gonad shields should be used for paediatric patients at all times when the gonads are within 5 cm of the collimated beam, except when their use will obscure relevant information which will reduce the diagnostic value of the image. It is estimated that the use of shielding will reduce the dose to the gonads by as much as 90%.[13] Utilising paediatric gonad shielding protocols should be practised by all imaging departments.

Varying the projection or position of the patient relative to the radiation beam can also be used to reduce the paediatric dose. For example the use of the postero-anterior (PA) projection for chest X-ray examination instead of the antero-posterior (AP) projection can minimise the dose to the thyroid gland, which has been reported as a very susceptible gland for the induction of cancer. The use of the PA projection in female patients also reduces the radiation dose to the breast, which is radiosensitive since they will be receiving attenuated radiation (exit dose) rather than entry dose. Positioning children for upper extremities necessitates that the reproductive organs are not subjected to either primary or scatter radiation. Measures should be taken to protect the sensitive organs by accurate positioning to keep the organs away from the radiation beam. This simple measure of maximising the distance between the radiation source and the reproductive organs, if carried out during the examination, will help reduce the dose.

The use of an appropriate distance between the radiation source and the patient is effective in reducing radiation dose. This method is based on the inverse square law, which means that when the distance between the radiation source and the patient increases, the radiation intensity greatly decreases. If the distance is doubled, then the dose is reduced to a quarter of the original value. Therefore, practitioners can reduce the dose to paediatric patients by keeping them as far away as possible from the radiation source (X-ray tube), according to the regulations.

Filtration of the primary radiation beam is another method of reducing patients' skin exposure due to the absorption of the lower energy (or soft radiation) photons from the beam. This process makes the emerging beam from the X-ray tube 'harder' (more penetrating), leading to a reduction in absorbed dose for the patient. Modern X-ray units come with preinstalled aluminium filters inserted between the exit port and the collimator. However, some equipment has the facility for extra filtration to be added when the procedure demands.

Dose reduction can also be obtained through good communication between practitioners and the parents, comforters and carers of paediatric patients. Practitioners should take time to explain to parents or carers what they intend to do, so that the parents' or carers' anxiety may not be passed on to their children or wards. They should be provided with lead aprons and possibly gloves (when the hands will be in the radiation field) if they are required to hold their children. This aspect can only be carried out effectively with good communication skills.

Fluoroscopy and CT are procedures which contribute to the high radiation dose for paediatric patients because of the increased exposure utilised.[14] In fluoroscopy or 'screening', use of a short exposure time is recommended and a low dose rate mode should be selected on the image intensifier. Practitioners should keep the patient's anatomy as close as possible to the image intensifier. In CT, doses may be minimised by selecting a low mA value and restricting volume coverage.

Finally, we should not forget the role digital imaging can play in reducing the radiation dose to children. Most departments are now equipped with either computed radiography (CR) and/or direct digital radiography (DDR) and the sensitivity of both systems should result in reduced patient doses, since lower exposures can be achieved relative to the old film-screen system. In addition, fewer repeat examinations should occur because of the post-processing capability of the CR and DDR systems. However, the use of higher exposures commonly called 'exposure creep' coupled with the capability to post-process over-expose images to obtain acceptable results can contribute to an increase in dose to paediatric patients. Care must be taken to ensure that manufacturer's exposure indices are used, while also following departmental protocols.

Safeguarding in pregnancy

Bearing in mind that the fetus is very sensitive to radiation, the exposure of the pregnant woman should be avoided wherever possible. One of the safety methods include the use of the '10-day rule' introduced in 1970 by the International Commission on Radiological Protection (ICRP). The rule states that examinations which involve the abdomen and pelvis of women of child-bearing age should be carried out within 10 days of the onset of the last menstrual period. This rule was easy to apply and prevents irradiation of an unknown pregnancy. However, evidence obtained from research in relation to the low sensitivity of the embryo to radiation showed that children exposed *in utero* at Hiroshima and Nagasaki to various doses and at various developmental stages, did not show excess mental retardation up to the 8th week from conception, but had maximum mental retardation between the 8th and 15th weeks and a consequent decline after the 15th week. This fact coupled with the misunderstanding of the application of the 10-day rule by clinicians, which involved cancellation of non-urgent X-ray examinations for women of reproductive age, necessitated another rule – the '28-day rule' – to be introduced. The '28-day rule' stipulates that radiological examination of the abdominal or pelvic area should not be carried out if the woman has not menstruated within the past 28 days. Whether it is the '10-day rule' or the '28-day rule' that is applied, the aim is to reduce the potential risks to the unborn child in the womb. The current practice is to apply the '10-day rule' to 'high dose' procedures such as pelvi-abdominal CT and barium enema studies, which deliver high radiation dose to the gonads. Although we have considered the protection required for an examination of the abdomen and pelvis of a pregnant woman, there is no reason why a pregnant woman should not have chest and extremity examinations. The required protection should ensure that the beam is well collimated and a lead apron is used to protect the abdomen and pelvis wherever possible.

Safeguarding radiation workers

Protection of radiation workers (staff) from the effects of ionising radiation is equally important. It should be noted that efforts made to protect patients will also reduce the dose to the staff. Time, distance and shielding are the principal protection methods for staff, in-line with the ALARA principle.

Keeping the exposure time as short as possible will limit the duration of exposure. This will also reduce the amount of scattered radiation produced. During fluoroscopy, staff should not expose themselves directly to the X-ray beam. Reducing radiopharmaceutical handling time and the contact period with patients who have been injected with radio-isotope material should be adhered to in nuclear medicine.

Maintaining a safe distance from the radiation source to reduce dose is a function of the inverse relationship between radiation dose and distance. The minimum distance from the radiation source for safe operation of exposure is recommended as 2 metres. This method should be used during fluoroscopy, mobile radiography, nuclear medicine and other high dose procedures.

Shielding is an inherent part of a controlled area in an imaging room or radiotherapy treatment unit. This is in the form of barrier construction with materials capable of reducing the radiation doses in the surrounding areas to levels below the recommended public dose limit of 0.3 mSv. Protecting staff against primary radiation in X-ray or radiotherapy rooms incorporate walls made of either concrete or lead ply (plasterboard), while doors have lead lining. Additionally, a lead screen containing a lead glass window to allow the operator to view the patient during the operation of the equipment completes the protective devices. In radiotherapy, due to the high voltage, the practitioner can only operate the equipment from outside the room while viewing the procedure through a closed circuit television system. An interlock system terminates the exposure when the door to the treatment room is opened during operation of the unit.

Protection against secondary or scattered radiation, which arises from either the patient or from the X-ray and treatment tables is obtained through the use of various types of lead protective shielding. These include lead aprons, gloves, thyroid shields and lead glasses (for interventional procedures). The specification of the lead content for each type of apron varies between 0.25 mm and 0.5 mm, since the higher the lead content, the heavier the apron and less comfort for the staff wearing it. Lead aprons should be checked regularly for cracks as these reduce their protective ability.

Staff who work with ionising radiation on a regular basis are normally monitored, wearing radiation badges containing films or thermoluminescent (TLD) discs. The badges are processed at regular intervals in order to calculate radiation exposure. In instances where dose values reach a certain level, an investigation must be undertaken and action taken to reduce future doses. Staff should wear their radiation monitoring badges at all times. Staff who declare a pregnancy have to be protected to ensure that radiation exposure to the fetus is reduced to the level which is set for members of the public. This is to limit the chance of teratogenesis. In order to be able to monitor the dose received, monthly monitoring of pregnant staff should be carried out and the badge should be worn below a lead apron when one is used to enable the measurement of the radiation exposure received by the fetus.

ESTIMATION OF RADIATION RISKS FROM IONISING RADIATION PROCEDURES

Certain tissues of the body (especially rapidly dividing cells) are more sensitive than others to the effects of radiation damage. According to ICRP publication No. 60, the following tissues are particularly sensitive to stochastic effects: testicles or ovaries (hereditary genetic defects),

Table 9.1 Probability coefficients of tissues to radiation

Tissue	Risk coefficient (10^{-2} per Sv)
Gonads	1.0 (hereditary disorder)
Colon	0.85
Lung	0.85
Bone marrow	0.50
Breast	0.20
Liver	0.15
Thyroid	0.08
Skin	0.02

bowel, lungs, bone marrow, breast, liver, thyroid and skin (carcinogenesis). In addition, the lens of the eye is regarded as a radiosensitive organ because of the risk (deterministic) of cataract formation.

ICRP 60 provides probability coefficients of tissue sensitivity to radiation (Table 9.1). The higher the probability coefficient, the greater the sensitivity. In order to estimate the risks due to ionising radiation in medical procedures, we need to know the radiation doses given to the individual organs and tissues of the body. These doses are combined to give an 'effective' or 'whole body' dose expressed in millisieverts (mSV).

Measurement of patient doses such as entrance surface dose, dose area product and CT dose index as well as effective doses from more common procedures may be carried out during the course of patient examinations. This is effected through a protocol which provides national medical imaging reference levels (DRLs) as dose indicators for departments to compare their performance with. If departments find that their doses are above the 75% level within the range of doses given nationally, then they should take steps to reduce them to more acceptable values.

MANAGING ACCIDENTS AND OVEREXPOSURES

It is possible that even with the best laid plans, a radiation incident can occur. As we know, ionising radiation is a highly emotive subject and any radiation incident, however minor, will cause some concern. The flowcharts in Figures 9.2 and 9.3 demonstrate the actions to take during incidents of radiation overexposure of patients and staff, and the handling of radioactive material spill, loss or theft.

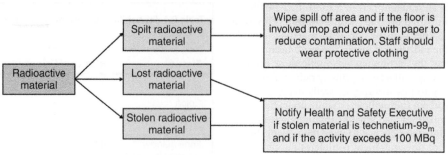

Figure 9.3 Flowchart for the management of radioactive spill, loss or theft.

KEY POINTS

- Ionising radiation consists of natural and artificial sources
- Ionising radiation hazard is caused by its ionising capability
- The biological effects of ionising radiation depend on the amount of exposure, the duration of the exposure, age and size or volume irradiated
- Deterministic effects are caused by doses above the threshold value
- Stochastic effect has no dose threshold but is chance related
- The possibility of cancer induction exists even with low doses
- Small doses of radiation can produce serious damage to the developing embryo and fetus
- Risk of cancer in children is very high due to their high sensitivity to radiation
- Safeguarding of members of the public and radiation workers is essential in order to prevent deterministic effects and minimising stochastic effects

- Regulations for safeguarding individuals from the effects of ionising radiation are based on ICRP recommendations and Directives from the European Eunion
- IRR 1999 recommends safety standards for employers to follow for the protection of members of the public and workers when the use of ionising radiation is involved
- IR(ME)R 2000 is designed for protecting patients during the case of radiation exposure
- The three principles of justification, optimisation and dose limitation to be followed in all uses of ionising radiation have been recommended by the ICRP
- In practical safeguarding a second set of three principles of time, distance and shielding is appropriate for keeping doses ALARA
- Protecting staff involves using the second triad of time, distance and shielding in addition to evaluation of doses received to determine if they are within the recommended level

Chapter 10

Non-ionising radiations and ultrasound

Martin Vosper

INTRODUCTION

The previous chapter covered the physical effects of ionising radiations such as X-rays, which are so important in medical imaging or radiotherapy departments and which loom large in the minds of patients attending for examination or treatment. Less well-known perhaps are the possible effects of the so-called 'non-ionising' radiations found especially in magnetic resonance imaging (MRI). The possible hazards of non-ionising radiations are a subject of ongoing research and the reader may have come across the occasional 'scare stories' which feature in newspapers. Headlines have featured mobile phones and overhead power lines at various times. But reassuringly, the effects of MRI are generally minor and temporary, so long as these procedures are carried out with proper regard to published safety guidance. This does not mean that we can be complacent – deaths have occurred in MRI on rare occasions when safe operating practice has not been observed.

What do we mean by non-ionising radiations? Classically, they include wave-like electromagnetic emissions with energy and power. These consist of radiowaves, microwaves and visible light. A further category includes static (constant) and time-varying (changing) electric or magnetic fields. All of these sources, unlike X-rays, are not regarded as energetic enough to remove electrons from atoms, although they may excite atoms. Thus, they would not be expected to break chemical bonds or damage DNA. This short chapter will focus on these radiations, as well as on medical ultrasound (US), which is not traditionally regarded in physics textbooks as a *non-ionising radiation* source but is important in medical imaging.

In this chapter we will consider the *biological effects* of non-ionising radiations and ultrasound, which although they result in changes to the human body, may not result in harm. We will also explore *biological hazards,* which are a source of possible harm. As with X-rays, which were discussed in Chapter 9, it is important to minimise risk by reducing the magnitude and likelihood of harm. This is achieved via published safety guidelines which set out recommended exposure limits and practices. Although these documents are not necessarily regulations, there is an expectation that they should be adhered to within the overall framework of health and safety in clinical practice. Failure to abide by published safety guidelines could be regarded as negligence in a court of law, in an instance where harm resulted to patients or staff.

MAGNETIC RESONANCE IMAGING (MRI)

Here we will introduce the theoretical basis of the biological effects and hazards which may be found in MRI. Patient safety and good operating practice in MRI is covered in more depth within Chapter 21. Health workers are often surprised to learn that injury or even death can occur as an immediate result of an MRI scan, although there is thought to be no risk of cancer. A patient is immersed in a powerful static (or unvarying) magnetic field, up to 60 000 times the amplitude of the Earth's field. The patient is also subjected to time-varying magnetic fields and bombarded with pulsed radiofrequency electromagnetic waves in the MegaHertz (MHz) frequency range. In addition, he or she may be startled by 'rat-a-tat' sounds which may reach over a 100 decibels level when heard at close range during a scan. There is in fact a wider range of biological effects to be found in MRI than in any other medical imaging procedure. Although this makes interesting physics, it can result in discomfort or even harm to the patient. Table 10.1 summarises the sources of the main non-ionising radiation effects in MRI.

Static magnetic fields

The effects of the main magnetic field of an MRI scanner increase directly with field strength. So-called 'high field' magnets of 3 Tesla are increasingly common in MRI. Effects such as feelings of nausea and vertigo, as well as visual disturbances (called magnetophosphenes – 'flashing lights' before the eyes) are more common in high field strength scanners but are typically absent in low field scanners. These changes may cause slight discomfort but are temporary and will disappear when the patient leaves the scanner. Reports of slight headaches are inconsistent. Nausea and visual disturbances are most pronounced when the patient moves within the field. A few published articles have reported a phenomenon known as 'mag lag', this being a loss of memory and concentration, affecting both patients and staff. However, this 'mag lag' effect is unproven but has even been noted in a wooden 'mockup' of an MRI scanner! It is a good precaution to prepare patients for the above-mentioned possible minor effects.

Much more serious is the so-called 'projectile effect', which causes ferromagnetic materials (such as iron, cobalt and nickel) to line-up parallel to the magnetic field (experiencing a 'torque' or twisting force) and to be attracted to its strongest point. This can cause objects such as scissors or even oxygen cylinders to be propelled at up to 40 miles per hour (65 km/hour) as they fly across the scanner room towards the magnet isocentre, with dangerous consequences for anyone in their way. Internally within the patient's body, ferromagnetic shrapnel, surgical clips or intraocular foreign particles can move and cause injury. It is for this reason that most metal surgical implants inserted since the 1980s have been of non-ferromagnetic titanium alloy. The static magnetic field will also 'switch off' cardiac pacemakers at a field strength of a little over 5 gauss (0.5 milliTesla, mT). Although the projectile effect is well known, fewer people are aware that the static magnetic field causes some changes in the cardiac ECG waveform and in blood pressure. The waveform becomes much more 'spikey' and irregular and in particular, the T-wave amplitude is raised. This is caused in part by the 'magnetohydrodynamic' effect of electrical potential in flowing blood, but subsides when the patient is removed from the scanner.

MRI is not recommended in the first trimester of pregnancy. This is because some animal experiments have suggested reductions in birth weight or length following exposure to strong or time-varying magnetic fields. The evidence is not always conclusive and might not be applicable to humans – however, there are possible mechanisms by which cells and ions in a developing embryo might be affected by powerful magnetic fields. It is reassuring to note that no published study of pregnant MRI staff or patients has yet indicated any significant effect of MRI on the child *in utero*, or after birth. It should also be remembered that in the case of a clinical emergency, MRI

Table 10.1 Non-ionising radiation effects in MRI	
Source of effect	**Effect**
Static (unvarying) magnetic field	Force exerted on ferromagnetic objects
	Alteration of cardiac pacemaker function
	Altered cardiac ECG waveform
	Nausea and vertigo at high field
	'Flashing lights' affecting vision at high field
	Loss of concentration and memory (?)
	Effects on the embryo *in utero* (?)
Changing (time varying) magnetic fields	Induced electric fields and currents
Radiofrequency electromagnetic waves	Tissue heating

would be regarded as a less harmful option during the first trimester of pregnancy than CT, which carries a large ionising radiation dose.

Time-varying magnetic fields

Magnetic fields of changing amplitude are applied across a patient during the course of an MRI scan. These induce electric fields and currents in body tissues, which are proportional to the frequency and rate of change of the applied time-varying magnetic fields. The electrical permittivity and conductivity of tissue also influences the magnitude of the induced currents. Larger currents can be expected in highly conductive tissues, tattoos (which may contain metal particles) or metal implants. As MRI technology has developed, the amplitude and rate of change of the time-varying magnetic fields has increased and patients are more commonly experiencing tingling, twitching or spasm during scan procedures. This indicates that induced electrical conduction is occurring in nerves and muscles. However, these currents are an order of magnitude lower than those that would be needed to cause heart muscle fibrillation. The nerve and muscle stimulation appears to be unaffected by body age, size and fat content. The induced currents in metal pigment-containing tattoos and surgical implants might contribute to heating – in fact burns have been reported to patients' tattooed skin. The strength of induced currents in tissues is increased if conductive 'loops' are created, e.g. if the patient's legs are touching or the hands are clasped together. This has even been known to cause skin burns. Incidentally, the time-varying magnetic fields cause parts of the scanner to flex and bang during MRI, creating a lot of noise and requiring patients to wear ear protection at levels above 85 decibels (dB).

Radiofrequency electromagnetic radiation

Radiowaves of about 21–127 MHz frequency (at 0.5–3 Tesla magnetic field) are directed into a patient during an MRI scan. As the radiowaves pass through the patient, electrical resistivity effects cause tissue heating. The energy transfer to the patient's body is expressed in Watts per kilogram (W/kg) and is termed the specific absorption rate (SAR). The heating effect increases with the radiowave frequency, which in turn is proportional to magnetic field strength, since the frequency needed for magnetic resonance increases with it. Heating also depends on the number and strength of the radiowave 'pulses', as well as on the patient's size and weight. Particular care is needed in infants and other patients with a reduced thermoregulatory capacity and SAR limits are set automatically by MRI scanners to ensure that core body temperature cannot rise by more than 1 °C. Tissues such as the eye and testes might be especially vulnerable to temperature rises. Although data is limited in humans, animal experiments have indicated that deep tissue temperature rises might reach 4 °C in some circumstances.

MRI safety guidelines

The International Commission on Non-Ionising Radiation Protection (ICNIRP) and International Electrotechnical Commission (IEC) have set limits for whole body temperature rises in MRI. The ICNIRP levels are illustrated in Table 10.2.

Temperature rises are controlled by restriction of SAR levels in scanners, especially by restricting the magnitude and number of RF pulses. Table 10.3 details the SAR limits set by the ICNIRP. It can be seen that the whole body limits are less than those for the trunk or extremities.

The ICNIRP have set normal, controlled and research limits for static magnetic field exposure to patients and volunteers of 4 Tesla, 8 Tesla and above 8 Tesla, respectively. Little is known about the effects of fields above 4 Tesla on infants or fetuses. Most clinical MRI scanners do not exceed 3 Tesla. It should be noted that the field strength of each MRI scanner has a set value in practice, determined by its design features – this field cannot be varied to suit individual patients. It is recommended that effects such as vertigo are reduced by restricting the speed at which patients are brought into or out of an MRI scanner.

There are ICNIRP and IEC limits for patient and volunteer exposures to time-varying magnetic fields. In terms of the IEC definitions, the normal limit (no physiological stress risk) is set at 80% of the value for peripheral nerve stimulation. The 'first level controlled operating mode' (at which there may be physiological stress) is set at 100% of the value for peripheral nerve stimulation, while a 'second level controlled mode' (at which there may be significant risk) exceeds it. These definitions correspond to the ICNIRP operating modes mentioned above. Additional limits exist to prevent cardiac fibrillation.

In view of the previously mentioned effects of static magnetic fields on pacemakers and ferromagnetic implants, all regulatory agencies recommend that strict screening and

Table 10.2 ICNIRP limits for whole body temperature rise in MRI	
Operating mode	**Temperature rise limit**
Normal mode – patients and volunteers	0.5°C
Controlled mode with monitoring – patients and volunteers	1°C
Research/experimental mode – volunteers	>1°C

Table 10.3 ICNIRP limits for specific absorption rate in MRI

Operating mode	SAR limit (Watts/kg)		
	Whole body	Trunk	Extremities
Normal mode – patients and volunteers	2	10	20
Controlled mode with monitoring – patients and volunteers	4	10	20
Research/experimental mode – volunteers	>4	10	>20

control of patient and public access to an MRI scanner area must be applied. It must be remembered that most MRI scanners are of a 'superconducting' category and are 'on' 24 hours a day, 7 days a week. In fact they cannot be turned off without a costly 'quenching' away of liquid helium. A controlled area exists around the scanner, set at the 0.5 mT (5 gauss) magnetic field strength contour and no patient, member of the public (or staff member) can enter this unless they have been MR-safety screened by a trained operator using a questionnaire. This field strength limit is chosen to avoid effects on pacemakers or other implanted medical devices. Additionally, access to the controlled area is by lockable doors or other physical restrictions. The UK Medicines and Healthcare products Regulatory Agency (MHRA) also define a 3 mT (30 gauss) inner controlled area, into which no ferromagnetic object may be brought, in order to avoid the 'projectile effect'.

MEDICAL ULTRASOUND

Safety, good practice and patient centred care in ultrasound are explored in Chapter 19. But here, we will briefly introduce the physical means by which high energy sound waves can cause *biological effects* and potentially *biological hazards*. Although a wide range of effects have been claimed for medical ultrasound at various times, few of these have been proven conclusively. Ultrasound is a very safe method of examination when undertaken in accordance with published safety guidelines.

Sound is not traditionally classified as a 'non-ionising radiation' in science textbooks but is covered in this chapter, since (like MRI) it provides an alternative medical imaging method to the use of ionising X-rays or gamma rays. Sound waves are not electromagnetic radiations or fields – they consist of vibrations that pass through matter and cause the substance of that matter to compress and rarefy. The particles (atoms and molecules) in the human body are made to agitate relatively slowly by an ultrasound wave, but the wave itself travels through the particles much faster, at speeds of over 1000 metres per second in fluid or soft tissue and over 3000 metres per second in

bone. Ultrasound refers to sound waves with a frequency greater than 20 kHz and in fact, sound frequencies in the 1–20 MHz range may be used in medical imaging. The body presents 'opposition', partly in the form of *acoustic impedance*, to the passage of sound waves and as a result energy is transferred from the sound waves to the body, especially in the form of heat. Rigid tissues such as bone provide more opposition than soft tissues and thus they will heat up more. Also tissues adjacent to bone, or to the ultrasound probe, will experience temperature rises, due to heat conduction. We saw above that many effects of MRI involve the whole of the patient's body within the scanner, but in ultrasound, the effects are localised to those body parts directly within the ultrasound beam. The intensity of the beam falls away as energy is transferred to tissues and thus body parts closer to the ultrasound probe or *transducer* will tend to receive more energy than those which lie deeper.

The physical mechanisms are complex but ultrasound energy transfer to body tissues will be increased by:

- A high power output from the transducer (probe)
- Use of a broad beam
- Use of a stationary transducer (e.g. in Doppler studies)
- A long scanning time
- A high sound frequency
- Tissues being close to the transducer
- Tissues being dense or rigid (such as bone)
- The presence of microbubbles in fluids (e.g. due to the use of bubble-producing contrast media).

As with MRI, new developments are leading to an increase in power outputs for scanning. In the case of ultrasound, this relates to the use of techniques such as elastography, harmonic imaging and colour flow studies. This means that operators must be vigilant about keeping power outputs within recognised levels. This can be achieved by monitoring thermal indices (TI) and mechanical indices (MI), as will be discussed below.

Heating effects

As mentioned above, the passage of ultrasound through the human body creates a heating effect. Tissues which have a low heat capacity, a low thermal conductivity and poor blood perfusion can be expected to heat up more. The developing embryo or fetus in the womb is especially vulnerable to temperature rises, both because tissues are developing and because the unborn child has a poor capacity to dissipate heat. Tissues at risk from heating in fetuses, infants and adults include bone (and tissue adjacent to it), brain and the eye. The 'thermal index' (TI) is an indication of the magnitude of the acoustic power being applied compared with that acoustic power which would cause a tissue temperature rise of 1 °C. So $TI = W/W_{deg}$, where W is the applied power and W_{deg} is the power needed to cause a 1 °C temperature rise. In adults, local temperatures of less than 43 °C can normally be tolerated in tissues, but the developing embryo or fetus may be at risk of harm if the temperature reaches 41 °C for about 5 minutes. The International Electrotechnical Commission (IEC) publish standards for reporting acoustic outputs, but do not specify maximum permissible TI values. The IEC do specify that the temperature of the ultrasound probe should not exceed 43 °C when in contact with body tissue. In reality, it is hard to predict actual temperature values at depth in particular tissues or patients. As a result, the use of thermal indices (which are displayed by ultrasound scanners during operation) is designed to restrict likely temperature rises in patients to levels below those which could cause harm. It is the sonographer's responsibility to pay attention to TI values during scanning. Thermal indices for bone and soft tissue may be displayed separately by scanners. The average thermal indices for bone may be up to 4 times greater within pulsed Doppler ultrasound scans than B-mode ultrasound. But the average thermal indices for soft tissue are only marginally greater within Doppler scans. The British Medical Ultrasound Society (BMUS) recommend that during obstetric ultrasound, thermal indices should not exceed 3.0 and scans need to be time-limited above a value of 0.7. It should be noted overall that the routine use of medical diagnostic ultrasound is unlikely to result in hazardous heating levels.

Cavitation effects

Sound waves exert an 'acoustic pressure' on tissues, which is the difference between atmospheric pressure and the local pressure caused by the ultrasound beam. This pressure can be positive (during compression) or negative (during rarefaction). Negative pressure is used within the definition of the mechanical index (MI) which is another measure displayed by ultrasound scanners during operation. As used in practice, MI is proportional to peak rarefaction and is a dimensionless quantity. MI values are smallest at higher ultrasound frequencies. The MI is important, since large values increase the likelihood of 'cavitation'. What do we mean by cavitation? This term refers to processes by which high energy sound waves can cause bubbles to form, oscillate, expand and collapse. During the collapse of bubbles, there may be very high local temperatures and pressures (within a tiny volume), causing mechanical damage to cells and even the formation of free radicals. Free radicals are very chemically reactive atoms, ions or atomic groups that have a lone unpaired electron. Cavitation effects are unlikely in most body tissues at diagnostic ultrasound energies, unless bubble-forming ultrasound contrast media are present. Bubble collapse could potentially damage cell membranes and capillary walls. Fortunately, cavitation is most likely to occur in *extracellular* fluid and thus any free radicals formed are unlikely to affect cellular DNA (remember that free radical damage to DNA is a major cause of risk resulting from the *intracellular* absorption of X-rays; see Chapter 9). In addition, cavitation within a cell would result in immediate cell death. Cells need to survive with mutated DNA for cancer to be initiated and thus there is unlikely to be a cancer risk from cavitation in ultrasound. The lungs are potentially an at-risk tissue for cavitation effects, due to the presence of air and fluid. The British Medical Ultrasound Society (BMUS) indicates that during obstetric ultrasound, mechanical indices above 0.3 might risk minor damage to the fetal lungs and values above 0.7 carry a risk of cavitation when using ultrasound contrast media.

Streaming

Acoustic streaming is thought to be a relatively minor factor as far as the biological effects of ultrasound are concerned. It arises in fluid due to differences in radiation pressure across an ultrasound beam, both with depth and width. This can result in a movement of fluid. In theory, streaming might affect molecular transport but evidence is weak *in vivo*.

Miscellaneous developmental effects

Since ultrasound is routinely used in pregnancy, a number of research studies have examined the possible effects of ultrasound on fetal and child development. The likely main mechanism for any effects would be heating *in utero*. There is no conclusive evidence yet of any significant effect on birth weight, dyslexia, attention deficit, speech development, neurological development, hearing, sight, left-handedness or school performance. Research is affected by the fact that complicated pregnancies (which might potentially result in subsequent effects) can often be accompanied by more ultrasound scans. Some published studies have suffered from methodological weaknesses. Thus, despite occasional 'scare stories' in the press and media about the use of ultrasound in pregnancy, definitive evidence of harm is lacking.

KEY POINTS

- Magnetic resonance imaging (MRI) employs a static magnetic field, time-varying magnetic fields and radiofrequency fields, all of which cause biological effects
- Most biological effects related to MRI are reversible and transient – however, death is a potential hazard in some circumstances and extreme care must be taken in safety-screening patients and staff
- The main effects of MRI are a 'projectile' producing force on ferromagnetic objects, as well as nerve stimulation and tissue heating
- As far as is known, there are no long-term effects on the fetus, although some (possibly inapplicable) evidence from animal studies advises caution in the first trimester of human pregnancies

- Ultrasound employs high frequency sound waves, which can cause biological effects at high power outputs
- The operator has a key responsibility for controlling ultrasound exposure levels, particularly by monitoring thermal and mechanical indices
- The main effects of ultrasound are tissue heating and cavitation (bubble oscillation and collapse), the latter being of more concern in the presence of ultrasound contrast media
- Although many studies have looked for long-term effects on the fetus, no conclusive detriment has been shown

Section | 4 |

Physical and medical aspects
of patient safety

Chapter | 11 |

Drugs and contrast agents

Andrew England

INTRODUCTION

The path from understanding a disease to treating it is generally long, difficult and expensive. Drug discoveries and innovations have rapidly changed the face of modern medicine and brought hope and relief to millions of patients. Today, drugs are a core part of radiology and radiotherapy practice. The desire to improve image quality, demonstrate organ function, optimise radiation dose, while ensuring patient comfort has expanded the range of drugs required. Healthcare professionals (HCPs) need to have an understanding of the drugs that they may wish to administer, as well as commonly prescribed medications and their possible interactions with the imaging process. Not only has the range of drugs available rapidly expanded but there have been significant changes to the prescribing of drugs. Patient Group Directions (PGDs), since their introduction in 2000, now provide a legal framework in which HCPs can supply and administer medicines to patients who fit the relevant criteria.[1] Medical imaging and radiotherapy practitioners now have the opportunity to become *supplementary prescribers* and prescribe any medicine, including controlled drugs, for any condition within their own competency under an agreed clinical management plan. Ever since the early 1920s, when sodium iodine was observed in the kidneys on abdominal radiographs for patients being treated for syphilis, the use of contrast agents with radiology has rapidly expanded. Nowadays, contrast agents span almost the full spectrum of radiological imaging modalities and there have been rapid developments in the fields of ultrasound (US) and magnetic resonance imaging (MRI) contrast agents. With such a dependence on the use of drugs and contrast agents there is clearly a need for practitioners to have a thorough understanding of these areas.

BASIC DRUG PHARMACOLOGY AND PHYSIOLOGY

Drugs are chemicals which interact with proteins in the body, thereby affecting a physiological function. Once drugs are absorbed into the systemic circulation they bind with certain proteins and this alters the functions of the target cell. In oncology, certain chemotherapy drugs bind to proteins on the surface of the cancer cells stimulating the cells to die. No drug is specific enough to interact with just one type of cell or protein and this limitation generates adverse or 'side' effects. There are many different types of proteins within the human body; each protein has a specific function and acts only on a specific type of cell. For example antibodies are proteins that defend the body from germs, enzymes are proteins which speed up chemical reactions. Proteins also act as drug targets; in order for the drug to have an effect it needs to be bound to a protein. This is often described as a 'lock and key system'; the drugs are the key and the protein is the lock. Once a drug binds to the protein it can generate two cellular responses: (1) it can change the response of the cell or (2) it can stop a normal response of the cell. Drugs that change the normal functioning of a cell are called *agonists*, e.g. phenylephrine, which is a decongestant and causes vasoconstriction of nasal blood vessels, thereby decreasing mucosal oedema.

Drugs which cease the normal function of a cell are called *antagonists*, e.g. chlorpheniramine, which blocks histamine receptors and is crucial in the management of allergies, e.g. hayfever. Once a drug is bound to a protein, then it exerts a therapeutic effect on the body – this is also termed the *pharmacodynamics*. An explanation of a selection of common drugs and their treatment areas are given in Table 11.1.

Pharmacokinetics is the process by which a drug is absorbed, distributed, metabolised and eliminated by the body. Different drugs will display different pharmacokinetic properties and will differ on how much of the drug is absorbed into the blood or across the cell membrane, how the drug is distributed around the body, how it is metabolised or broken down after administration and how the drug is finally excreted from the body. Ultimately, the pharmacokinetics of a drug influences how much is available to affect the relevant biological system; this is termed the *bioavailability* of a drug. Every drug has a range of dosages that can effectively treat a condition while still being safe. This is the range between the lowest dose which has a positive effect and the highest dose before we see any negative effects; this is known as the *therapeutic window* of a drug. A drug will generally produce the same end-result and the same side-effects across most people. Although the quantity of these effects either adverse or therapeutic will be different, some people may experience a shorter action of the drug or a more intense side-effect. Variations in both the therapeutic and adverse effects of drugs are thought to occur due to differences in pharmacokinetics and pharmacodynamics between different ethnicities, ages, genetic make-ups and disease states.

SAFE ADMINISTRATION OF DRUGS

The safe administration of any drug is paramount; it is for this reason that HCPs must have a factual knowledge of the drug; the reasons for its use, intended action,

Table 11.1 Common drugs and their main treatment areas

Drug group	Generic name	Method of action	Use in radiology/ radiotherapy
Antiemetic	Metoclopramide	Dopamine antagonist – blocks dopamine receptors in a specific part of the brain that have been activated by nerve messages from the stomach, which have detected an irritant. If the dopamine receptors were activated, they would send messages to the brain's vomiting centre, which in turn would send messages back to the gut, causing the vomiting reflex	Prevention or cessation of vomiting following a reaction to the administration of an iodinated contrast medium
Non-steroidal anti-inflammatory drug (NSAID)	Ibuprofen	Ibuprofen works by acting on a group of compounds called prostaglandins. These are often called local hormones and one effect is to cause inflammation. Ibuprofen inhibits the synthesis of prostaglandins by interfering with the action of an enzyme (protein) called cyclo-oxygenase.	Anti-inflammatory drug often used as an analgesic after radiological uterine artery embolisation (UAE)
Antihypertensive	Furosemide	Furosemide is a loop diuretic. It works by increasing the amount of salt and water that the kidneys remove from the blood. This decreases the overall blood volume and in turn blood pressure	In computed tomographic urography (CTU) and some nuclear medicine studies, it increases urine production and in combination with iodine-based contrast agents or radioisotope, improves visualisation of the renal tract
Anticoagulant	Heparin	Heparin binds to the enzyme (protein) antithrombin III, which in turn inactivates thrombin and other proteases that are involved in blood clotting	Heparin is used to prevent blood clots during arterial and venous radiological interventional procedures, e.g. angioplasty

any common adverse reactions, any special precautions when administrating and the normal dose ranges. Before administration it is important that the practitioner takes into account any history of allergies, any previous adverse reactions and any relevant changes to the condition of the patient. Allergy history should always expand beyond a simple check of drug allergies and include a history of allergies to foods, pollen and any family history of allergies. Patients with a past history of allergies are more likely to experience additional allergies and must therefore be monitored more closely. Consideration to any changes in the condition of the patient is also important; it would be unwise to administer an oral contrast to a patient with nausea or with a deteriorating conscious level.

Appropriate care should then be undertaken when preparing any drug for administration. An initial check must be made to ensure that the drug has been prescribed in the UK, this may be part of a PGD. When retrieving the drug it is important to ensure that it has been stored in an appropriate facility, e.g. contrast warmer or fridge and prevented, where necessary, from exposure to direct sunlight. Drugs should always be prepared in a clean well-lit area with hand-washing facilities available. The drug label should be checked when removing the drug from the storage area and when preparing the drug for administration. Label checks should include the name of the drug, dosage and expiry date. Departmental protocols often dictate that drugs should be checked with an appropriately trained colleague and this should be recorded. Caution must always be taken when preparing drugs that are kept in similar containers, e.g. ampoules of normal saline and lidocaine or drugs that have similar names, e.g. amitriptyline and amlodipine. Hands must always be washed before preparing any drug; in cases requiring oral administration, hands should not touch individual tablets or capsules. Aseptic techniques should be closely adhered to when preparing drugs for administration using a needle and syringe. Care should also be taken when measuring out the dosage of the drug under preparation, in this instance a thorough understanding of the unit of measurement is necessary. Frequently, protocols define drug quantities as a mass, e.g. 20 mg of Buscopan, yet these are stored as liquid ampoules and this would normally translate into a 1 mL dosage.

Drug delivery routes are also key factors to consider when planning drug administration. Traditional delivery routes include oral and intravenous administration; these have always been limited in certain situations, e.g. a vomiting or an unconscious patient (oral) and for long-term home administration (intravenous). Within radiology practice, drug delivery routes are often dictated by the relevant body area or organ under examination, but administration can span the full spectrum to include enteral, topical and parenteral routes (Table 11.2).

Table 11.2 Drug administration routes currently available

Route	Sub-route	Drug example and indication
Enteral (*passing through the intestine*)	Tablets and capsules	Oral paracetamol for headache
	Sublingual (*under the tongue*)	Glyceryl trinitrate spray for angina
	Buccal (*between the gum and cheek*)	Midazolam for status epilepticus
	Nasogastric/gastrostomy	Nutrison as an enteral feed
Topical (*applied to the surface of a body part*)	Transdermal	Nicotine patches for smoking cessation
	Ophthalmic	Chloramphenicol eyedrops for conjunctivitis
	Otic	Prednisolone eardrops to reduce inflammation in otitis externa
	Nasal	Fluticasone nasal spray for allergic rhinitis
	Vaginal	Misoprostol for the induction of labour
	Rectal	Diazepam suppositories for the treatment of convulsions
Parenteral (*not through the alimentary canal*)	Intradermal/subcutaneous	Enoxaparin (Clexane) for the prophylaxis of deep-vein thrombosis
	Intramuscular	Pethidine for pain control
	Intravenous	Buscopan as an antispasmodic used during CT colonography

CONTRAST AGENTS

Contrast agents or contrast media have been around for almost as long as medical imaging. Their purpose is to enhance the structural and functional information that is provided by radiological imaging. Their use was originally restricted to imaging modalities which used ionising radiation. Today, both magnetic resonance imaging (MRI) and ultrasound (US) examinations frequently make use of contrast agents. Contrast agents can now be introduced by virtually all drug delivery routes, with oral and intravascular being the most frequently used. Water-soluble iodine-based contrast dominates intravascular administration; however, a significant contribution is made by barium sulphate for the radiological evaluation of the luminal gastrointestinal (GI) tract. Barium studies are based on either the conventional radiographic or fluoroscopic examination of the GI tract following the enteral administration of large insoluble particles of barium sulphate suspended in water.

Barium sulphate (BaSO$_4$)

Barium sulphate is an inert white powder which is insoluble and has a high density (atomic number, 56). Owing to its high density, barium sulphate is highly radio-opaque and this makes it an ideal agent for X-ray based examinations its further advantages are that it is neither absorbed nor metabolised within the GI tract. If direct visualisation of the luminal GI tract is required then barium compounds are superior to any water-soluble iodine-based agents. In addition, barium has been proven to provide superior coating and delineation of the gastrointestinal mucosa and is also less expensive. Barium sulphate does have limitations; barium is a heavy metal and is therefore highly toxic when absorbed. With its extremely low solubility, patients are protected from absorbing harmful amounts of barium when it is used clinically. However, when barium is administered, great care must be taken to ensure that barium in not inadvertently instilled into the peritoneal cavity. Contraindications therefore preclude administration in suspected bowel obstruction or perforation, severe ulcerative colitis, toxic megacolon and pregnancy.

After administration, barium sulphate ultimately leaves the body relatively unchanged in the faeces. The timeframe for this can vary between patients and as such, patients should be advised that their stools may have a chalky white appearance for several days following the procedure. Retained barium can also generate problems with future imaging procedures. Concentrations of barium sulphate used in fluoroscopy procedures can cause artefacts on abdominal CT scans if any barium is retained. Where possible, a sufficient time period should be allowed to elapse between the barium examination and any planned CT procedures. In some situations, sufficient clearance of barium may be verified by a pre-procedural abdominal radiograph.

Barium sulphate falls into the group of *positive* contrast agents. Positive contrast agents, when examined using fluoroscopic (X-ray) imaging appear opaque in areas where they have been introduced. On the contrary, contrast agents which lower the density of the area in which they are introduced produce lucent areas relative to surrounding structures and are termed *negative* contrast agents, e.g. air/CO_2.

Air/carbon dioxide

Air and carbon dioxide (CO_2) are negative contrast agents and are used in the imaging of the GI tract. In addition, CO_2 does have a role as an intra-arterial angiographic contrast agent for patients with significant renal insufficiency. Air/CO_2 can be introduced into the GI tract either by oral ingestion of carbex, direct insufflation using a rectal catheter or via nasogastric/jejunal tube. In modern fluoroscopic examinations negative contrast agents are rarely used in isolation. They are usually combined with a positive (barium) contrast agent to provide a double-contrast examination (meal or enema). This combination of a positive (barium sulphate) and a negative (air/CO_2) contrast agent yields superior medical imaging capabilities, especially when attempting to identify subtle mucosal abnormalities, e.g. polyps.[2] The improved accuracy of a double-contrast technique also applies when imaging the stomach (barium meal). Nowadays, single contrast examinations are rarely undertaken, except when acute confirmation of the presence and location of a bowel obstruction is required. In this case, rectal administration of a water-soluble contrast agent (Gastrograffin) retains superiority over barium, since surgery is likely and there is a risk of possible contrast contamination of the peritoneal cavity. Many centres opt for a multi-slice CT investigation of acute bowel pathologies and this modality has largely replaced single contrast examinations.

For routine double-contrast barium enema (DCBE), examination dilatation of the GI tract using rectally administered room air is painful and can induce spasm. Many practitioners now opt to use CO_2 as this is reabsorbed from the colon quicker; this helps achieve less patient discomfort both during and after the procedure.[3] Smooth muscles within the bowel wall oppose the distension of the colon; insufflation with a gas results in a degree of procedural pain which can vary from moderate to severe, depending on the patient. The use of a short-acting antispasmodic, e.g. Buscopan, can reduce patient discomfort, motion artefact from peristalsis and can also allow greater colonic distension, which can assist the overall medical imaging yield.

Iodinated contrast agents

Iodine-based contrast agents have revolutionised the investigation of many diseases. Intravascular iodinated contrast agents fall into four types: ionic monomers, ionic dimers, non-ionic monomers and lastly newer non-ionic dimers. Ionic monomers are considered part of the first-generation of contrast agents and consist of a tri-iodinated benzene ring with a carboxyl group and two organic side chains (Fig. 11.1). Ionic monomers have the highest osmolality (>7 times that of plasma) of all contrast agents and fall into the group of high-osmolar contrast media (HOCM). Ionic monomers have the lowest viscosity of all contrast agents but the high osmolality leads to a higher incidence of adverse reactions. Conray is an example of ionic monomers and contains iothalamate meglumine. It still has some use clinically but for intravascular administration; it has largely been replaced with one of the three other agents.

Ionic dimers have a similar osmolality to non-ionic monomers. They are ionic and dissociate but carry twice the number of iodines as the non-ionic monomers, so half the number of molecules are needed to achieve the necessary iodine concentration; again, they contain significant high concentrations of sodium as cations, so the incidence of adverse reactions is higher than with non-ionic agents. Ionic dimers are formed by joining two ionic monomers and eliminating one carboxyl group (Fig. 11.2). They have intermediate osmolality and viscosity between ionic and non-ionic monomers. The only commercially available ionic dimer is ioxaglate (Hexabrix).

Non-ionic monomers are termed low-osmolar contrast media (LOCM) since they do not ionise into anions and cations. In order to achieve this, a tri-iodinated benzene ring is made water soluble by adding a hydrophilic hydroxyl group to the organic side chains (Fig. 11.3). They have intermediate viscosity and an elevated hydrophilicity, with three atoms of iodine per molecule. Common non-ionic monomers include iohexol (Omnipaque), iopromide (Ultravist) and ioversol (Optiray) and in most instances, they are the most commonly administered intravascular contrast agents.

Non-ionic dimers combine the best of both worlds; dimeric properties without any dissociation and as such, produce an even lower osmolality than the non-ionic monomers and ionic dimer. Non-ionic dimers are formed by joining two non-ionic monomers and have the lowest osmolality and contain six iodine atoms for every one particle in solution (Fig. 11.4). A trade-off is the high viscosity, which can limit their clinical utility. This can be reduced by warming the contrast to body temperature before administration. Large volume injections can be problematic, especially in patients with a small gauge cannula and fragile veins. Examples of non-ionic dimers include iotrolan (Isovist) and iodixanol (Visipaque).

The pharmacokinetic properties of water-soluble iodinated contrast agents are such that they are distributed in the extracellular fluid only with virtually no protein binding and are not metabolised. Iodinated contrast agents are excreted almost exclusively by the kidneys by passive glomerular filtration and have associated nephrotoxic effects. In normal patients, elimination of iodine takes place rapidly; after 2 hours approximately half of the injected dose is recovered in the urine. For those with severe renal impairment removal is slower, approximately half of the injected dose is recovered in the urine between 16 and 84 hours after injection. For patients with end-stage renal failure, there is long-lasting retention of injected contrast medium because of the slow compensating alternative of biliary elimination. Concentration of iodine (mg/mL) can vary between products and the overall contrast volume administered usually varies between examinations and patient types. Practitioners must have a clear understanding of the type of iodine-based agent, the concentration

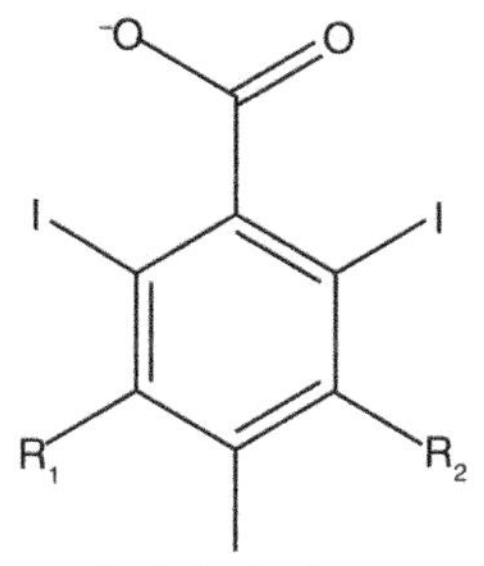

Figure 11.1 An ionic monomer.

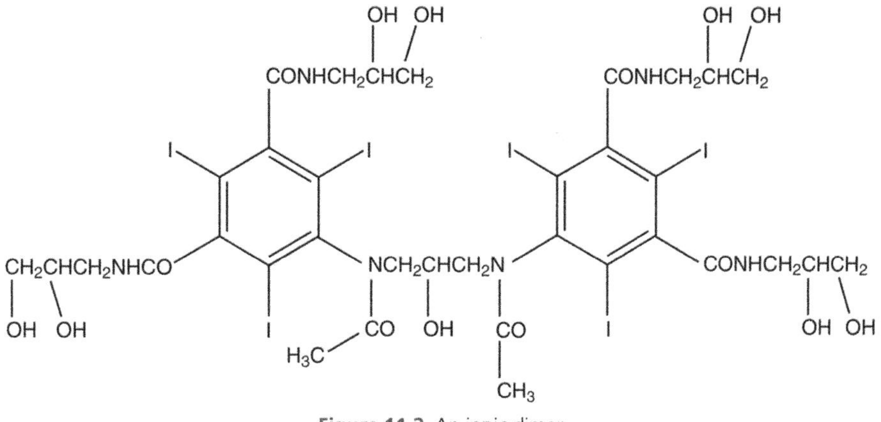

Figure 11.2 An ionic dimer.

and volume required for each examination. For some situations volumes may be weight specific, e.g. paediatric examinations.

ADVERSE REACTIONS TO CONTRAST AGENTS

Many patients who are injected with intravascular iodinated contrast agents experience some subjective sensations such as warmth, flushing and altered taste.[4] Often, patients are advised about the possibility of experiencing these sensations immediately before injection. In rare instances, failure to advise a patient may adversely affect the imaging procedure, e.g. failure to undertake respiration instructions or induce motion artefacts. With the administration of any drug comes the risk of side-effects. Iodinated contrast agents are no exception, the majority of any side-effects are mild. Nonetheless, severe or life-threatening reactions can occur and practitioners must observe patients both during and after any contrast injections. In addition, HCPs involved in the administration of contrast agents must be aware of

the potential risk factors, strategies to minimise side-effects, and how to promptly recognise and manage any reactions.

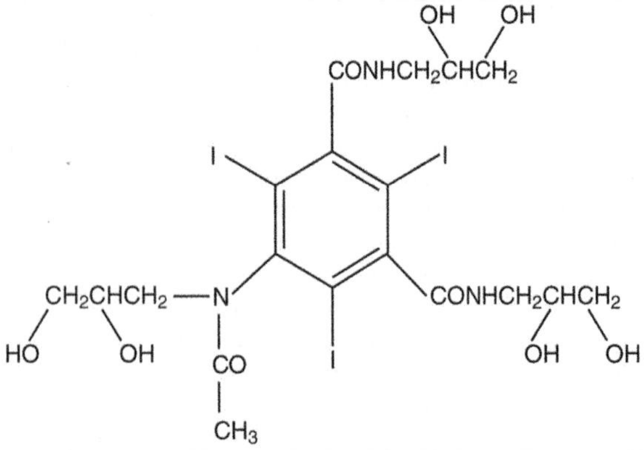

Several classification systems exist for side-effects or reactions relating to iodinated contrast agents. The simplest of these systems splits the side-effects into non-renal and renal; non-renal, e.g. itching or hives are generally independent of the administered dose, whereas renal effects are dependent on the dose of contrast agent administered.

Non-renal adverse reactions

Non-renal reactions are those typically associated with an anaphylactic reaction and include but are not limited to urticaria, pruritus, nausea, vomiting, oedema, bronchospasm, syncope and ventricular tachycardia and cardiac arrest. In order to prevent a non-renal side-effect, patients first need to be screened and found to be at an increased risk of reaction. These are commonly patients with a history of a previous moderate or severe iodine reaction or those with asthma or any other allergy requiring medical treatment. Such patients may be flagged up by the referring clinician and for this reason, it is important that the referral system has an alert facility. Careful screening of each patient prior to administering the contrast agent may also highlight patients at heightened risk. In such situations, practitioners may wish to consider an alternative medical imaging test or the prophylactic use of a corticosteroid. For high-risk patients, premedication with either prednisolone or methylprednisolone, administered 12 and 2 hours before contrast administration, may help.[5] Regardless of risk factors and choice of contrast agent, all patients should be kept within the respective department for a minimum of 30 minutes following administration. Drugs and equipment for resuscitation should also be available and checked at regular intervals.

If a contrast reaction does occur within 1 hour of administration, then it is defined as an *acute* reaction. Such reactions can be further classified as mild, moderate or severe (Table 11.3) and as such, continual patient observation following contrast administration is recommended. If a reaction does

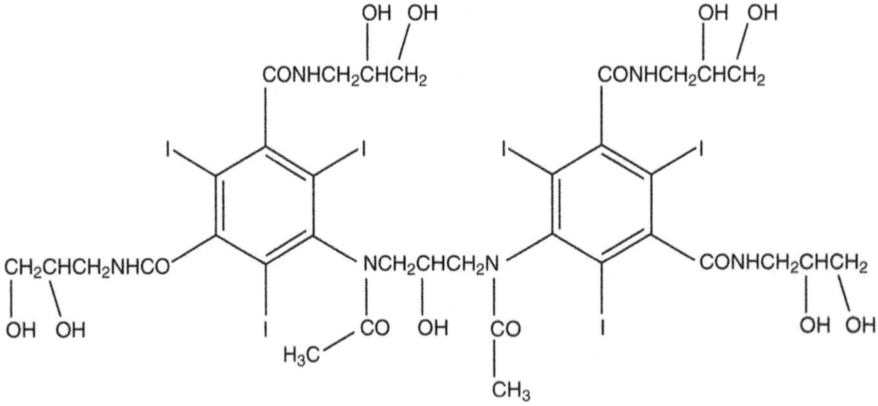

Figure 11.3 A non-ionic monomer.

Figure 11.4 A non-ionic dimer.

Table 11.3 Classification system for contrast media reactions based on ESUR Contrast Media Guidelines

Classification	Signs/symptoms
Mild	Nausea, mild vomiting
	Urticaria
	Itching
Moderate	Severe vomiting
	Marked urticaria
	Bronchospasm
	Facial/laryngeal oedema
	Vasovagal attack
Severe	Hypotensive shock
	Respiratory arrest
	Cardiac arrest
	Convulsion

European Society for Urogenital Radiology. ESUR Guidelines on Contrast Media. 2008.

occur, then medical advice is generally advised; if moderate or severe, then intervention, often by the administration of emergency drugs, is frequently necessary.

A reaction which occurs between 1 hour and 1 week after contrast administration is considered to be a *late* adverse reaction. Headaches, nausea, vomiting, fever and musculoskeletal pain have all been reported in this time period. *Very late* adverse reactions generally occur more than 1 week after contrast medium administration. It is accepted that the true incidence of late and very late reactions may be underreported, as patients may self-manage or seek treatment outside of the imaging department. If a non-renal reaction does occur, then a note should be placed within the Radiology Information System (RIS) and if possible, in the patient's case notes. Patients should also receive counselling regarding any future examinations involving iodine-based contrast agents.

Renal adverse reactions

Iodine-based contrast agents are eliminated from the body via renal filtration. Administration of iodine can cause renal toxicity and have a resultant effect on renal function. Contrast-induced nephropathy (CIN) is defined as a decline in renal function within 3 days following intravascular administration of contrast media with the absence of an alternative reason.[6,7] A CIN-related decline in renal function is generally classified by a rise of greater than 25% in

serum creatinine (SCr).[8] Some patients are clearly more at risk and patients with elevated SCr levels should be flagged up at the time of referral. In addition, any patient who has a history of raised SCr levels, metformin controlled diabetes, referral for catheter angiography or a history of possible renal impairment, should have their renal function checked before any intended contrast media administration.

If a patient is referred with renal insufficiency, then they are usually managed using locally derived protocols. These may include the use of an alternative medical imaging test, withholding metformin for 48 hours before the examination and terminating any other nephrotoxic drugs. Hydrating the patient is also valuable and should start 6 hours prior to the examination, this can be orally where possible or by intravenous infusion of saline. A low or iso-molar contrast agent should be used and hydration should continue after the examination. Theoretically, there should be some benefit from administering a contrast agent which is iso-osmolar (e.g. Visipaque). One RCT showed a 31% rise (>10%) in SCr for patients who received a LOCM compared with 15% of patients who showed a rise following an iso-osmolar agent.[9] More recent evidence[10] suggests that the relative risk of CIN from iso-osmolar contrast agents is no different than for LOCM. Despite this, some departments still opt to administer iso-osmolar contrast agents in high-risk patients. Finally, renal function can be checked after 48 hours and if acceptable, metformin can then be restarted.

Many departments rely on SCr levels as indicators of renal function, however, an estimated glomerular filtration rate (eGFR) is more likely to be a reliable indication of renal function. By using eGFR, the effects of age, gender and race on SCr levels can be taken into account. One study[11] showed that 15% of outpatients had a normal SCr level but had estimated GFR of ≤50 mL/min per 1.73 m^2. Chronic kidney disease (CKD) has been described[12] as GFR levels of ≤60 mL/min per 1.73 m^2 from which there are subcategories (Table 11.4). It has been shown that the risk of CIN rises slowly for patients with eGFR of ≤60 mL/min per 1.73 m^2. For most patients, any decline in renal function will be transient. However, patients with eGFR of <30 mL/min per 1.73 m^2 are at higher risk of requiring dialysis after contrast administration.[13] Care should be taken when administering contrast agents in patients with eGFR levels of <60 mL/min per 1.73 m^2. There are two common formulas for calculating eGFR: the MDRD[14] and Cockcroft–Gault[15] equations.

There have been discussions regarding pharmaceutical preparations which may provide protection from CIN. Current evidence suggests that the use of renal vasodilators, receptor antagonists of endogenous vasoactive mediators or cytoprotective drugs do not offer any consistent protection from CIN.[16] Care must be taken to avoid an osmotic or fluid overload when administering iodine-contrast agents to haemodialysis patients. There is no need to alter the timing of haemodialysis sessions around contrast administration or introduction extra dialysis sessions.

Table 11.4 Classification of chronic kidney disease (CKD)

| CKD stage | GFR (mL/min per 1.73 m²) | Serum creatinine levels μmol/L[a] | | | | Description |
| | | Age 60 | | Age 80 | | |
		M	F	M	F	
1	>90	<94	<73	<90	<70	Normal/↑ GFR
2	60–89	95–135	74–105	91–129	71–100	Mild reduction in GFR
3	30–59	136–250	106–193	130–237	101–183	Moderate reduction in GFR
4	15–29	251–450	194–358	239–440	184–340	Severe reduction in GFR
5	<15 (or dialysis)	>470	>359	>441	>341	Renal failure

[a]Ethnic groups other than African American. GFR, glomerular filtration rate. (Reprinted by permission from MacMillan Publishers Ltd: Levey AS, Eckhardt KU, Tsukamoto Y, Levin A, Coresh J et al. 1969. Definition and classification of chronic kidney disease: a position statement from Kidney Disease: Improving Global Outcomes (KDIGO), Kidney International, The Nature Publishing Group.)

Metformin controlled type II diabetes

There is heightened concern regarding the administration of iodine-based contrast agents in patients with type II diabetes treated with metformin (Glucophage). In a patient with normal renal function, metformin is entirely excreted by the kidneys and remains relatively unchanged in the urine. For some patients, the administration of an iodine-based contrast may cause transient renal impairment, which may restrict the excretion of metformin and allow levels to accumulate in the body. If metformin accumulates in sufficient quantities, then this may cause lactic acidosis, which in some cases may be fatal.[17] Strategies for preventing metformin-induced lactic acidosis include the exclusion of metformin either before and/or after contrast administration. For patients with normal renal function, some departments will only cease metformin for 48 hours post-examination. This practice may further depend upon the examination type, concentration and volume of contrast administered. If the decision is made to withdraw metformin for any period of time then it is important that this information is relayed to the responsible clinician. For a patient with well-managed type II diabetes the stoppage of metformin is unlikely to lead to any adverse events.

Contrast extravasation

The extravasation of a contrast agent during intravenous administration is undesirable. Most injuries from extravasation are in fact minor; severe injuries which can include skin ulceration, soft tissue necrosis and compartment syndrome are rare. Management of extravasation usually focuses on prevention by identification of risk factors.[18] Reductions in the incidence of contrast extravasation can be achieved by using an appropriately sized cannula placed in an appropriately sized vein. Test injections with normal saline are mandatory as is the use of non-ionic contrast media. If extravasation does occur, then management for the majority of cases will be conservative by elevating the affected limb, placing ice packs around the site and careful monitoring. Compartment syndrome has been reported following contrast extravasation[19] and a medical opinion should be sought in all cases. Patients should be advised to report any pain or discomfort at the injection site during administration with the effects of extravasation being dependent on the location and volume of extravasated contrast.

Miscellaneous adverse reactions

There are several other factors which must be considered when administering iodinated contrast agents. Patients may be at risk of thyrotoxicosis when contrast is administered to an elderly patient with Graves' disease or those with thyroid problems. Iodinated contrast media should not be administered to patients with manifest hyperthyroidism and thyroid stimulating hormone (TSH) blood levels should be checked where indicated.

Concern has also been raised about the administration of iodinated contrast agent in patients with multiple myeloma. A systematic review[20] identified seven retrospective studies reporting iodinated contrast administration in 476 myeloma patients for a total of 568 imaging studies. The frequency of acute renal failure was 0.6–1.25%, as against a comparable frequency of 0.15% in the general population receiving iodinated contrast. Although the administration of contrast media to myeloma patients is not totally risk free, it can be performed in well hydrated patients if the clinical need arises.

For patients with catecholamine producing tumours (e.g. phaeochromocytoma), administration of an iodinated contrast medium can induce a life-threatening hypertensive crisis. In such patients, before intravenous injection of iodinated contrast medium α-and β-adrenergic blockade with orally administered drugs is recommended. For catheter angiography, the addition of α-blockade with intravenous phenoxybenzamine should also be considered.

It is safe to administer iodinated contrast media during pregnancy but ESUR guidelines recommend that thyroid function of the neonate (TSH) should be checked during the first week of life.[21,22] In addition, there are frequent requests for advice for women who are breast-feeding and who are receiving iodinated-based contrast. This increase is most likely a result of the increase in CT pulmonary angiograms in postpartum women with suspected pulmonary embolus. Current advice suggests that breast-feeding may continue normally after the administration of iodinated contrast.[23]

MANAGING CONTRAST REACTIONS

Contrast medium reactions are relatively infrequent and range from 5% to 12% for HOCM and from 1% to 3% for LOCM.[24] There have also been a few cases of reactions to oral contrast agents,[25,26] however the bulk of all reactions are from intravascular administrations. Management will largely depend on the severity of symptoms and local policies. For all but the most minor of reactions medical advice should be obtained; if any intervention is warranted then this should be commenced under medical supervision.

Urticaria (skin rash) results from an anaphylactoid reaction to the contrast agent. These are generally self-limiting and do not require any intervention. Occasionally, oral chlorpheniramine can be administered in cases which are moderate to severe. Bronchospasm is again an anaphylactoid type reaction but generally requires more urgent attention. Vital signs, e.g. oxygen saturation, pulse and blood pressure should be monitored and where necessary, the airway secured. An inhaler such as salbutamol can be administered followed by oxygen at 6–10 L/min. In severe cases, the drug epinephrine (1:1000) can be given by subcutaneous or intramuscular injection. For facial or laryngeal oedema, the airway must be secured if necessary and vital signs monitoring started. Oxygen should be administered (6–10 L/min), if symptoms are severe, then epinephrine (1:1000) can be given by subcutaneous or intramuscular injection. If the patient is also hypotensive, then intravenous epinephrine (1:10 000) can be given by slow injection.

Hypotension and tachycardia can also present as a vasodilation response to the administration of a contrast medium. In this situation, the patient's legs should be elevated and vital signs monitoring should commence promptly. Oxygen should be administered at 6–10 L/min with intravenous fluids given rapidly. Treatment with the intravenous administration of epinephrine (1:10 000) can be started (by a slow injection). Hypotension and the opposite bradycardia can be a vasovagal response to the administration of a contrast

medium. The management is similar to cases of hypotension and tachycardia but epinephrine should be replaced by a slow intravenous injection of atropine (0.6–1 mg).

There are a group of non-anaphylactoid reactions which include cardiac arrhythmias, hypertension, seizures and pulmonary oedema. Cardiac arrthymias are a result of ionic abnormalities and chemical variations following the administration of a contrast medium. Treatment must be directed by an appropriate medical team and vital signs monitoring should also include an ECG. Hypertension can result from the histamine release of catecholamine and again management should start with the monitoring of vital signs. Blood pressure can be lowered by sublingual administration of nitroglycerine or intravenous phentolamine. Seizures can also result from ionic abnormalities and chemical variations. Early intervention by a medical team is mandatory; seizures may be stopped by administering either diazepam or midazolam. If seizures persist, then it may be necessary to start a phenytoin infusion. Pulmonary oedema can manifest following contrast injection as a result of osmolar changes which can cause large fluid volume shifts. At-risk patients include those with a history of asthma, pulmonary hypertension and asymptomatic or mild cardiac failure. Administering a low or iso-osmolar contrast medium, together with the smallest possible volume may help prevent an attack. If not, early involvement of the medical team is essential; the patient's airway should be secured and oxygen administered at 6–10 L/min. A diuretic such as furosemide (20–40 mg) should be given by slow intravenous injection and morphine (1–3 mg) can also be given intravenously.

ULTRASOUND CONTRAST AGENTS

For many years, ultrasound was considered a modality not amenable to the use of contrast agents. Now we have access to intravenous ultrasound contrast agents, which are small gas bubbles covered by a stabilising shell and have a size, typically in the order of neurons.[27] Ultrasound pulses are applied with a frequency near to the resonance frequency of the gas bubbles causing the microbubbles to increase and decrease in diameter.[28] This produces strong echoes in regions which are perfused with the microbubbles. Within radiology, the focus is on imaging in oncology, gynaecology and vascular disease. Ultrasonic contrast agents can be subdivided into three distinct groups:

- *Tissue-specific contrast agents* that improve image contrast resolution through differential uptake. Such agents are injected intravenously and are taken up by specific tissues or bind to specific targets, e.g. venous thrombosis
- *Contrast agents for vascular enhancement* – traditional sonographic detection of flow is limited by factors such as tissue motion, low blood volumes or slow velocities and the attenuation properties of the intervening tissues.[29] Vascular ultrasound agents work by enhancing the

backscatter Doppler flow signals when using both colour and spectral imaging. Microbubbles seen within small blood vessels can provide an indicator of tissue perfusion

- *Targeted contrast agents* are gas-encapsulated microbubbles that, when coated with a specific target ligand molecules, can adhere to molecular markers of disease. The contrast agents seek to identify the molecule of interest through ligand-receptor binding and then act as an echo responder for detection using an ultrasound scanner. Most of this work is still in its infancy. Reports have demonstrated that microbubbles can be successfully conjugated with specific ligands allowing the evaluation of blood clots,[30] peripheral lymph nodes,[31-33] malignant tumours[34] and cardiac transplantation rejection.[35]

CONTRAST AGENTS IN MAGNETIC RESONANCE IMAGING (MRI)

In MR imaging, the soft tissue contrast between structures is based on the T1 and T2 relaxation times when subjected to an external magnetic field after an external radiofrequency pulse. MRI is attractive as an imaging modality because in addition to anatomical information, MR can demonstrate physiological processes such as flow, perfusion and diffusion. The main gadolinium-based MR contrast agents work by increasing the relative contrast between tissues and causing a reduction in the T1 relaxation time of the enhancing structure. Other MR contrast agents are based on the elements manganese or iron, which appear either bright or dark. The majority of available gadolinium-based agents are generic and can be used in the imaging of the central nervous system and for nonspecific body imaging.

Gadolinium is useful as an MR contrast agent, since it has seven unpaired electrons and a relatively long electron-spin relaxation time. As such, gadolinium has the ability to alter the relaxation times of adjacent protons. The effect of gadolinium on the T1 and T2 relaxation times is similar but since the T1 relaxation times of tissues are longer than the T2 time, the predominant effect of gadolinium is to shorten T1 relaxation times. Tissues which have taken up gadolinium therefore appear bright on a T1-weighted MR sequence.[36] Gadolinium has an impeccable safety record; however, concern has arisen in recent years from reports highlighting a very rare association between the use of gadolinium and the incidence of nephrogenic systemic fibrosis (NSF). The pathogenesis of gadolinium-induced NSF remains unclear with the only documented link being the use of gadolinium in patients with severe renal impairment. Many clinicians now avoid the use of gadolinium in patients with CKD classifications of 4 or 5 or GFR <29 mL/min per $1.73\,m^2$. Common extracellular fluid gadolinium contrast agents include the brands Magnevist, Dotarem, Omniscan, Prohance and Gadovist.

There are several targeted or organ-specific MR contrast agents including the manganese-based agent Teslascan, which is used in the imaging of the liver. Small particles of iron oxide can also be used as a superparamagnetic MR contrast media and they appear predominantly dark on MRI. These newer negative MR contrast agents exhibit strong T1 relaxation properties and due to a strong variation in local magnetic field, they enhance T2 relaxation, which darkens the contrast media containing structures. There are two distinct types of superparamagnetic agents: superparamagnetic iron oxide (SPIO) and ultra-small contrast agents superparamagnetic iron oxide (USPIO). SPIO agents have been used as darkening contrast agents in liver imaging, e.g. ferumoxide (Endorem). Endorem is used for detecting liver lesions that are associated with alterations in the reticuloendothelial system (RES). Endorem is taken up by macrophages found only in healthy liver cells and causes a reduction in their signal intensity. If hepatic lesions are present, then there will be an enhancement difference between healthy (dark) and abnormal tissues (bright).

Generic gadolinium-based agents distribute through the extracellular fluid space following injection. Vasovist and MultiHance are gadolinium based blood-pool contrast agents. They stay within the intravascular space because of their much larger molecular weight. Blood-pool agents are therefore useful in studies which require prolonged imaging and can be also used to assess perfusion in areas of ischaemia and show the extent of tumour neovascularity. USPIO blood-pool contrast agents include the drugs Supravist and Clariscan.

Enteral MR contrast agents (orally or rectal administered) are now available and include the gadolinium-based (Magnevist enteral), manganese-based (LumenHance) and the perfluorooctylbromide (Imagent-GI). Research is also now focusing on other non-parentally administered MR contrast agents especially for the airways. Trials using inert hyperpolarised gases are underway evaluating contrast-enhanced MR imaging of the respiratory air spaces.

MISCELLANEOUS CONTRAST AGENTS

Clear delineation of the oesophageal lumen is frequently required when undertaking cross-sectional imaging by either CT or less commonly, MRI. Oral liquid based agents either fail to completely opacify the whole of the oesophagus for the required period of time. Weak barium preparations in the form of a paste are a superior substitute, can be used to outline the oesophagus and can be useful in both the investigation of benign and malignant oesophageal disease. Carboxy-methyl cellulose sodium paste containing 2% barium sulphate has been used for CT examinations[37] and gadopentetate dimeglumine barium paste has been reported in MR studies.[38]

In abdominal CT, positive oral contrast agents can clearly delineate the luminal GI tract but can create difficulties when attempting to evaluate subtle bowel wall abnormalities. Weaker oral contrast agents which utilise barium are attractive because they are inert, are not absorbed, do not effect peristalsis or have any osmotic effect and allow the assessment of bowel wall pathologies. VoLumen is such an agent and uses a low density (0.1%) barium sulphate contrast agent specifically designed for multi-slice CT examinations. VoLumen contains sorbitol, which is a non-absorbable sugar alcohol that promotes luminal distension and restricts the reabsorption of water while allowing excellent visualisation of the bowel wall mucosa.[39]

ANTIMICROBIAL DRUGS

Antimicrobials are a group of chemicals which either kill or prevent the growth of bacteria, viruses, fungi and protozoa. In some instances, some antimicrobials are produced by bacteria themselves, e.g. penicillin. Within radiology, antimicrobials may be applied topically as an antiseptic agent, e.g. Betadine, prior to a percutaneous procedure or given intravenously to prophylactically prevent infection (gentamycin or cefortaxime). Within oncology, patients often require antibiotics prior to surgery to prevent infection; their use is also extended to those patients with compromised immune systems following chemotherapy.

Antibiotics have historically been viewed as 'wonder drugs' since they revolutionised the treatment of serious bacterial infections. Prior to the 1940s, bacterial infections such as endocarditis were almost universally fatal together with either pneumonia or meningitis.[40] Although there are well over 100 different antibiotics available today, the majority come from a few types of drugs.

Viruses are much harder to treat than bacterial infections because the virus lives inside the cell. It is difficult for our immune system to see the virus and attack them. Several drugs have been developed recently to treat common viruses (tamiflu and relenza), however the management of viral infections still focuses on their prevention by vaccination. Most antiviral drugs work by inhibiting the development of the virus instead of destroying the pathogen. This is commonly achieved by interfering with DNA production and preventing the virus from replicating.

Antifungals are a group of drugs used to treat infections caused by fungi. Two of the most common fungal infections are tinea (ringworm) and candidiasis (thrush). The method of action for most antifungals is to act on the walls of the cell and make them permeable. The contents of the cells subsequently leak out and the fungi die. Most fungal infections affect the skin and mucous membranes, so drug application is topical, using creams, pessaries and powders. If the infection persists, then these can be administered orally and for even more deep-routed infections, by an intravenous route.

Protozoa are one-celled organisms that can cause human infections ranging in severity from mild to very severe. Parasitic protozoa are typically found in ticks, fleas and mosquitos but can also be found in water contaminated by waste products, e.g. faeces. Common protozoan infections include malaria and the gastrointestinal tract conditions of amoebiasis and giardiasis. Generally, protozoan infections are confined to underdeveloped sub-tropical and tropical countries where sanitation is generally poor. Treatment is by the administration of antiprotozoal drugs, e.g. metronidazole, which can be used to treat protozoan infections of the GI tract (amoebiasis) and GU tract (*Trichomonas vaginalis*).

Antiseptics are antimicrobials which, when applied to living tissue (skin/mucous membranes), reduce the possibility of infection. There are distinct types: bactericidals (which kill microbes) and bacteriostatic (inhibit bacterial growth). Common radiological antiseptic preparations include iodophors (Betadine) and chlorohexidine gluconate (Hibiscrub). Both agents can be used for preparing the skin prior to percutaneous procedures and can also be used as a surgical scrub for hand-washing. Alcohol-based agents (60–90% ethyl or isopropyl) are also effective antiseptic agents but cannot be applied to the mucous membranes. Towels or small pads impregnated with alcohol are commonly used as a skin prepping agent prior to venepuncture.

ANTICONVULSANT DRUGS

Seizures or convulsions are abnormal discharges of electrical activity within the brain. Seizures generally include a period of unconsciousness and rapid uncontrollable shaking. A prolonged seizure must be treated, as there will be increased requirements for both oxygen and glucose within the brain, which may lead to permanent neurological damage. Most convulsions cease within 30 seconds but those that persist are given the term *status epilepticus* and require urgent treatment.

In the pre-hospital environment or where vital signs monitoring are not available, rectal diazepam or buccally administered midazolam can be used. Both of these are benzodiazepines which enhance the effects of the neurotransmitter gamma-aminobutyric acid (GABA) resulting in a sedative, anticonvulsant and muscle relaxant effect. If the seizures persist or monitoring is available, then many clinicians will opt for intravenous injection of lorazepam; this is also benzodiazepine but is more potent and has a longer action. If seizures still persist, then the drug phenytoin can be administered by an infusion. Phenytoin acts by suppressing abnormal brain activity by reducing electrical conductance among brain cells.

CARDIOVASCULAR DRUGS

There are a wide range of cardiovascular drugs available. Common applications are for the management of hypertension, angina, myocardial infarction, arrhythmias and hypercholesterolaemia.

Hypertension

Several classes of drugs are currently available for the treatment of hypertension. In order to achieve a clinically acceptable reduction in blood pressure, treatment will frequently require a combination of drugs. Antihypertensive drugs include diuretics, ACE inhibitors, α-and β-blockers, angiotensin II receptor antagonists, calcium channel blockers and direct renin inhibitors.

Angiotensin-converting enzyme (ACE) inhibitors such as captopril and lisinopril block the conversion of angiotensin I into angiotensin II. This helps lower arteriolar resistance and reduces the amount of water reabsorbed by the kidneys. This combination results in a lowering of blood volume and blood pressure. Drugs called angiotensin II receptor antagonists, such as losartan, work in a similar manner to ACE inhibitors but may be indicated if there are unpleasant side-effects from the use of an ACE inhibitor.

Calcium channel blockers such as nifedipine cause a reduction in cardiac contractility and the relaxation of vascular smooth muscles. This produces dilation to the coronary and peripheral arteries, and blood pressure is lowered because there is both less resistance in these wider dilated arteries and a lower cardiac output. Nifedipine has traditionally been administered sublingually during percutaneous arterial interventions in order to acutely reduce blood pressure and help achieve haemostasis at the end of the procedure. The use of sublingual nifedipine can be associated with severe headaches. More recent research has suggested that captopril is just as effective but carries a low incidence of any adverse effects.[41]

β-blockers (atenolol) work by reducing the nerve impulses to the heart and blood vessels. This makes the heart beat slower and with less force, thereby lowering blood pressure. α-blockers (prazosin) work in a similar manner but only affect blood vessels. They cause a dilatation of blood vessels which lowers vascular resistance and in turn blood pressure. Direct renin inhibitors are a newer group of pharmaceuticals used for the treatment of hypertension. Aliskiren is an example and is currently licensed for the treatment of hypertension. These drugs may show additional advantages in terms of renoprotection when compared with alternative anti-hypertensive medications.

Diuretics are another group of antihypertensive drugs which can lower blood pressure by increasing urine production and lowering the overall blood volume. There are three main types of diuretic: loop, potassium-sparing and thiazide. Loop diuretics include furosemide and work by blocking the absorption of sodium, chloride and water from the filtered fluid in the kidneys. As water is not reabsorbed there is marked increase in urine production and a lowering of the overall circulating blood volume. Potassium-sparing diuretics (amiloride and trimterene) work in a similar manner to loop diuretics but do not encourage the secretion of potassium into the urine. Low potassium levels or hypokalaemia may cause cardiac arrhythmias and muscle weakness and, in severe cases, they can be fatal. Thiazides (bendroflumethiazide and cyclopenthiazide) are a further class of diuretic which lowers blood pressure by inhibiting the reabsorbtion of sodium and chloride ions from the beginning of the distal convoluted tubule.

Cardiac arrhythmias

Arrhythmias are disturbances in the normal rate or rhythm of the heart. They range from the occasional ectopic beats that may be experienced in healthy people to complete disorganisations of cardiac activity seen in ventricular fibrillation (VF). Antiarrhythmic drugs generally work by modifying the pattern of ion channel opening and closing during the cardiac action potential. They are grouped into four main classes, based on the Vaughan–Williams classification system.[42] Sodium channel blockers such as disopyramide and procainamide are grouped into Class 1. They work by blocking open Na+ channels and this prolongs the action potential and slows down conduction, this widens the QRS segment on an ECG. Class 2 anti-arrhythmic drugs are β-blockers (atenolol and propranolol) that work by slowing the heart down and thus reducing its overall workload. Membrane stabilising drugs (amiodarone and sotalol) are in Class 3 and are used to treat a fast and irregular heart rate. These drugs show similar properties to β-blockers and K+ channel blockers and prolong phase 3 of the action potential. Calcium channel blockers (dihydropyramide, phenylalkylamine and benzothiazepine) are Class 4 drugs and block voltage-gated calcium channels in the cardiac muscle. This leads to a reduction in cardiac muscle contraction and overall contractility. This decreases the cardiac afterload and thereby reduces the overall workload on the heart. Other antiarrhythmia drugs include adenosine and digoxin. Adenosine improves the pumping action of the heart by slowing down conduction and allowing the heart to fill with blood correctly. This drug does not remove the arrhythmia but helps improve the cardiac output. Digoxin causes a transient heart block and can be used to successfully terminate supraventricular and atrial tachycardias. With any anti-arrhythmic drug, there is always the possibility of making things worse; current practice is to only treat arrhythmias if they pose a threat to life.

Angina

Angina is characterised by severe chest pain which results from a lack of oxygenated blood reaching the heart muscle (myocardium). Angina is generally caused by a narrowing or spasm of the coronary arteries. Treatment focuses on reducing the pain relating to angina, preventing the condition worsening and reducing overall risk of a myocardial infarction. The treatment of angina focuses on the use of nitrates, statins, anti-platelet agents, β-blockers and ACE inhibitors. Glyceryl trinitrate (GTN) belongs to a group of drugs called *nitrates* which contain the chemical nitric oxide. Nitric oxide is a naturally occurring chemical, which has the effect of making blood vessels relax and dilate. By dilating the coronary arteries, there is less resistance to blood flow so more blood can reach the heart muscle. Another nitrate is the drug isosorbide dinitrate and this can also be used during arterial interventional procedures. Small arteries may go into spasm when mechanically irritated by the internal manipulation of catheters and guidewires. This is termed an iatrogenic vasospasm and usually resolves spontaneously after removal of the instrumentation but can be assisted with a vasodilator.

Statins (simvastatin) are group of drugs which are used to lower cholesterol and prevent further narrowing of the coronary arteries. Statins work by inhibiting the enzyme HMG-CoA reductase, which plays a major role in the production of cholesterol in the liver. Statins have been proven to lower low density lipoproteins (LDL) and in turn, decrease related cardiac events by 60% and stroke by 17%.[43]

Aspirin has a role in the management of angina but it is a diverse drug and can act as a mild analgesic, antipyrexial and an anti-inflammatory drug. For the treatment of angina, aspirin displays useful anti-platelet properties and inhibits the production of thromboxane, which normally binds platelet molecules together to create a patch over the damaged walls of blood vessels. This group of bound platelets can obstruct blood flow or move and cause an embolus. By administering low-dose aspirin, the incidence of myocardial infarction, stroke and thrombosis can be reduced.[44] Other anti-platelet drugs are available and again work by reducing platelet accumulation, binding and thrombus formation. Adenosine diphosphonate (ADP) receptor inhibitors such as clopidogrel inhibit platelet aggregation and stop the cross-linking of platelets by fibrin. Clopidogrel is used in the treatment of myocardial infarction, acute coronary syndrome and to prevent a vascular event in patients with symptomatic atherosclerosis. A benefit from clopidogrel has been also demonstrated following carotid artery stenting. A study reported fewer neurological events, without any increase in bleeding complications, when administering dual anti-platelet therapy (aspirin and clopidogrel) both before and after carotid artery stenting.[45]

Myocardial Infarction

Thrombolytic therapy may be used in the treatment of an acute myocardial infarction. Thrombolysis may also be initiated for an acute peripheral artery occlusion where drug delivery is by angiographic catheters implanted directly within the thrombus. Direct catheter placement allows the accurate infusion of thrombolytic drugs. This treatment unfortunately carries a major risk of haemorrhage and patients should be screened for risk factors prior before treatment. There are two key types of thrombolytic agent: streptokinase and plasminogen activators. Streptokinase is a binding protein, which can activate human plasminogen. Plasmin is produced in the blood to break

down fibrin, which is a major component of thrombus. Plasmin is needed to break down a blood clot once it has sufficiently stopped bleeding. The extra production of plasmin produced by streptokinase helps break down unwanted clots. Streptokinase needs to be delivered close to the start of symptoms in order to achieve the best results. Tissue plasminogen activator (TPA) is a protein involved in the breakdown of blood clots. It is an enzyme which catalyses the conversion of plasminogen into plasmin (the major enzyme responsible for clot breakdown).

ANALGESIA AND SEDATION

There are numerous analgesia drugs available to help alleviate pain. Deciding on an appropriate analgesia strategy can be difficult and will depend on the type, onset, duration, severity and underlying aetiology of the pain. In order to promote consistency, the World Health Organization (WHO) devised a conceptual framework for the prescription of analgesia drugs.[46] This 'analgesia ladder' was initially set up to help manage cancer-related pain but has been applied to a wide range of medical conditions. The WHO analgesic ladder promotes a stepped approach to the prescribing of analgesics which are taken from the following subgroups:

- Non-opioid analgesics: paracetamol and NSAIDs (ibuprofen, diclofenac)
- Weak opioids: tramadol and codeine
- Strong opioids: morphine, pethidine, fentanyl
- Adjuvants (drugs which were not originally designed for pain management but have demonstrated pain lowering effects).

For every step on the analgesic ladder, non-opioid analgesics provide a basis for the management of pain. Paracetamol and NSAIDs should, where necessary, be prescribed with a weak or strong opioid analgesic. This pain management technique is known as multi-modal analgesia and is based on the theory that pain is best managed by a combination of several analgesic agents, this being more effective than the use of a single analgesic. Evidence has demonstrated that when using a multi-modal approach, pain relief is better, smaller quantities of painkillers are required and there are less side-effects.[47] Analgesic drugs can be split into non-opioid (non-narcotic) and opioid (narcotic). The principle distinction between the two is that dependence on opioids can develop with long-term use and they can also cause central nervous system depression.

Non-opioid analgesics

Non-steroidal anti-inflammatory drugs (NSAIDs), which include ibuprofen, diclofenac and aspirin together with paracetamol fall into the non-opioid analgesic group.

Aspirin and other NSAIDs inhibit prostaglandin production around the body. Prostaglandins are produced as part of the body's inflammatory response to injury. Prostaglandin production is successfully inhibited by blocking the cyclooxygenase enzymes (COX-1 and COX-2). By blocking the enzymes, NSAIDs reduce the sensation of pain and reduce inflammation. This mechanism can, however, lead to unwanted gastrointestinal side-effects. In view of the potential for gastrointestinal side-effects, paracetamol has become a useful alternative. Paracetamol has no COX-1 or COX-2 action but it does selectively inhibit the cyclooxygenase (COX-3) enzyme in the brain and spinal cord which is thought to be its method of action for reducing pain.

Opioid analgesics

Opioid analgesics include: codeine, morphine, fentanyl and pethidine. These drugs are available in a wide range of formulations, including modified-release (MR) preparations, transdermal (TD) patches, buccal tablets, granules for suspension and parenteral preparations. The analgesic effects of opioids cause a decrease in the perception of pain, a decreased reaction to pain and an increase in pain tolerance. Opioids block pain signals by binding to opioid receptors around the body in the central and peripheral nervous system. Opioids do not interfere with the detection of pain but they reduce the feeling of pain via pathways in the spinal cord and by decreasing activity in the brain. There are many different types of opioid receptors in the body; the activation of each different type leads to a different effect. The activation of μ and κ-opioid receptors leads to analgesic effects but there are additional side-effects. Activation of a κ-opioid receptor can cause sedation and increased urine production. The activation of the peripheral μ-receptors in the gastrointestinal tract may lead to constipation.

Nitrous oxide

Nitrous oxide (N_2O) is a colourless non-flammable gas which can be used for the safe and effective relief of pain in short procedures, e.g. wound dressing changes, suture removal. By inhaling Entonox (50% nitrous oxide/50% oxygen), short-term pain relief comparable with strong opiates can be achieved. Nitrous oxide acts by dulling the pain receptors in brain. If used on its own, it will cause a loss of consciousness but when combined with 50% O_2 and administered by a demand valve, its analgesic effect is achieved without loss of consciousness. The use of nitrous oxide within radiology can provide short-term analgesia during biopsy procedures, biliary catheter placements and peripheral angiography.[48]

Sedation

Complex radiological interventional procedures frequently require the combined use of a sedative and analgesic drug to ensure patient comfort and cooperation. The level of sedation required to successfully undertake a procedure will depend on multiple factors. These include the type and length of procedure and existing anxiety and pain levels. The Ramsay Sedation Scale[49] is used clinically to monitor the level of sedation, for most radiology-based procedures, conscious sedation is required where the patient can still respond to verbal commands.

Within radiology, the primary sedative agent is the benzodiazepine midazolam. This is highly suitable, since it reduces patient anxiety, provides a sedative effect, causes antegrade amnesia and produces minimal respiratory and cardiovascular depression. Midazolam has no analgesic effects, so must be combined with an appropriate analgesic agent (pethidine or fentanyl). Care must be taken when administering midazolam to elderly patients who may have decreased hepatic clearance. Midazolam administration to this group of patients may lead to an increased risk of respiratory depression and agitation. If this happens, then reversal can be achieved using the antagonist Flumazenil. Midazolam being a benzodiazepine works by exerting an effect on gamma-amniobutyric acid (GABA). GABA being the brain's quieting or tranquillising neurotransmitter.

Diazepam is also a benzodiazepine drug and again enhances the effects of GABA. It is commonly administered orally and due to its short duration of action can be used to help reduce anxiety before interventional procedures and MRI examinations. For MRI examinations, patients with severe anxiety and/or claustrophobia may be prescribed oral diazepam. This practice should only be undertaken in collaboration with the radiology/radiotherapy department, as this will be safer and can form part of a specific anxiety/claustrophobia imaging care pathway.

In recent years, the drug propofol has received massive popularity as both a sedative and an induction agent for general anaesthesia. Advantages are its rapid onset and offset, which leads to an extremely quick recovery time and very little 'hangover effect'. Propofol is not without limitations, the main side-effect being respiratory and cardiac depression. Neither the infusion rate nor the size of the bolus necessary to achieve airway obstruction and apnoea can be predicted. Even in moderate sedation, airway obstruction can be common in susceptible patients. Many believe that propofol should therefore only be administered by anaesthetic trained practitioners and its use is often restricted.

ANTIEMETICS

Nausea and vomiting are common symptoms, especially in patients with cancer. Even minor symptoms of nausea can be debilitating and for this reason, the management of nausea and vomiting is extremely important. Ideally, the identification and treatment of the underlying cause may allow total resolution of symptoms. This may take time and subsequently, initial management focuses on the use of anti-sickness or antiemetic drugs. Nausea and vomiting result from the activation of protective physiological mechanisms, which exist to help eliminate toxins from the body. There are four principal sites which can activate the vomiting centre in the brainstem: (1) the gastrointestinal tract when there is either stasis or irritation of the gastric mucosa; (2) the chemoreceptor trigger zone (CTZ) in the base of the fourth ventricle – activation is usually mediated by the presence of chemicals, e.g. opioids or biochemical abnormalities; (3) raised intracranial pressure, resulting from cerebral metastases or traumatic haemorrhage can directly act on the cerebral cortex and cause activation of the vomiting centre; (4) changes in the vestibular apparatus can also cause the vomiting centre to become stimulated, e.g. motion sickness. The pharmacological treatment of nausea and vomiting usually starts with first-line antiemetic drugs and moves on to second-line if they prove to be ineffective.

First-line antiemetics

A prokinetic antiemetic such as metaclopromide or domperidone can be administered if there is gastric stasis or a functional outflow obstruction. Both drugs are dopamine receptor antagonists and stop signals from the CTZ to the vomiting centre. Being prokinetic antiemetics, they also increase the rate of gastric emptying and increase peristalsis. They have also been shown to decrease the sensitivity of receptors in the pharynx and upper GI tract to noxious stimuli. If nausea and vomiting result from chemical causes, then a D2 antagonist, e.g. Haloperidol can be prescribed. Haloperidol works by blocking activity at the CTZ and restricting the messages sent to the vomiting centre. Cyclizine is an alternative for organic bowel obstruction, raised intracranial pressure, opioid-related nausea and motion sickness-related causes. Cyclizine works by blocking histamine and muscarinic receptors in the vomiting centre. This prevents the vomiting centre from receiving nerve messages from the vestibular apparatus (useful in the prevention of nausea and vomiting due to motion sickness). Cyclizine also prevents the vomiting centre from receiving messages from the CTZ, which may be stimulated by agents in the blood, e.g. opioids or anaesthetics. If nausea and vomiting results from raised intracranial pressure, mechanical bowel obstruction or motion sickness, then a vomiting centre-targeting antiemetic can be prescribed, e.g. promethazine.

Second-line antiemetics

Second-line antiemetics may be initiated if the first-line drugs fail to produce adequate symptom control. Methotrimeprazine again exerts an antihistamine effect but has a broader spectrum activity and can act on a range of receptor sites. This drug is useful if the cause of nausea and vomiting is unclear or there are multiple mechanisms implicated. There is an associated sedative effect when using methotrimeprazine. It is recommended that treatment must commence with low doses. Ondansetron is a $5HT_3$ antagonist and blocks the effect of the release of serotonin by enterochromaffin cells in the gut wall caused by certain chemotherapy drugs or abdominal radiotherapy. In some situations, it may be necessary to try to directly treat the underlying cause of the nausea and vomiting. Dexamethosone is a potent steroid which can be used to reduce peri-tumoral oedema and can help reduce intracranial pressure and this helps alleviate any associated nausea and vomiting.

ANTISPASMODICS

Antispasmodics are a group of drugs which can help alleviate some symptoms which are caused by spasm of the gastrointestinal tract, e.g. colicky abdominal pain and bloating. The GI tract is partially controlled by an extensive network of nerves which help to regulate the motility of the gut. The nerves work by controlling the smooth muscle that is present in the walls of the bowel. These muscles, which are responsible for gut movements, are stimulated by nerves which are triggered by different chemicals produced by the body. The chemicals produce either a contraction or relaxation response. Contractions cause food to move along the GI tract and in some conditions, when there are too many contractions of the smooth muscle it can cause pain and symptoms of bloating. When air or CO_2 is introduced as part of a radiological procedure, it is these muscles which resist dilatation and cause pain. Antispasmodic drugs are used to treat abdominal pain and assist bowel distension during radiological procedures. There are two main groups of drugs which can exert antispasmodic effects on the bowel. Antimuscarinics include atropine sulphate, dicycloverine hydrochloride and hyoscine butylbromide (Buscopan) and work by blocking muscarinic receptors. These are a class of receptors found in the gut that cause the smooth muscle to contract. Blocking the receptors reduces the amount of contractions and should help to relieve some of the symptoms. Since muscarinic receptors are also found in other parts of the body, the administration of antimuscarinics can have other effects, e.g. a dry mouth, blurred vision.

Hyoscine butylbromine (Buscopan) is an antimuscarinic and therefore an indirect smooth muscle relaxant. It is commonly used in DCBE and CT colonography procedures and predominantly acts on the intramural parasympathetic ganglia. For many years, great care was taken to avoid the administration of Buscopan in patients with a history of closed angle glaucoma and/or cardiac failure. This guidance was often considered controversial, the rationale being the possibility of a rise in intraocular pressure following injection. For patients with undiagnosed closed angle glaucoma, it is universally agreed that the administration of Buscopan could cause serious visual problems. Undiagnosed patients are more at risk than those with a history of treated glaucoma; patients with treated glaucoma should therefore not be excluded. There is, however, wide variation in practice, with contraindications varying between institutions. More recent reports[50] suggest that patients should be asked about any Buscopan allergies and any recent cardiac-related problems (cardiac instability, such as those recently admitted with acute coronary syndrome, recurrent cardiac pain at rest, uncontrolled left ventricular failure and recent ventricular arrhythmias). If these do not generate contraindications then Buscopan should be administered and advice given not to drive for 30 min and to wait until any blurred vision has resolved. Medical attention must be sought urgently if the patient develops acute pain in either one or both eyes. If Buscopan is felt to be contraindicated, then the alternative agent is glucagon. Glucagon acts directly on smooth muscles and diminishes the tone and motility of the stomach, duodenum, small and large bowel. Studies have shown that Buscopan provides better distension of the colon than glucagon and it is cheaper and a more easily prepared.[51]

Direct smooth muscle relaxants, which include alverine citrate, mebeverine hydrochloride and peppermint oil are also useful. In a Japanese study,[52] peppermint oil was substituted for Buscopan in double-contrast barium enema procedures. The authors concluded that rectally administered peppermint oil was both safe and effective and could be used as a buscopan substitute.

LOCAL ANAESTHETICS

Local anaesthetic drugs work by causing a temporary block to conduction along nerve fibres. These drugs have revolutionised the practice of interventional procedures both surgically and radiologically and have removed the need for a general anaesthetic in many instances. Different types of local anaesthetics are available, which vary in their potency, duration of action and ability to penetrate tissues. Local anaesthetics can be administered by many routes, including topical application and by subcutaneous infiltration. Local anaesthetic agents can also be used to achieve peripheral nerve blocks, intravenous regional anaesthesia (Bier's block), plexus blocks, epidural and spinal anaesthesia.

The precise dosage of local anaesthetics depends on the site and type of procedure. Local anaesthetic drugs cause dilation of blood vessels and therefore may increase bleeding and absorption of the anaesthetic leading to a shorter anaesthetic effect. To counter this, some local anaesthetics contain a vasoconstrictor such as adrenaline, which helps diminish local blood flow, slows the rate of absorption and lengthens the anaesthetic effect.

KEY POINTS

- Drug action is primarily based on either *agonists*, which when binding to a cell receptor cause a response, e.g. morphine is an agonist and binds to a κ-receptor causing an analgesic effect – or *antagonists*, e.g. Buscopan, which decrease the function of a cell causing the relaxation of bowel smooth muscles

- The *therapeutic window* of a drug is the range between the lowest dose which has a positive effect and the highest dose before we see any negative effects

- The preparation and administration of drugs must adhere to local and national guidance

- Introduction of oral and rectal negative contrast agents can cause discomfort. Improvements in comfort, distension and medical imaging yield can be achieved using CO_2 and an antispasmodic agent (e.g. Buscopan)

- Intravascular administration of contrast agents is common. Reactions are rare but must be considered before, during and after the administration of both iodine and gadolinium-based agents

- Practitioners must have an understanding on the typical management strategies for contrast reactions. In all but the very mildest cases, advice from the supervising clinician should be sought

- Contrast-induced nephropathy (CIN) is generally transient; patients most at risk are those with a history of renal impairment and diabetes

- Serum creatinine levels are useful and easily acquired indicators of renal function. eGFR levels, which incorporate age, gender and ethnicity are believed to be superior in indicating renal impairment

- Antimicrobial drugs can be used to both prevent and treat infections which can result from bacteria, viruses, fungi and protozoa

- Status epilepticus increases the brain's requirements for both oxygen and glucose. If they are not stopped this may lead to permanent neurological damage. Treatment usually starts with buccal midazolam or intravenous lorazepam (if monitoring available)

- Cardiovascular drugs are commonly used to treat hypertension, angina, myocardial infarction, arrhythmias and hypercholesterolaemia. For many cardiovascular diseases, there may be an overlap of applications for a drug, e.g. β-blockers can act as antihypertensive and anti-arrhythmic drugs and can also help in the treatment of angina

- Analgesics can be split into opioid and non-opioid drugs; the principle difference between the two is that dependence on opioids can develop and they can also cause central nervous system depression. For cases of moderate to severe pain, analgesia is multi-modal and usually consists of a non-opioid taken together with a weak or strong opioid drug

- Sedation is frequently required for radiological interventional procedures to ensure patient comfort and compliance. Administering sedation carries the risks of cardiac and respiratory depression and patients must be carefully monitored in order to ensure their safety. Sedation can also be used for MRI examinations for paediatrics or extremely anxious/claustrophobic patients and this should be in collaboration with the medical imaging department

- Antispasmodic drugs are crucial for GI imaging procedures which require bowel distension. Buscopan is the most widely used antispasmodic but there are safety issues surrounding its use in patients with possible narrow angle glaucoma

- Nausea and vomiting are both debilitating symptoms and can lead to dehydration. Practitioners will need to have an understanding of the underlying cause of the symptoms in order to identify the appropriate anti-emetic drug

- Developments in local anaesthetic drugs have allowed minor surgical procedures to be undertaken in the radiology department with the patient awake or under conscious sedation

Chapter | 12 |

Cancer chemotherapy drugs

Ciara M. Hughes, Stephanie R. McKeown

INTRODUCTION

Cancer is a disease characterised by uncontrolled cell division. Through a very highly controlled mechanism, cells and tissues develop and increase in number, which results in normal growth and development. Cell division occurs through a process called the cell cycle. Once we reach adulthood, suppressor genes responsible for cell growth stop this division. However, in some cell types, cell division can continue in order to replace cells that turnover rapidly such as blood cells and the mucosa of the gastrointestinal tract.

Sometimes the complex controls of cell division become modified (mutated) and this results in a loss of the cell's ability to tightly control their growth. This often requires mutations in several key control genes before a cell becomes out of control; when this occurs the cell numbers increase and a tumour develops. Tumours are three-dimensional structures that require nutrients and oxygen provided by blood vessels growing into the tumour mass (angiogenesis). A tumour is therefore a complex mass of several cell types as well as the out-of-control tumour cells. As the tumour control mechanisms are abnormal, there is a greater tendency for more mutations to occur. Consequently, tumours become more malignant (i.e. more highly mutated/out of control) as they grow. More malignant cells are also more likely to become independent of their tissue of origin and move round the body via the blood and lymphatic systems. These cells have the potential to develop into secondary tumours in sites distant from the original primary tumour. This metastatic spread is often the cause of death in cancer patients.

Cancer treatments aim to eradicate the primary tumour through surgical removal, sterilisation by exposure to high dose radiation or the use of cytotoxic chemotherapy drugs. Only the last of these options can target cells that have metastasised to sites distant from the primary tumour.

THE CELL CYCLE

Many approaches to cancer chemotherapy involve interfering with cell division and so an understanding of the normal cell cycle is essential. The cell cycle is a sequence of events during which a cell duplicates its contents and then divides into two. There are two main periods: interphase, when a cell is not dividing, and the mitotic phase when the cell divides. Cell proliferation is regulated through the five phases of the cell cycle, see Figure 12.1.

- G0 – the cells are at rest
- G1 – growth of the cell and duplication of organelles
- S – synthesis of new strands of DNA
- G2 – growth and assembly of microtubules and centrioles necessary for cell division
- M – mitosis – division of cellular and nuclear content to produce two daughter cells.

During the G1 phase, the cell is metabolically active and replicates most of its organelles and cytosolic components. Cells may leave the cell cycle during this phase and enter the G0 phase where they carry out their normal function as differentiated cells and therefore do not divide, hence

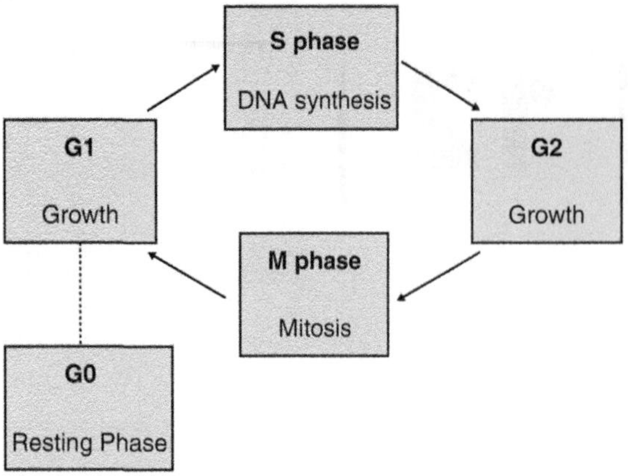

Figure 12.1 The cell cycle: a sequence of events during which a cell duplicates its contents and then divides into two.

they are said to be resting. Cells that leave the G1 phase and enter the S phase undergo a period of DNA replication so that when the cell divides, each daughter cell will have a full complement of DNA.

During the G2 phase, growth of the cell continues and enzymes and proteins are synthesised in preparation for cell division. Growth and assembly of microtubules and centrioles necessary for cell division also occurs.

The cells then move into the mitosis phase, which can be further divided into four stages: prophase, metaphase, anaphase and telophase. During prophase, the chromosomes condense and shorten. As DNA replication has already taken place during the S phase of the cell cycle, each chromosome now contains a pair of identical double stranded chromatids, i.e. the cell contains double the normal amount of genetic material. During this phase, the spindle, a ball-shaped network of microtubules, forms. The function of the spindle is to allow separation of the chromatids to opposite ends of the cell later in the process. During metaphase, the chromatids line up along the centre of the cell and during anaphase, these chromatids separate and chromatids from each pair move to opposite sides of the cell along the spindle. These chromatids will form the chromosomes for the new daughter cells. During telophase, the chromosomes uncoil, a nuclear envelope forms around the two areas of genetic material and the spindle breaks up.

DNA replication

DNA carries all of the genetic information required for protein synthesis and to regulate most of the activities that take place within our cells. DNA is arranged in two long strands which coil around each other to form a double helix. Each strand is composed of millions of nucleotides and each nucleotide is made up of three parts; a nitrogenous base (there are four bases – adenine and guanine, which are purines and thymine and cytosine which are pyrimidines);

a five-carbon sugar called deoxyribose and a phosphate group. The phosphate group and sugar form the backbone of the DNA and the bases project inward. The two strands are held together by bonds between complementary base-pairs (i.e. between adenine and thymine or between cytosine and guanine). The sequences that these bases are arranged in will code for a particular protein. When a cell is at rest, these strands of DNA condense into chromosomes. In order for the DNA to replicate during the S phase of the cell cycle, the DNA uncoils and becomes separated into two strands. This uncoiling is controlled by an enzyme called topoisomerase. New bases (pyrimidines and purines) pair up with the bases along the uncoiled strands and new complementary DNA strands are formed.

Protein synthesis occurs when the cell is not dividing. Again, DNA uncoils and separates into two individual strands; however, during this process, messenger ribonucleic (mRNA) acid is formed by complementary base-pairing under the control of an enzyme RNA polymerase. DNA therefore acts as a template for the formation of this mRNA. This process is known as *transcription*. The mRNA then leaves the nucleus and enters the cytoplasm of the cell where it attaches to ribosomal RNA (rRNA). Then, during a process known as *translation*, the rRNA reads the code on the mRNA and along with transfer RNA (tRNA), they select appropriate amino acids to be joined together to form proteins.

Cell cycle control and mitosis

There are checkpoints during this process which stop cell division if there has been damage to the DNA. This action is controlled by tumour suppressor genes such as P53. It may be possible to repair the damage, however if the damage cannot be repaired, then the cell dies by a process known as apoptosis. During apoptosis, enzymes are produced which damage the cell by disruption of the cytoskeleton and nucleus, leading to DNA fragmentation and shrinkage of the cytoplasm. Phagocytes then ingest the dying cell. This process should inhibit the formation of mutated cells which may lead to malignancy. However, abnormalities within the tumour suppressor genes would allow cells with damaged DNA to multiply leading to tumour formation.

There are also genes that code for growth factors which stimulate cells to divide. These genes, e.g. the ras gene, are known as proto-oncogenes. Damage to these genes will also result in cells growing uncontrollably. These mutated genes are known as oncogenes.

CANCER CHEMOTHERAPY DRUGS

Chemotherapy is the treatment of cancer with an antineoplastic (i.e. anti-tumour) drug or with a combination of drugs. The aim of cancer chemotherapy is to *selectively* kill the tumour cells while having limited effect on normal tissues. As these drugs kill cells, they are termed cytotoxic. Over the past 40 years, most of the currently used cancer chemotherapy drugs have been developed. Until recently, most have been designed to kill cells which are actively progressing through the cell cycle. However, this means that they also harm healthy cells that divide rapidly under normal circumstances such as those in the bone marrow, gastrointestinal tract and hair follicles. This results in the most common side-effects of chemotherapy such as decreased production of blood cells (myelosuppression); decreased production of white blood cells, which leads to immunosuppression, inflammation of the lining of the digestive tract; and alopecia (hair loss). More recently, research has focussed on targeting other specific features of tumours (these are discussed below).

As cytotoxic chemotherapy affects cell division, tumours with high growth fractions (such as acute myelogenous leukaemia and the aggressive lymphomas, including Hodgkin's disease) are more sensitive to chemotherapy, as a larger proportion of the cells are undergoing cell division at any time. Malignancies which grow at a slower rate, such as lymphomas, do not respond as well to chemotherapy. As chemotherapy targets dividing cells, it has little or no effect on quiescent cells (G0, cells in the resting phase of the cell cycle) which remain viable; consequently, they can re-enter the cell cycle following chemotherapy and repopulate the tumour. This explains why few cancers are curable with chemotherapy drugs and highlights the importance of early detection. For example, a small 1 cm breast tumour may contain 1 billion cancer cells before it can be palpated. Even if chemotherapy kills 99% of these cells and the lump is no longer palpable, 10 million cancer cells would remain and these may begin to divide. However, one of the aims of drug therapy is to lower the cancer cell number sufficiently to allow the patient's immune system to control or eliminate the remaining cells. As only a fraction of the cells in a tumour die with each treatment (known as fractional kill), repeated doses must be administered to continue to reduce the size of the tumour. Therefore, chemotherapy regimens deliver drug treatment in cycles, with the frequency and duration of treatments limited by the cumulative toxicity to the patient.

There are a number of strategies in the administration of chemotherapeutic drugs. Chemotherapy may be used in an attempt to cure the patient or it may aim to prolong life or to alleviate symptoms. Combined modality chemotherapy is the use of drugs with other cancer treatments such as radiation therapy or surgery. Most cancers are now treated in this way. Combination chemotherapy involves treating a patient with a number of different drugs simultaneously. The drugs used often differ in their mechanism of action and side-effects, which reduces the chances of resistance developing to any one agent and, as side-effects are not accumulative, they are less likely to compromise attaining the required treatment dosage. Neoadjuvant

chemotherapy may be provided preoperatively. Theoretically, this should shrink the primary tumour allowing surgery or radiotherapy to be more effective. Adjuvant chemotherapy (postoperative treatment) can be used when there is little evidence of cancer remaining but there is risk of recurrence. This can help reduce the chances of developing resistance if the tumour does develop. It is also useful in killing any cancerous cells which have spread to other parts of the body. This is often effective as the newly growing tumours are fast-dividing, and therefore very susceptible to chemotherapy. Palliative chemotherapy may be provided simply to decrease tumour load, ease pain, improve quality of life and increase life expectancy.

The majority of cancer chemotherapeutic drugs can be divided into: alkylating agents, antimetabolites, cytotoxic-antibiotics, plant alkaloids and related drugs, drugs which regulate hormonal control of tumours, drugs specific for the control of the tumour microenvironment and molecular targeting drugs (Table 12.1).

Alkylating agents

This drug group works by chemically modifying the cell's DNA. They are named alkylating agents because of their ability to alkylate, i.e. attach an alkyl ($C_nH_{2n+}1$) group with guanine bases on DNA forming covalent bonds. Each alkylating agent attaches in a different way. They form bonds independently of the stage of the cell cycle. However, once the cell attempts to divide, the attached drug prevents the DNA from uncoiling and separating, causing breakages in the DNA strands and this results in a block in cell division and consequent inhibition of tumour growth. Classical alkylating agents include the 'nitrogen mustards' such as mechlorethamine, cyclophosphamide, chlorambucil and ifosfamide. Cisplatin, carboplatin, oxaliplatin are all considered alkylating-like agents. These drugs do not have an alkyl group but they contain platinum and bind to DNA to prevent cell division. Blood cells are particularly sensitive to alkylating agents and so they are often used to treat lymphocytic leukaemia. They are also used to treat a variety of solid tumours. Side-effects such as alopecia, sterility, neurotoxicity and nephrotoxicity may also occur. In addition, epithelial cells of the GI tract may be damaged leading to nausea, vomiting and diarrhoea. There is also a risk of developing non-lymphocytic leukaemia following treatment with these drugs, although this will not occur until some considerable time after treatment; usually after at least 5 years.[1,2]

Antimetabolites

Antimetabolite drugs have a similar chemical structure to some of the essential building blocks of cells and therefore can interfere with the metabolism of the tumour.[3] The rapidly growing tumour requires large amounts of nutrients to create the component cellular structures such as

Table 12.1 Summary drug table: cancer chemotherapy drugs

Drug group	Examples	Mechanism of action	Common clinical use	Side-effects
Alkylating agents	Classical: cyclophosphamide. Non-classical: cisplatin	Damage DNA by forming covalent bond across the DNA strands attaching to the guanine base	Leukaemia, lymphomas, soft tissue carcinoma, solid tumours, myeloma, adenocarcinoma	Infertility, bone marrow suppression, non-lymphocytic leukaemia
Antimetabolites	Methotrexate, mercaptopurine, fluorouracil	Act as false versions of the building block for DNA and inhibit the synthesis of these building blocks	Leukaemia, colorectal cancer, solid tumours, mesothelioma, non-small cell lung cancer	Nausea, diarrhoea, bone marrow suppression
Cytotoxic antibiotics	Doxorubicin, dactinomycin, bleomycin	Intercalates between DNA strands inhibiting DNA replication. Topoisomerase inhibitor	Leukaemia, lymphomas, squamous cell carcinoma, breast cancer	Bone marrow suppression, nausea, diarrhoea, cardiotoxicity, lung fibrosis (bleomycin)
Plant alkaloids and related drugs	Taxanes: docetaxel. Vinca alkaloids: vincristine	Inhibit tubulin and so inhibit the formation of microtubules including the mitotic spindle	Taxanes: ovarian, breast and non-small cell lung cancer Alkaloids: leukaemia, sarcoma, lung and breast cancer	Peripheral neuropathies, cardiac arrythmias, myelosuppression, neuropathy
Drugs which regulate hormonal control of tumours	Oestrogen receptor antagonists: tamoxifen. Aromatase inhibitors: anastrozole. Anti-androgens: bicalutamide	Block the effect of hormones in the tissue or reduce the production of hormones	Breast and ovarian cancer, prostate cancer	Nausea, diarrhoea, fatigue, dizziness, fluid retention, hot flushes
Drugs specific for the tumour microenvironment: Bioreductive drugs	Tirapazamine, Banoxantrone	Damage to DNA under hypoxic conditions. Cause DNA strand breaks or inhibit topoisomerase	Not licensed – in clinical trials	Limited adverse effects to normal tissue
Molecular targeting drugs: Monoclonal antibodies, Tyrosine kinase inhibitors	Avastin, Herceptin, Imatinib	Block receptors for growth factors. Inhibit protein kinases which can become uncontrolled within cancer	Lymphoma, leukaemia, breast, colorectal, renal, small-cell lung cancer, leukaemia	Cytokine release syndrome, nausea, diarrhoea, liver toxicity

proteins and nucleic acids. As described previously during the S phase of the cell cycle, a complete copy of the cell's DNA is made as a pre-requisite for cell division. This requires incorporation of billions of purine (adenine and guanine) and pyrimidine (cytosine and thymine) bases that make up the genetic code. If the tumour cell incorporates an antimetabolite in place of the required component, the cell's genetic code is compromised, which is usually fatal to the cell.

There are three main types of antimetabolite drugs. Some drugs act directly on pathways of purine and pyrimidine synthesis or block their incorporation into DNA. 5-Fluorouracil is a thymidylate synthase inhibitor which blocks the synthesis of the pyrimidine thymidine.[4] Mercaptopurine and thioguanine are examples of purine analogues that can become incorporated into the DNA in place of hypoxanthine and guanine, leaving the tumour cell unable to divide.[5]

Methotrexate, pemetrexed and pralatrexate are examples of folic acid analogues. Folic acid analogues are drugs which block the synthesis and action of tetrahydrofolate, which is a co-factor in a number of essential synthetic pathways in the cell. Folic acid is required for the formation of thymidine and for purine base synthesis. Methotrexate inhibits the enzyme dihydrofolate reductase, which is required to convert dihydrofolate to the active tetrahydrofolate. As tetrahydrofolate is essential for the production of purines and pyrimidines, methotrexate therefore inhibits the synthesis of DNA.[6] Bone marrow toxicity is the main dose limiting adverse effect caused by antimetabolite drugs, however GI disturbance and hepatotoxicity may also occur.

Cytotoxic antibiotics

Antibiotics are naturally occurring substances produced by microorganisms for protection against other invading microorganisms such as bacteria by inhibiting growth. These substances have been extracted and in some cases modified to produce antibiotics for human use. Some of these drugs are used very successfully to treat common bacterial infections in people. However, many are too toxic against normal cells but have been developed for use as anti-tumour drugs as severe side-effects are more acceptable when balanced against patient's lives. These drugs work in several different ways mainly to interfere with DNA structure and function. Several act as agents which intercalate nucleic acid structure, i.e. they fit (intercalate) between the bases, changing the structure of the DNA strands and so compromise efficient functioning.

Anthracyclines are derived from *Streptomyces* bacteria. An example of an anthracycline, doxorubicin, forms hydrogen-bonds within DNA and intercalates between the bases. Therefore once the cell tries to divide, the DNA strands cannot separate to allow replication. Doxorubicin also interferes with topoisomerase II activity. As described previously, topoisomerases are the enzymes that unwind and wind DNA in order for DNA to control the synthesis of proteins and to facilitate DNA replication. If doxorubicin inhibits this enzyme, then DNA is prevented from uncoiling and so the process of DNA replication is inhibited. Doxorubicin is used to treat leukaemia, lymphoma and solid tumours. The main limiting adverse effect of these drugs is cardiotoxicity. Other adverse effects include alopecia, nausea, vomiting and reduction in blood cell counts.

Some cytotoxic antibiotics such as mitomycin C form covalent bonds to produce DNA cross-links, inhibiting DNA replication. The main adverse effects of mitomycin C are myelotoxicity and nephrotoxicity. Bleomycin also forms covalent bonds with DNA and is thought to chelate metal ions (primarily iron), producing a pseudoenzyme that reacts with oxygen to produce superoxide and hydroxide free radicals. A free radical is any atom or molecule that has a single unpaired electron in an outer shell. Excess free radical production damages cellular structures, causing DNA strand breaks, damage to cell membranes due to lipid peroxidation and oxidation of other cellular molecules. This fragmented DNA is therefore unable to replicate. This drug may produce limited myelotoxicity and can also cause fatal lung fibrosis in some patients.

Plant alkaloids and related drugs

These drugs are derived from plants and mainly block cell division by preventing microtubule function. Microtubules form the spindle cytoskeleton during mitosis and so are vital for cell division. The main examples are vinca alkaloids and taxanes.

Vinca alkaloids are derived from the Madagascar periwinkle plant. They bind to specific sites on tubulin, inhibiting the assembly of tubulin into microtubules during the metaphase of the cell cycle. This inhibits the formation of the mitotic spindle and so arrests mitosis in metaphase. Examples of vinca alkaloids include vincristine, used for paediatric leukaemias, lymphomas and solid tumours, and vinblastine, which is used to treat Hodgkin's lymphoma and testicular cancer. Adverse reactions include increased susceptibility to infection and neurotoxicity.

Taxanes include the natural product paclitaxel, which was originally isolated from the bark of the Pacific Yew tree. Docetaxel is a semi-synthetic analogue of paclitaxel. Taxanes enhance stability of microtubules inhibiting their breakdown, and so prevent the separation of chromosomes during anaphase and the completion of mitosis. This causes cells to die by apoptosis or return to the resting phase of the cell cycle.[7,8] Paclitaxel is used for ovarian and breast cancer and for Kaposi's sarcoma. Docetaxel is used in the treatment of breast cancer, small cell lung cancer and prostate cancer. Adverse effects include hypersensitivity reactions, bone marrow suppression, peripheral neuropathy, hair loss and cardiac arrhythmias.

Podophyllotoxin is a plant-derived compound primarily obtained from the American mayapple used to produce two cytostatic drugs, etoposide and teniposide. They prevent the replication of DNA during the S phase by inhibition of topoisomerase II. This results in double strand breaks and cell death due to apoptosis.[9] They are mainly used in small cell lung cancer and testicular cancer and teniposide is also used in acute childhood leukaemias. Adverse effects include nausea and vomiting, hair loss and bone marrow suppression.

Drugs that regulate hormonal control of tumours

Tumours deriving from tissues that are normally under the control of steroid hormones may be sensitive to hormone antagonists, i.e. drugs that block the normal action of the natural hormone. These drugs are less toxic than other chemotherapy drugs, although they still have appreciable side-effects. Normally, steroid hormones bind to cytoplasmic receptors. This results in their transfer to the nucleus where they bind to specific factors that control transcription, resulting in a change to protein production and so elicit an effect on the cell. Glucocorticoids naturally suppress cell division in lymphocytes and as such, their value in cancer therapy is mainly in the treatment of lymphomas and leukaemias. Examples are dexamethasone and prednisone.

Antioestrogen drugs are used to treat tumours which are dependent on oestrogen for their growth. These drugs block oestrogen receptors and so interfere with growth stimulation pathways. One such drug, Tamoxifen, is widely used for breast cancer.[10,11] Aromatase inhibitors block the enzyme aromatase which converts adrenal androgen to oestradiol. Anastrozole and letrozole are examples of this group of drugs which are used in the treatment of postmenopausal women with breast and ovarian cancer.

The anti-androgen bicalutamide is an effective drug which is used in the treatment of locally advanced prostate cancer. It prevents activation of the androgen receptor by binding to it and so reduces upregulation of androgen responsive genes.[12] Another option is luteinising hormone-releasing hormone agonists such as goserelin acetate, which is used to suppress production of the sex hormones (testosterone and oestrogen), particularly in the treatment of breast and prostate cancer. Goserelin acetate stimulates the production of the sex hormones testosterone and oestrogen in a non-physiological manner. This causes the disruption of the endogenous hormonal feedback systems, resulting in the downregulation of testosterone and oestrogen production.[13]

Drugs specific for the tumour microenvironment

In order for tumour cells to survive, they need oxygen and nutrients. An initial clone of aberrant cells cannot grow beyond about 200–400 microns unless it can stimulate the development of a blood supply. Dividing endothelial cells are rare in adults, however within the tumour microenvironment, there is an increased ability to stimulate the growth of endothelial cells and therefore new blood vessels (angiogenesis) into the tumour. The capillaries formed are leaky and subject to vascular collapse which leads to areas low in oxygen (hypoxia), a feature only found in tumours and not in healthy tissue. Various drugs have been developed which target this vascular pattern within tumours, many of which are monoclonal antibodies and so are described under molecular targeting drugs within this chapter.[14]

Drugs that target tumour vasculature

Members of the combretastatin family possess varying abilities in causing disruption to the blood vessels in tumours. Combretastatin binds to tubulin inhibiting polymerisation and so prevents cancer cells from producing microtubules.

Microtubules are essential to cytoskeleton production, intercellular movement and formation of the mitotic spindle used in chromosome segregation and cellular division. The anti-cancer activity from this drug results from a change in shape in vasculature endothelial cells which balloon in shape resulting in necrosis of the tumour core as the delivery of oxygen and nutrients by the blood vessels is reduced. The tumour edge is supported by normal vasculature and remains mainly unaffected, therefore these drugs are more effective in combination with other chemotherapy drugs.[15]

Bioreductive drugs

Tirapazamine is an experimental bioreductive drug that is activated by reductase enzymes to a toxic radical only under hypoxic conditions. Thus, tirapazamine is activated to its toxic form preferentially in the hypoxic areas of solid tumours which makes it tumour specific. Cells in these regions are resistant to killing by radiotherapy, as oxygen is required for radiation to induce cell death. In addition, most anticancer drugs are not effective in hypoxic regions, as they require the cell to be undergoing cell division to have an effect, whereas hypoxic cells are at rest.[16] Thus, the combination of tirapazamine with conventional anticancer treatments is particularly effective. Conventional drugs will attack the dividing cells within the tumour, while tirapazamine activates within the hypoxic cells forming reactive radicals which cause breaks to DNA strands resulting in cell death.[17] Banoxantrone is another example of a bioreductive drug which is in clinical trials.[18,19] This drug has a strong affinity to DNA and also acts as a topoisomerase II inhibitor, therefore once bound to DNA this drug will inhibit DNA unwinding when the cell attempts to replicate, causing DNA strand breaks and cell death. These drugs have limited systemic toxicity; however, although several drugs have entered clinical trials, none have been licensed.

Molecular targeting drugs

Targeted cancer therapies are drugs or other substances that block the growth and spread of cancer by interfering with specific molecules involved in tumour growth and progression. By focusing on molecular and cellular changes that are specific to cancer, targeted cancer therapies may be more effective than other types of chemotherapy and less harmful to normal cells. Many of these therapies focus on proteins that are involved in cell signalling pathways which form a complex communication system that governs basic cellular functions. Most targeted therapies are either small-molecule drugs or monoclonal antibodies.

Monoclonal antibodies

Drugs have been developed which block growth factor receptors on the cell surface. Growth factors are usually proteins or hormones which regulate cellular processes such as promoting cell differentiation and maturation. They do so by binding to a receptor on the surface of a target cell. A monoclonal antibody will therefore block these receptors and inhibit the action of the growth factors. These antibodies can promote apoptosis or inhibit cell growth by binding to their target.

Vascular endothelial growth factor inhibitors such as Avastin slow the growth and development of tumours by inhibiting the growth of blood vessels within the tumour, starving the tumour of oxygen and reducing tumour growth. However, clinical trials have shown that they do not seem to significantly increase the survival time for most cancer patients and therefore are generally used in combination with more traditional anti-cancer chemotherapies.[20,21]

The human epidermal growth factor receptors (HER receptors) are proteins that are embedded in the cell membrane that regulate cell growth, survival, adhesion, migration and differentiation functions. In some cancers, notably some breast cancers, HER2 is over-expressed, and, among other effects, causes breast cells to reproduce uncontrollably. Trastuzumab (Herceptin) is a monoclonal antibody which targets HER2 overexpression by attaching to HER2 receptors and blocking HER2 growth response.

Monoclonal antibodies have been developed which cause lysis of B lymphocytes. Examples are rituximab and alemtuzumab. These drugs attach to a protein on B lymphocytes which is involved in activation and growth of the lymphocyte cell. These drugs are used for the treatment of leukaemia. The most serious adverse effect is known as cytokine release syndrome, which includes fever, nausea and allergic reactions such as rashes, itching and bronchospasm.

Small molecule inhibitors

Some tumours express/over-express specific proteins, which allow for targeting. Tumours vary in their gene expression and so only sub-populations will be sensitive to this targeting. Imatinib, used for the treatment of chronic myeloid leukaemia and for gastrointestinal stromal tumours, is the first member of this new class of agents that act by specifically inhibiting a certain enzyme that is characteristic of a particular cancer cell, rather than non-specifically inhibiting and killing all rapidly dividing cells. This targeted therapy modalities acts through tyrosine kinase inhibition. Protein kinases are enzymes which phosphorylate (add a phosphate to) proteins and by doing so, regulate the activity of these proteins. They are involved in the control of cell division. Protein kinases can become mutated and cause unregulated growth and division of the cell allowing development of a tumour. Protein kinase inhibitors, such as imatinib, inhibit the protein and so reduce the uncontrolled growth.

Interferons

Interferons are cell signalling proteins involved in the immune system. They have potent effects on cellular proliferation. They can be used as a treatment for leukaemia and solid tumours. Their effect on cancer cells is thought to be due to inhibition of cellular growth, induction of apoptosis and recruitment of immune cells. Adverse effects include flu-like symptoms, nausea, thyroid disfunction and elevation of liver enzymes.

CHEMOTHERAPY ADMINISTRATION

Administering the correct dose of chemotherapy is essential. If the dose is too low, the drug will not be effective against the tumour, whereas, at excessive doses, there will be increased toxicity to the patient. The dose is normally adjusted for the patient's body surface area, a measure that correlates with blood volume. The BSA is usually calculated with a mathematical formula using a patient's weight and height. Most chemotherapy is delivered intravenously, although a number of drugs can be administered orally (e.g. melphalan, busulfan, capecitabine).

Depending on the patient, the cancer, the stage of cancer, the type of chemotherapy and the dosage, intravenous chemotherapy may be given on either an inpatient or an outpatient basis. For continuous, frequent or prolonged intravenous chemotherapy administration, various systems may be surgically inserted into the vasculature to maintain access such as the Hickman line or the peripherally inserted central (PICC) line. These have a lower infection risk, and remove the need for repeated insertion of peripheral cannulae.

ADVERSE EFFECTS OF CANCER CHEMOTHERAPY

Adverse effects of chemotherapy drugs are the main limitation to the dose of drug which can be delivered to cancer patients. In some cases, patients have to withdraw from drug therapy due to the adverse effects suffered. Chemotherapy drugs have a range of side-effects that depend on the type of medications used. The most common medications mainly affect the fast-dividing cells of the body, such as blood cells and the cells lining the mouth, stomach and intestines.

Most chemotherapy drugs cause myelosuppression, which is reduction in the production of blood cells due to their effects on the bone marrow. This leads to a decrease in the number of white blood cells, red blood cells and platelets. Granulocyte colony-stimulating factor (G-CSF) and granulocyte-macrophage colony-stimulating factor (GM-CSF) are cytokines that function as white blood cell growth factors which therefore stimulate stem cells to produce granulocytes (neutrophils, eosinophils and basophils) and monocytes. They can be used to stimulate the production of white blood cells following chemotherapy, allowing higher-intensity treatment regimens. Anaemia and thrombocytopenia, when they occur, can be treated with a blood transfusion. Treatments for anaemia also include hormones to boost blood production (erythropoietin) and iron supplements. This will also alleviate the symptoms of fatigue, which often accompanies anaemia. The reduction in the number of platelets in the blood can result in bruises and bleeding. Extremely low platelet counts may be temporarily boosted through platelet transfusions. In severe myelosuppression, a bone marrow cell transplant may be necessary.

Depression of the immune system may occur due to the reduction in white blood cells, which can result in potentially fatal infections. Patients often suffer from infections due to naturally occurring microorganisms in their own gastrointestinal tract and skin, which may result in systemic infections, such as sepsis or as localised infections, such as herpes simplex or shingles.

Nausea and vomiting are common side-effects of chemotherapeutic medications. This can also produce diarrhoea or constipation. Malnutrition and dehydration can result when the patient does not eat or drink enough, or when the patient vomits frequently resulting in weight loss. Patients are advised to eat frequent small meals and drink clear liquids or ginger tea. This is a temporary effect, and frequently resolves within a week of finishing treatment. The effect on the GI tract can be so severe that it can compromise patient compliance with the drug regime. However, these side-effects can be reduced or eliminated with antiemetic drugs.

A class of drugs called 5-HT$_3$ antagonists are the most effective antiemetics in the management of nausea and vomiting in patients with cancer. These drugs block serotonin receptors in the central nervous system and gastrointestinal tract that cause nausea and vomiting. Approved 5-HT$_3$ inhibitors include dolasetron, granisetron, and ondansetron.

The 5-HT$_3$ inhibitor, palonosetron, also prevents delayed nausea and vomiting, which occurs during the 2–5 days after treatment. These drugs are available by injection, as orally disintegrating tablets or as transdermal patches. However, they can also cause constipation, diarrhea, dry mouth and fatigue.[22]

Hair loss due to destruction of the cells within the hair follicles is another temporary side-effect of chemotherapy. Psychological support is provided to patients as are wigs; however, hair usually starts growing back a few weeks after the last treatment.

In a small proportion of patients, development of second primary tumour can develop after successful chemotherapy or radiotherapy. This may be due to damage to the DNA within other cell types as a result of treatment, which then have the potential to divide and form tumours. The most common neoplasm is acute myeloid leukaemia.

Some types of chemotherapy are gonadotoxic and so may cause infertility.[23] Chemotherapies with high risk include procarbazine and other alkylating drugs such as cyclophosphamide, ifosfamide, busulfan, melphalan, chlorambucil and chlormethine. It is possible for younger patients to cryopreserve semen, ovarian tissue, oocytes or embryos before chemotherapy treatment.

Other common side-effects include red skin (erythema), dry skin, damaged fingernails, a dry mouth, water retention and pain. Damage to specific organs such as cardiotoxicity, hepatotoxicity, nephrotoxicity may also occur with some drugs.

RESISTANCE TO CANCER CHEMOTHERAPY

Cancer cells may develop ways of avoiding the effects of chemotherapy. Drug resistance can be acquired due to adaptation to continued exposure or by mutation of the cell. A drug may have difficulty reaching the tumour cells due to variation in vasculature or fluid pressure within the tumour. Tumour cells also have the ability to develop pumps which are membrane bound proteins that can move the drug out of the cell or they can metabolise the drug within the cell to make the drug inactive. Mutations may occur in genes, such as the P53 gene. As previously described, this gene allows apoptosis to occur, therefore mutations within this gene will lead to a decrease in tumour cell death in response to chemotherapy. Tumours may also over-express genes, which suppress apoptosis or for DNA repair, which will also lead to resistance to some chemotherapy drugs. Mutations may occur at the binding sites for drugs, which will inhibit the effect of the drug. Attempts to overcome resistance mainly involve the use of combination drug therapy using different classes of drugs with minimally overlapping toxicities to allow maximal dosages.[24]

KEY POINTS

- Cancer occurs when cells mutate and divide uncontrollably
- Cancer chemotherapy aims to interfere with cell division within tumour cells, however this leads to toxicity to normal cells while under cell division such as those in the bone marrow, hair follicles and GI tract
- Cancer chemotherapy is limited by a lack of specificity and as a result of the toxicity to normal tissues suboptimal doses of chemotherapy are often given
- Treatment has improved with the introduction of antiemetic drugs and GM-CSF which allow patients to tolerate a higher dose of chemotherapy drug
- The introduction of treatments which selectively target cancer cells, such as monoclonal antibodies, will improve the therapeutic outcomes and limit toxicity to the patients
- Targeted therapies show great promise in the development of new treatments for cancer

Chapter | 13 |

Radiotherapy-related treatment reactions

Bridget Mary Porritt, Terri Gilleece

INTRODUCTION

Radiotherapy, in terms of planning, delivery and verification has evolved dramatically over the last 100 years. From the days of the pioneering work of Marie Curie with Radium in the 1900s, to development of Cobalt-60 units through to the medical Linear Accelerator in the 1940s, the evolution in equipment has facilitated dramatic improvements in delivery techniques and verification. This has enabled the maximising of dose to tumour tissue and minimising of dose to normal tissue and sensitive structures.

This chapter explores the concept of acute and late radiotherapy-related side-effects. Despite every effort being made to minimise toxicity to normal tissue, inevitably the toxic effects of radiotherapy will present themselves in the form of side-effects. These can be acute or long lasting and if not managed effectively, can result in treatment gaps, which can have negative effects on overall treatment outcome and debilitating effects on long-term quality of life.

The term radiotherapy encompasses a wide range of techniques from external beam, which may include: intensity modulated radiotherapy (IMRT), hyper-fractionated, hypo-fractionated, adjuvant, neo-adjuvant, stereotactic, image guided to intra-cavity or brachytherapy. Whether treatment is given with a palliative or radical intent will impact upon the effects expected. It is important that these be distinguished, as both have individual associated side-effects. External beam radiotherapy can also be given alone or in combination with chemotherapy and as such, patients may experience radiotherapy-related effects but also chemotherapy effects dependent on the agent(s) used.

MEASUREMENT OF RADIOTHERAPY SIDE-EFFECTS

How in fact do we measure these effects? There is a vast range of toxicity tools available which can be used objectively by the patient to score the physical symptoms they are experiencing or subjectively by members of the healthcare professions, who assign a score to the symptoms reported by a patient to them. There are some differences interprofessionally in interpretation of side-effects. Some professionals will prefer to record symptoms descriptively in free text, others will prefer to quantify and assign a score. Such discrepancies may lead to inconsistencies in toxicity data. Considering that such data may be discussed with a patient to inform them of the potential risk of developing certain effects with a certain treatment method; it is important that further work be done to improve and standardise the way in which toxicity is recorded. The use of toxicity tools should not be restricted to research activity but used daily as routine practice.

But what does this score mean? Will a treating team follow a care pathway when an RTOG score of 2 for bowel symptoms is reported, for example? Will a tried and tested management approach be adopted in a consistent manner throughout a department? In my experience, I would be inclined to say that such scripted management is rare and certainly not available for all acute effects. Management can differ from centre to centre and vary within from healthcare professional to healthcare professional.

Practitioners are ideally placed to assess and record toxicity and thus contribute to the evolution of evidence-based management. This concept of role extension is not something new. For many years now, radiotherapy practitioners have been practising outside what is considered the normal remit of a radiotherapy practitioner. In fact, radiotherapy practitioners have historically undertaken regular review of patients having radiotherapy treatment from the perspective of ensuring fitness to continue with a prescribed course.

As the workload of oncologists has increased, the weekly review of the radiotherapy patient has been recognised as an area where radiotherapy practitioners could step in and take on this responsibility. Such change needs to be supported clinically and academically, ensuring practitioners are armed with appropriate knowledge and skills. There is also the consideration of how other professions view responsibility being shifted away from them. We are by no means suggesting that a radiotherapy practitioner take full responsibility for management of radiotherapy induced side-effects but that they are able to fully engage with the multidisciplinary team and effectively contribute to the monitoring and management of a patient. As workloads continue to increase, surely the sharing of responsibility and thus knowledge and experience can only be a positive for both professions and patients?

THE CONCEPT OF 'SURVIVORSHIP' AND LATE EFFECTS

As healthcare professionals, we strive for what is best for the patient. As cancer patients become cancer survivors and survival statistics improve, it becomes all the more important to ensure that late effects are managed effectively. The fact that we describe cancer patients now as cancer survivors suggests a change in our thinking. Perhaps now, we acknowledge our responsibility in caring for a patient/survivor beyond the routine follow-up term. It is important that the individual and collective voices of patients affected by their treatment are heard. For many years now, organisations such as Radiotherapy Action Group Exposure (RAGE) have fought to publicise late effects of radiotherapy treatment by campaigning for national standards and raising awareness of radiation injuries. Much work has been undertaken by The Macmillan Late Effects Group working with expert patients, carers and professionals who want to make a difference. Combined with the influence of high profile cases of people damaged by radiotherapy, this helped to put

'survivorship' on the agenda. The Macmillan Health and Well Being Survey (2008) highlighted the impact of cancer treatment and the need for long-term support. Results showed: 40% of survivors were unaware of long-term side-effects; 78% have experienced physical health problems in the last 12 months; 40% with emotional problems have not sought help and 71% of those who finished treatment 10 years ago have experienced physical health problems in the last 12 months.

The radiotherapy community are all too aware of the importance of managing symptoms in order to give patients the best quality of life possible. The National Cancer Survivorship Initiative (NCSI) is a partnership between the Department of Health and Macmillan Cancer Support and is supported by NHS Improvement. The aim of the NCSI is, by 2012, to have taken the necessary steps to ensure that those living with and beyond cancer get the care and support they need to lead as healthy and active a life as possible, for as long as possible.

It is essential that radiotherapy patients are prepared for 'life after treatment'. As healthcare professionals, it is our duty to educate ourselves and peers on the subject of late effects. We must be able to recognise when there is a problem and know the appropriate action to take.

AN OVERVIEW OF RADIOBIOLOGY FOR RADIOTHERAPY

Radiotherapy – what does it mean? It is basically the application of ionising radiation to treat malignant disease with either a palliative (to relieve symptoms) or radical (to cure) intent.

What do we mean by ionising radiation? Ionising radiation is radiation having sufficient energy to cause ionisation. In very basic terms, ionisation is the removal of electron(s) from an atom. Photons (X-rays) are most commonly used for radiotherapy. Electrons are also used for the treatment of more superficial tumours. The use of protons, neutrons (heavy ion particle therapy) is rare in the UK, as there is currently only one radiotherapy centre (Clatterbrideg Cancer Centre NHS Foundation Trust) providing such treatment. However, cutting edge proton facilities are to be located at the Christie Hospital NHS Foundation Trust Hospital in Manchester and University College London Hospitals NHS Trust, reaching full capacity by 2017.

A photon is a discrete bundle (or quantum) of electromagnetic energy. Electromagnetic waves are cyclical fluctuations of magnetic and electric fields. The atom is said to be ionised when an electron is completely removed. When an electron moves from one orbit to another, it is said to be in an excited state. These free electrons can then go on to interact with other atoms close by causing in effect, a kind of chain reaction.

Effects of ionising radiation on the cell

To understand how the body is affected by radiation, we must go back to the workings of the cell. Cells are organised into structural and functional units. A membrane separates the inside from the external environment. Inside are a number of different organelles with specific functions. The genetic material in the form of DNA is held within the nucleus. The cell cycle describes the way in which a cell grows and a cell's sensitivity to radiation depends upon which phase of the cycle the cell is in. The most sensitive phase is the mitotic phase.

Cancer in a way, arises as a result of the disruption of cellular balance. A population of cancer cells grow outside the restrictions and controls of a normal cell cycle.

Cell death is achieved by the production of irrevocable damage to DNA. The type of damage achieved when ionising radiation hits tissue can be put into three categories:

1. Lethal damage – is irreversible and leads to cell death
2. Sub-lethal – this can be repaired unless additional sub-lethal damage is added
3. Potentially lethal – this can be modified by environmental changes.

Once hit by ionising radiation, the cells will respond to DNA damage by either DNA repair mechanisms or cell cycle regulation. It is not just damage to the nucleus that can lead to cell death, but also damage to the cytoplasm and cellular membrane. The repair mechanisms are controlled by the cell cycle checkpoints. After the cell has recognised it has been damaged, it has to make the decision of whether to give in and commit suicide via apoptosis, or to repair the damage.

- DNA repairs – cell proliferates
- DNA is mis-repaired – cell mutates
- DNA cannot be repaired – cell dies.

The repair of damage between fractions (radiotherapy treatments) is extremely useful as normal tissues and tumours often differ in their ability to repair any damage incurred.

In an ideal world, we would like to give a dose of this ionising radiation without complication, in essence kill the tumour cells and cause no other harm. However, the complicated interaction processes occurring when tissue interacts with ionising radiation, means this is tragically impossible.

In order to initiate tumour cell death, a sufficient dose of ionising radiation must be given. What dose to give has been studied for many years and our understanding is based on the radiobiological effectiveness model. The model is used today to predict what dose is needed to maximise tumour cell kill and minimise normal tissue damage.

Radiobiological effectiveness (RBE) and tumour cure probability (TCP)

By examining cells under laboratory conditions, you can measure the proportion of cells of a particular type that survive different doses of radiation. From this, a radiobiological effective dose can be calculated. This provides the radiotherapy treatment team with essential information. The knowledge of what dose it takes to kill a tumour is essential – however of equal importance, is the knowledge of what dose will kill a normal cell.

Tumour control probability curves are plots of cure rate versus dose. Curves are typically sigmoid in shape, with minimal chance of cure at low doses, then a rapid rise in cure rate once a particular dose is achieved, which slows as dose increases further. The rate of normal tissue complications follows a similar curve to tumour control, ideally shifted to the right (fewer complications than tumour control). The ratio of tumour control to normal tissue complications is the *therapeutic index* or *therapeutic ratio*.

Oxygen effect

Cells irradiated in the absence of oxygen are more resistant to radiation. *Why?* The oxygen molecules react with free radicals to produce chemically unrepairable peroxy radicals. ($R\bullet + O_2 = R\bullet O_2$) – Oxygenated cells suffer more DNA damage.

The degree of sensitisation by oxygen can be quoted as an oxygen enhancement ratio (OER). OER = ratio of doses needed to produce a given biological effect in the presence or absence of oxygen.

Tumour hypoxia is accepted as a cause of radiotherapy failure. Over the years, work with hypoxic manipulation, particularly in bladder cancer, has demonstrated promising results. The BCON (bladder carbogen nicotinamide) study compared radical radiotherapy with and without carbogen and nicotinamide. The carbogen used was a mixture of 98% oxygen and 2% carbon dioxide. Nicotinamide is the amide of nicotinic acid (vitamin B_3/niacin); it acts as a chemo- and radio-sensitising agent by enhancing tumour blood flow, thus reducing tumour hypoxia. The study findings were that differences in overall survival, risk of death and local relapse were significantly in favour of the radiotherapy + carbogen and nicotinamide. This represents a new treatment option, however future work needs to be done to further improve outcome for bladder cancer by investigating this approach in conjunction with radiosenitiser agents.

Dose and fractionation

Some frequent questions asked by patients are:

- 'Why am I having a different number of treatments to X in the waiting room?'
- 'Why can't I have my treatment at weekends?'

Fractionated radiotherapy refers to radiotherapy treatment given in small equal doses (like a course of antibiotics). The breaking up of an overall dose enables higher doses to be given safely. It also takes advantage of the inherent differences between tumour and normal cells response to and recovery from a dose of ionising radiation.

The 4 Rs of radiobiology describe the factors modifying such response:

1. **Repair** of radiation induced damage within cells
2. **Repopulation** of irradiated area by surviving cells
3. **Redistribution** of cells within the cell cycle
4. **Reoxygenation** of the tumour

Using these principles, we can enhance the radiation effects on rapidly dividing tumour cells in comparison to more slowly dividing normal tissues. The outcome of treatment will depend on the dose delivered. This has led to the classical radiation schedule delivering one fraction per day (1.8–2 Gy per fraction), 5 days over 5–7 weeks.

The majority of treatment regimes consist of one daily radiotherapy treatment on weekdays only. Thus allowing a 2-day recovery period over the weekend, however, there are a number of non-standard radiotherapy regimes in use:

- Accelerated radiotherapy – is when conventional fraction sizes and overall dose is given but treating more often, e.g. twice daily with a number of hours in between each treatment
- Hyper-fractionation – reduced dose per fraction – this should result in reduction in induced late effects
- Continuous hyper-fractionated accelerated radiotherapy (CHART).

Effects on normal cells

Some normal cells will die within a short space of time after a dose of ionising radiation; one such example being the lymphocyte. In fact, some studies suggest that the lymphocyte count is affected for years after radiation therapy. The decrease in red blood cells is not as large, as red cell production (erythropoiesis) will compensate. Normal tissue, although affected by treatment in the same way, has the ability to recover. Stem cells replace the cells that are lost. With the effect that radiation has on peripheral blood counts, it is essential that patients receiving long courses of radiotherapy have a weekly blood count that is assessed by the treating team as part of the on-treatment review process.

Radiation-induced side-effects

Different cells are affected at different rates by radiation. Some damage will show itself during a course of radiotherapy and up to 6 weeks post-treatment. Such an effect is classed as an *acute* effect. Acute effects are related to the total dose given and length of time taken to give it. While others may present after 6 weeks post-radiotherapy and years later in some cases, such an effect is classed as a *late* effect. Late effects are very dependent on the dose per fraction. It is important to note that both acute and late effects can be present in the same tissue.

Sensitivity

Increased knowledge of the tumour microenvironment has led to dramatic changes in radiotherapy treatment delivery. The ability to specifically target a tumour with radiotherapy and no normal tissue, despite the advances in treatment technique is impossible. There is always a necessary volume of normal tissue included within the treatment volume. Every effort is made in terms of planning, delivery and verification to ensure that the correct dose is given accurately. This correct dose has to take into account what is an effective dose to achieve tumour cell kill and what is the tolerance of surrounding normal tissue. Encompassed within the treatment volume, we have to be aware of any sensitive structures. The term sensitive structures, critical structures and organs at risk are somewhat interchangeable.

Radiotherapy treatment regimes are evidence-based and the majority of patients experience the anticipated acute and late effects. However, there is a minority who seem to develop more severe effects early on in treatment than anticipated. In many ways, it would be advantageous to identify such patients prior to treatment being given. This leads us to the idea of individualised radiotherapy treatment. If it is known that a patient has a certain genetic make-up that only enables them to tolerate a lower dose of radiation, then those patients' management needs to take account of this, either by dose adjustment, early intervention to manage symptoms and careful consideration of any concurrent chemotherapy agents.

Radioprotectants

Agents that protect a patient from the effect of radiotherapy are known as 'radioprotectants'. Given prophylactically prior to treatment commencing, they can benefit the patient by reducing the severity of radiotherapy-induced side-effects.

A useful agent in head and neck radiotherapy is Amifostine. It is used therapeutically to reduce the incidence of neutropenia-related fever and infection induced by DNA-binding chemotherapeutic agents, including alkylating agents (e.g. cyclophosphamide) and platinum-containing agents (e.g. cisplatin). It is also used to decrease the cumulative nephrotoxicity associated with platinum-containing agents. Amifostine is also indicated to reduce the incidence of xerostomia in patients undergoing radiotherapy for head and neck cancer.

Radiosensitising agents

Chemotherapeutic agents have been developed that preferentially sensitise a tumour cell to the effects of ionising radiation. The agents used can increase normal tissue damage and radiotherapy related side-effects. However, the combination of chemotherapy agents and radiotherapy may overcome radioresistance and sensitise tumour cells allowing for improvements in treatment outcomes. Work continues in various tumour sites to establish effective chemo-radiotherapy protocols.

Example agents

Antimetabolites: these agents generate intracellular metabolites that interfere with nucleic acid synthesis and DNA replication. 5-Flurouracil (5FU) is an antimetabolite and works by inhibiting thymidylate synthase, which is the rate limiting enzyme in pyrimidine nucleotide synthesis. It needs to be given as a continuous i.v. infusion during a course of radiotherapy to achieve optimum radiosensitisation.

There is now a modern alternative to i.v. 5-Flurouracil – an oral pro-drug of 5FU called Capecitabine. This drug offers the patient an alternative to i.v. infusion, allowing patients to be treated on an outpatient basis.

Capecitabine is broken down in three stages in the liver and dihydropyrimidine (DPD) is a key enzyme in the metabolic catabolism. It is possible for a patient to be deficient in DPD which can have negative effects on their ability to tolerate Capecitabine. A link between deficiency in DPD activity and severe toxicity in response to 5FU treatment has been studied for many years.

ACUTE AND LATE EFFECTS OF EXTERNAL BEAM RADIOTHERAPY (EBRT)

The main aim of radiotherapy is to give a tumoricidal dose with minimum damage to surrounding normal tissue. It is impossible to deliver a dose of radiation without having some effect on normal tissue. From previous radiobiological studies, the tolerance doses for all tissues have been calculated and when planning treatment, the team must abide by these doses. In spite of this, it is accepted that radiotherapy treatment will cause a number of acute and late effects, the likelihood of which is dependent on the patient's individual radiosensitivity.

As more and more patients become cancer survivors, it is important to minimise the risk of long-term radiotherapy-induced side-effects. Early symptom reporting and recognition is essential in order to provide optimum intervention and management. Here, the radiotherapy practitioners come into their own by recognising, reporting, offering advice and managing treatment-induced side-effects.

Some practitioners have chosen to extend their role and are now able to prescribe under departmental patient group directives (PGDs). This enables the patients to be managed by a practitioner-led service, promoting efficacy and efficiency. Care of the patient should always be a team approach.

Some factors affecting toxicity:

- Total daily dose
- Total delivered dose
- Fractionation schedule
- Volume of organ at risk (OAR)/sensitive structure treated
- Radiation technique
- Beam energy and type (photons or electrons)
- Dose distribution
- Individual factors – skin type, prior treatment, i.e. chemotherapy, surgery.

The risk of developing a complication post-radiotherapy treatment has been calculated and tables of tolerance doses are available to use as reference. Most clinical oncologists will adopt a cautious approach when considering the prescribed dose to an organ at risk. Over the years the observation of manifestation of late effects has led to development of fractionation schedules. Work done has established normal tissue tolerance doses to therapeutic irradiation. Work done in clinical trials and continued adherence to ICRU 50 and 62 play an important role in increasing standardisation of practice across radiotherapy centres.

- TD 5/5 = the tolerance dose for the probability of a 5% complication rate within 5 years
- TD 50/5 = the tolerance dose for the probability of a 50% complication rate within 5 years
- NTC = normal tissue complication rate.

TOXICITY SCORING TOOLS

Assessment of toxicity is an essential part of evaluating the biological effect of treatment and enables the setting of dose limits for cancer treatments. It was back in the 1970s that the World Health Organization (WHO) introduced its advice for reporting results of treatment and specifically addressed the reporting of side-effects experienced. In the same decade, the Radiation Oncology Group (RTOG) and European Organisation for Research and Treatment (EORTC) combined to produce a tool covering the late effects of radiotherapy treatment.

A vast array of tools is available for the recording of toxicity experienced by a patient receiving radiotherapy. The majority of departments will now use the Common Toxicity Criteria (CTC), developed by the National Cancer Institute, as this tool is used in research trials and provides extensive descriptions covering all major anatomical sites. However, there is little consistency between departments across the UK; in fact there is little consistency among members of the multidisciplinary team in the same department.

The assessment of a patient should take a broad and holistic approach, not just looking at physical symptoms reported but also the psychological and emotional wellbeing of the patient. It is therefore the duty of all healthcare professionals to ensure that appropriate assessment tools are utilised and outcome documented. Such documentation can then go on to inform future practice.

MANAGEMENT OF RADIOTHERAPY-INDUCED SIDE-EFFECTS

Once a patient's symptoms have been acknowledged and assigned a score, how we then go on to manage them is of paramount importance. If managed poorly, a patient may have to miss some treatment, which may have serious consequences on overall outcome and cause undue emotional distress. A patient must be managed effectively, so as to enable them to complete a course of treatment with minimum effect on their quality of life. Support of the radiotherapy patient, irrespective of treatment site, technique and approach, is essential. Such support will be provided by the whole multidisciplinary team and in particular, by the treating team of radiotherapy practitioners.

The team involved in the daily delivery of radiotherapy are best placed to initially form an effective patient–practitioner relationship. Through daily interactions, they can establish whether the patient is experiencing treatment-related side-effects. With their oncology and radiotherapy knowledge, they can advise on appropriate skin care, dietary and lifestyle changes, correct timing and doses of medication. Moreover, as effective members of the multidisciplinary team they are aware of the limits of their scope of practice and able to refer on to appropriate members of the team.

Departments will vary in the management of induced side-effects. Their practice may be based on in-house research evidence or evidence from the wider research community. Oncologists in the same centre may adopt slightly different approaches in the management of a skin reaction, for example. It is essential that treating teams collaborate to produce coherent consistent management guidance based on the best available evidence. Again it is only by accurate documentation of side-effects experienced and management approaches adopted that evidence can be gathered to inform and improve future practice.

SOME EXAMPLES OF EXTERNAL BEAM RADIOTHERAPY-INDUCED REACTIONS

Skin reactions

Radiation erythema (skin reddening) is an inevitable deterministic effect of radiotherapy, given the large absorbed radiation doses required to treat tumours. Radiotherapy techniques aim to deliver penetrative high energy radiations which are 'skin sparing' and deliver most ionisation at depth rather than superficially within the body. The proliferative cell division within the epidermis renders it vulnerable to radiation but also provides it with a good capacity to recover. Skin effects include erythema as well as dry desquamation (itchy flaking skin) and moist desquamation (blistering and falling off of skin). These effects may occur in combination. Reactions tend to occur by about 2 weeks following the start of a course of radical radiotherapy but show strong recovery a month after the close of treatment. Areas where skin folds occur, such as the groin and axilla, are especially vulnerable to radiation-induced skin reactions. Although radiotherapy dose and technique are important, patient factors such as age, body habitus and general health status also seem to affect the severity of skin reactions, which may vary between patients receiving the same treatment regime. Procedures for the monitoring and measurement of skin reactions are diverse and may include recording of surface area of reaction, visual or technical assessment of severity and use of the patient's own perception of symptoms.

The recommended management of skin reactions varies between clinical centres but can usefully include mild washing, avoidance of frictional injury, use of moisturising cream, complementary therapies and avoidance of irritants such as wet-shaving or cosmetic products. Care of areas of moist desquamation must take account of the need to provide wound protection while avoiding further skin injury and permitting regular monitoring. Hydrocolloid or alginate dressings, which appear to provide a moist environment conducive to wound-healing, have been recommended by many authorities but practices are inconsistent.

Gastrointestinal reactions

The mucosal cells within the gastrointestinal tract are rapidly dividing and vulnerable to radiation effects. Their irradiation can result in acute or long-term symptoms such as increased bowel frequency, diarrhoea, nausea, vomiting and difficulty during defecation. Radiation proctitis may result in straining, small but frequent stools and blood staining. Altered absorption may result in fluid, electrolyte and nutritional deficits which will complicate treatment plans and further reduce health. Bowel problems not only render life even more unpleasant for radiotherapy patients but may be under-reported, due to feelings of embarrassment. Thus, good open communication with patients is vital as it will encourage them to log and discuss their symptoms.

Nausea and vomiting may be countered to some extent with antiemetic agents such as 5-hydroxytryptamine antagonists, but this practice is not universal. At-risk patients (such as those receiving total body irradiation, large treatment volumes or single palliative fractions) may be offered prophylactic antiemetics pre-treatment. Some authorities have advocated the use of mind–body therapies for enhancing relaxation and feelings of wellbeing during radiotherapy treatment. Dietary control of diarrhoea, using reduced fibre intake or 'elemental diets' (food divided into its constituent elements) has been advocated but not fully applied in practice. Drug treatments for diarrhoea have been trialled but may result in constipation and other side-effects.

Respiratory reactions

There are a number of factors which may cause patients to find it 'difficult to breathe' during a course of radiotherapy treatment. Fear of the process and feelings of claustrophobia within radiotherapy planning and treatment can lead to distress and 'panicky' breathing patterns. This again highlights how radiotherapy practitioners and other staff can usefully provide vital comfort, reassurance and information during the whole treatment process.

Radiotherapy to the upper airways can result in inflammation and swelling, which will constrict breathing. Radiation applied to the lungs can cause inflammation, swelling, fibrosis and fluid production; a set of outcomes termed radiation pneumonitis. These outcomes cause additional distress to cancer patients and some of the reactive lung changes may be permanent.

Psychological factors affecting breathing may be countered by radiotherapy staff using reassurance and relaxation techniques. Upper airways radiotherapy may necessitate tracheostomy in order to maintain the airway. Advice on posture and feeding mechanisms may be useful to prevent sensations of panic and choking caused by narrowing of the pharynx. Lung reactions may be countered to some extent by corticosteroids and antibiotics.

BRACHYTHERAPY REACTIONS

Brachytherapy is the treatment of disease using discrete sealed radioactive sources. It originated in 1901 with the use of Radium-226 and is therefore one of the oldest forms of radiotherapy. Over the years, more suitable radiation sources have been employed because Radium-226 has a complicated decay scheme with some high energy photon emissions and gaseous Radon-222 making radiation protection an issue.

There are advantages and disadvantages to this type of 'close' (brachy)therapy. A high dose can be delivered to the tumour while the surrounding and overlying tissues can be spared some or all of the effects of radiobiological interactions because of the steep dose gradient of the alpha and beta emissions of these sources. This dose distribution therefore reduces the side-effects to the patient. Brachytherapy treatment regimes can vary from a few minutes to 10 days, so compared with external beam radiotherapy

treatments, the schedules are usually preferable for the patient. On the negative side, the sources require insertion within body cavities, implantation into tissues or application to surface tissues (this latter technique has been largely replaced by electron beam treatments). Such techniques, whether permanent or temporary, can be problematic and uncomfortable for the patient.

Brachytherapy is a successful treatment method for a range of conditions.

- Intracavitary implant for pelvic tumours (cervix, body of uterus, vagina), oral cavity, naso-, oro- and hypopharynx
- Intraluminal implants for oesophagus, bronchus, bile ducts, vascular (non-malignant)
- Interstitial implants for prostate, lung, pancreas, brain
- Surface application of eye plaques for intraocular tumours, pinna, skin.

As with all forms of radiation treatments, side-effects are possible and vary according to the type of source, dose, treatment site and time since treatment. The best way to reduce side-effects from brachytherapy is with careful treatment planning techniques and to ensure that applicators and sources are correctly positioned. Bowel and urinary preparation can ensure that adjacent organs are removed from the proximity of high dose targets during pelvic brachytherapy. Metal 'buttons' or plates can be placed in areas to reduce the dose to surrounding tissues.

Acute side-effects

The most obvious side-effects from brachytherapy are pain, swelling and bruising around the site of implant. There will undoubtedly be inflammation, even with intracavitary implants, but this will be increased with intraluminal and interstitial work. The reactions will be obvious if surfaces are visible, e.g. Irridium-192 wire implants in the mouth or breast, but we must remember that the same intensity of reactions occur at all sites. Analgesia is prescribed to overcome this discomfort. If the area is accessible, ice packs can be applied. Pain and swelling should ease rapidly, and implants are usually removed without the aid of anaesthetics.

Late side-effects

Telangiectasia and permanent pigmentation of the skin are among the most common late side-effects. Again, attention should be paid to internal sites, as telangiectasia can result in bleeding around the site. If bleeding does occur, it is usually mild and intermittent, but it can cause considerable distress for the patient who has already had a diagnosis of cancer.

As radioactive sources are being implanted, it is possible that these may induce cancerous growths. This is of particular significance if brachytherapy is being employed for cardiac restenosis, as this is a non-malignant disease. The long-term implications of the use of intravascular brachytherapy are still unclear, as it is a relatively new technique.

The specific side-effects from the most common brachytherapy treatment regimes are discussed below.

Prostate

Brachytherapy for prostate tumours can result in a higher dose to the tumour than that administered during external beam radiotherapy (EBRT), typically 145 Gy to a Planned Target Volume (PTV) of prostate plus 2–3 mm margin compared to 64–74 Gy with EBRT. The organs at risk are the bladder, rectum and neurovascular bundle. The toxicity to these structures during brachytherapy is decreased in comparison to EBRT or surgery, therefore the risk of urinary incontinence and impotence is reduced. The most common side-effect of prostatic brachytherapy is grade 2 urinary symptoms. Table 13.1 lists the possible side-effects and methods of treatment.

Gynaecological malignancies

Cervical, vaginal and endometrial cancers can be treated with combinations of surgery, brachytherapy and/or EBRT, depending on the stage of disease.

Gynaecological brachytherapy reactions are described, but because brachytherapy is frequently given in combination, readers are advised to familiarise themselves with *all* common reactions to pelvic EBRT.

Bowel and rectum

Using metal filters or packing the rectum can reduce the brachytherapy dose to this structure. Some tenesmus, mild rectal bleeding and diarrhoea may occur at the time of treatment but should settle quickly with the help of medication such as loperamide and dietary advice.

Less than 3% will develop obstruction, bleeding, necrosis or fistula as late reactions. If a fistula does develop, it is usually at the site of the anterior rectal wall behind the posterior vaginal fornix. The treatment for proctocolitis is conservative administration of Predsol enemas, progressing to colostomy if other treatments fail.

Careful planning and the use of a rectal probe to give 'real' time dose rate can reduce the possibility of developing rectal complications.

Bladder

Bladder irritation is less likely than bowel side-effects. If it does occur during or immediately after treatment, it is usually mild and increasing fluid intake can relieve the symptoms. Cranberry juice is often suggested as it can alter the acidity of the urine, making it more comfortable for the patient to micturate.

Late bladder side-effects are usually mild and include frequency and telangiectasia. The latter can cause haematuria, which can be treated by diathermy. It is estimated

Table 13.1 Side-effects of prostatic brachytherapy

Site/symptom	Time post-implant	Side-effect	Treatment
Skin/perineum	Immediately	Bruising, pain/tenderness, haematoma (rare)	Cleanse gently Apply ice pack
Urinary	48–72 hours	Haematuria	Encourage oral fluids/i.v. hydration
	7–10 days (may take 6–10 months to resolve)	Dysuria, increase in nocturia, urinary retention, urinary incontinence	Rule out UTI Urinary catheter for 48 hours Analgesics Reduce caffeinated/alcoholic beverages Decrease liquid intake after 8 p.m.
Bowel/proctitis	3–4 weeks	Soft stools >3/day, diarrhoea, 'gassy' bowel movements, painless rectal bleeding	Low residue diet Loperamide hydrochloride Cortisone suppositories
Late proctitis	12 months	Mild intermittent rectal blood on bowel movement	Colonoscopy to rule out colorectal cancer or fistula (rare)
Painful ejaculation		Burning sensation during ejaculation/blood streaked semen	Patient information at time of implant Reassure patient
Passing seed with semen (rare)	Up to 2 months		Wear condom if patient is worried about this rare possibility

that the late effects to the bladder will affect around one in five patients. Again, careful planning and accurate imaging prior to treatment should eliminate the possibility of severe symptoms.

Infection

Cervical tumours are often infected. Dilatation of the uterine canal for the insertion of brachytherapy sources can spread the infection. Drainage of pus and administration of antibiotics are required.

Vaginal dryness/stenosis

The possibility of permanent dryness along with shortening and narrowing of the vagina should be discussed with the patient prior to consent for treatment. Oestrogen creams can address the issue of dryness and regular use of dilators can help maintain the patency of the vagina.

HORMONE THERAPY REACTIONS

Beatson, who noted that inoperable breast cancers sometimes regressed after oophorectomy, described the significance of hormone action on cancers of the reproductive system in 1896. In modern medicine, in addition to surgical interventions such as oophorectomy and orchidectomy, there is now a range of hormonal drugs to alter the hormone profile of the patient. We can either lower the plasma protein of hormones that are known to stimulate the tumour or give additive hormones that compete with the tumour dependent hormones during the synthesis process. However, just as natural hormone variations and imbalances (such as puberty and menopause) can cause unwanted side-effects, so too can hormonal drug treatments (Table 13.2).

IMMUNOTHERAPY REACTIONS

Immunotherapy is a form of treatment that utilises the body's own response mechanisms. These therapies can be used to either enhance the immune system response or suppress it. It is useful for many conditions, malignant and non-malignant. The form of immunotherapy we are probably all familiar with is vaccination, where antibodies are stimulated to provide protection against a disease, e.g. MMR vaccine. Immunotherapy is also commonly used to treat allergies.

Immunotherapy can be divided into two categories: *Active* where the body's own immune system is stimulated to fight a disease and *Passive*, which relies on antibodies

produced in a laboratory to initiate a response to the disease. The majority of immunotherapy agents employed for treatments are *specific* immunotherapies, where only one type of cell or antigen is targeted while non-specific immunotherapies have a more general effect on the immune system.

The most common form of immunotherapy used for cancer treatment is monoclonal antibody (MAb) therapy. MAbs were originally derived from murine (mouse) cells and were likely to cause allergic reactions in the patient. Since their initial development, the mouse antibody proteins have been replaced by human cells to give *chimeric* or *humanised* antibodies depending on the degree of humanisation that has been achieved (Table 13.3).

Side-effects of MAbs and precautions

Compared with the effects of cancer chemotherapy, the side-effects of MAb treatment are low, particularly since the development of chimeric and humanised forms. If side-effects do occur, they are usually mild and associated with allergic reactions that occur during or shortly after the first administration of the agent producing a Type I hypersensitivity reaction. Patients develop symptoms such as fever, chills, itching and skin rashes. In more severe cases, they can develop angio-oedema, bronchospasm and hypotension.

Patients should be injected while lying on a bed and drugs to relieve anaphylaxis should be at hand. As with all procedures, a full explanation should be provided before administration of the agent and the importance of the patient reporting any unusual sensations or discomfort should be emphasised. The patient must be observed carefully for any signs of allergic reaction during the administration of the agent. Manufacturer's advice and information is available for all drugs, the staff should familiarise themselves with these and ensure that the patient remains in the department for some time after the drug has been administered.

If a reaction does occur, the administration of epinephrine, antihistamines and corticosteroids may be required.

Long-term side-effects

While the greatest possibility of side-effects from MAbs occurs at the time of injection, MAbs can also have side-effects that are related to the antigens they target. Avastin targets new blood vessel growth, but this can have long-term repercussions causing bleeding or poor wound healing. MAbs that target epidermal growth factor receptors may cause acne-like skin rashes. With the range of agents increasing, staff should familiarise themselves with the possible long-term side-effects of each agent used in their department.

Table 13.2 Hormone therapy and reactions

Hormone type	Action	Drugs	Side-effects
Oestrogens	Prostate cancers: Action in males is to inhibit release of luteinising hormone (LH) reducing testicular androgens. Possible direct effect on prostate	Diethylstilboestrol	Loss of libido, shrinkage of genitalia, gynaecomastia
Anti-oestrogens	Action not fully understood, but binds competitively to oestrogen receptors (ER-positive), possibly reduces amount of free oestrogen	Tamoxifen	Hot flushes, nausea and vomiting have been the most commonly reported symptoms (25% of patients) for both pre and postmenopausal women. Premenopausal women also reported amenorrhoea, altered menses. There is a minor increased risk of endometrial cancer
Progesterone	Utilised in breast and endometrial cancers, but exact mechanism unclear, although there is thought to be an anti-oestrogenic effect	1. Megastrol 2. Medroxy-progesterone	(1) Weight gain, fluid retention, vaginal bleeding, amenorrhoea, nausea and thrombophlebitis. (2) Increased risk of blood clotting.
Antiandrogens	Prostate cancers. Androgen agonist suppresses testicular and adrenal androgens (used in combination with LHRH analogues)	1. Flutamide 2. Casodex	(1) Hepatotoxicity (monitor during 1st 3 months), gynaecomastia, insomnia, tiredness. (2) Hot flushes, pruritis, abnormal LFTs, somnolence, dry mouth, dyspepsia
Luteinising hormone releasing hormone (LHRH) analogues (Males)	Prostate cancers. LH and follicle-stimulating hormone (FSH) levels fall (after an initial surge) and the corresponding peripheral androgens and oestrogens decrease	Zoladex	Initial hormone surge can cause symptoms to increase (tumour flare); this should last no longer than 2 weeks. Hot flushes, gynaecomastia, loss of libido, nausea
LHRH analogues (females)	Advanced breast cancers. Has similar action as oophorectomy	Zoladex	Hot flushes, tumour flare, nausea
Aromatase inhibitors	Endocrine sensitive breast cancers (advanced or recurrent). Exhibits oestrogen depleting effects as it prevents oestrogen synthesis	1. Anastrazole (non-steroidal). 2. Letrozole 3. Exemestane (steroidal)	Hot flushes, osteopenia (higher fracture rate than with tamoxifen), arthralgia (can be severe at first, but improving with time), muscle stiffness, hair thinning. (3) Sweating and dizziness
Glucocorticoids (adrenal hormones)	Control carbohydrate and protein metabolism. Cytotoxic properties for acute leukaemias, lymphomas, breast cancers. Reduce cerebral oedema, vomiting, and spinal cord compression	Naturally occurring: cortisone and hydrocortisone Synthetic: 1. Prednisone 2. Prednisolone 3. Dexamethasone	Adrenal insufficiency, fluid retention possibly leading to cardiac failure, round (moon) face, GI upset, increase risk of infections and tissue reactions with associated healing problems, thinning and/or bruising of skin, muscle weakness, psychosis

Table 13.3 Cancer immunotherapy

Antibody	Name	Type	Target	Uses
Alemtuzumab	Campath	Humanised	CD52	Chronic lymphocytic leukaemia
Bevacizumab	Avastin	Humanised	Vascular endothelial growth factor	Colorectal cancer
Cetuximab	Erbitux	Chimeric	Epidermal growth factor receptor	Colorectal cancer
Gemtuzumab ozogamicin	Mylotarg	Humanised	CD33	Acute myelogenous leukaemia
Ibritumomab tiuxetan	Zevalin	Murine	CD20	Non-Hodgkin lymphoma
Panitumumab	Vectibix	Human	Epidermal growth factor receptor	Colorectal cancer
Rituximab	Rituxan, MabThera	Chimeric	CD20	Non-Hodgkin lymphoma
Trastuzumab	Herceptin	Humanised	ErbB2	Breast cancer

KEY POINTS

- Side-effects are an inevitable aspect of radiotherapy treatments but can be alleviated by appropriate care and consideration
- Radiotherapy practitioners are well placed to take part in the monitoring and treatment of side-effects
- There are clinical variations between hospitals in the treatment of side-effects
- Depending on the radiotherapy treatment regime and target volume, side-effects are of variable severity but can commonly include skin, respiratory and gastrointestinal changes

Chapter | 14 |

Moving and handling

Melanie Mansfield, Toni Meyer

INTRODUCTION

Patient moving and handling is a vital everyday element of patient care, as it must be performed safely and efficiently. In this chapter, you will learn how back problems can develop among staff due to lifting at work, as well as how to care for your back by following simple principles. We will consider the structure and biomechanics of the spine by reviewing basic anatomy, structure and functions of the spine. The legal matters which govern moving and handling in your workplace, including the components that form a manual handling risk assessment are outlined. There are some patient handling scenarios included for review, alongside common equipment use and procedures performed in medical imaging and radiotherapy environments. Unsafe and complex situations will be highlighted and at the end of the chapter, you will find advice on everyday back care and how to keep your spine healthy for life.

Back and neck pain affects 80% of people at some time during their adult lives. Musculoskeletal back strain and injury problems cause more pain, and more work days lost each year (120 million) than any other condition. It is estimated that back pain costs the NHS approximately £512 million per year in outpatient, inpatient and A&E treatment. About 3600 nurses alone are retired each year due to back pain. No official figures are recorded relating to unqualified staff and family carers. Back pain at work has the highest incidence in healthcare, construction, retail and food industries.

The really good news is that these conditions can be prevented, and looking after your back can be part of your work as a practitioner so that you can have a full and active life and a long career in healthcare. The introduction of specialist equipment and robust training systems means that staff should no longer have to be injured while doing their job.

 Why is Manual Handling so important to healthcare professionals?

- The statistics prove that we work in very high-risk professions
- The Law tells us we have to follow safe practice
- The HealthCare Professions Council, Code of Professional Conduct and Ethics govern our practice – including Manual Handling
- It is an integral part of providing patient care

Most back and neck problems develop over weeks, months or even years. This is why it is so important to care for your back every day, whether at work or at home, so that 'everyday back care' becomes a good habit. When something goes wrong, we tend to think the problem was caused by the last patient we moved, the last heavy object we pushed, pulled or lifted, even if it was several days or weeks ago. This is often not the case. This chapter will enable you to understand how to keep your spine healthy and how to find the causes of stress in your daily work and home routine.

Back pain is a costly problem to employers and society in general, but what does it mean for the individual? What does back pain mean for you as a health worker? Think for a moment how your life would be altered if you had back pain or suffered a back injury? What would it stop you doing? You only have one back – knees and hips can be replaced, backs cannot!

STRUCTURE AND BIOMECHANICS OF THE SPINE

Your spine is made of 33 vertebral bodies that stack on top of each other to form a continuous flexible column. In between the vertebral bodies are intervertebral discs, all of which are bound together with ligaments forming an 'S' shape. These ligaments are tough, non-elastic bands that help limit joint movement. In its natural or normal position, it is very strong. This 'normal' position will be referred to when we discuss moving and handling techniques later in the chapter.

Looking from the posterior aspect, the vertebral column is straight. From the side, the spine has three curves and a sacrum/coccyx region. The vertebral column can therefore be grouped into four regions;

1. Cervical (7) – This area is very flexible and a common location of injuries
2. Thoracic (dorsal) (12) – Ribs attach to 10 of these vertebrae. This area is not very flexible as it is the structural part of the spine
3. Lumbar (5) – This is the main load-bearing region in the back where the vertebral bodies are the largest. It is very flexible as they are the first moveable vertebral segments above the static pelvis, and a main and common site for injuries. The normal curvature of the region can change in standing and sitting positions
4. Sacrum and coccyx (9) – The 9 lowest vertebra become fused into two bones. The five sacral bones are convex, attaching to the pelvis and the four very small coccygeal bones are concave.

Bones, ligaments, nerves, discs and muscles

Your spine gives your body a structure and provides protection for the spinal cord. The spinal cord runs the entire length of the spine and a nerve root exits at each joint. The intervertebral discs act as a shock-absorbing pad that allows spinal movement. The discs do not have blood or nerve supplies, but nutrients are supplied and wastes are eliminated by the 'pumping' action of daily activity and motion. The two distinct parts are the annulus fibrosus and the nucleus pulposus. The nucleus pulposus is an incompressible watery gel contained within an elastic wall.

Nuclei are located more centrally in the discs between vertebrae at the top of the body. Near the lumbar region, nuclei are not located centrally. Herniation of the disc is more likely in inferior regions of the spine where the flexibility of the region and loading is greater. The annulus is a fibrous cartilaginous rim surrounding the nucleus, offering structural strength.

The disc is like a sponge; when healthy, it is full of fluid and can change shape rapidly as you bend and stretch. Keeping mobile and doing exercises at home and work (see below) helps to prevent the discs remaining in the same position for too long and giving a 'stiff' back. Regular exercise will help to keep your discs mobile and healthy.

There are three main columns of muscles associated with the spine: erector spinae (on the vertebrae themselves); longissimus dorsi and iliocostalis run parallel to the vertebral column. These muscles help to maintain an erect posture and are in constant use when we move and change position. Our muscles contract and relax to make us move. The back muscles get shorter and stronger as the body arches backwards and as the body bends forwards, they become long and weak. Back and abdominal muscles help to stabilise the spine when lifting and carrying (core stability). As your job as a healthcare professional involves moving, lifting and handling, it is extremely important to keep your muscles strong and in good condition.

BACK INJURIES

Why do some people tend to have low back strains and sprains more often? We do know some factors that tend to influence the development of this type of problem, but often these symptoms strike in unexpected situations. Most commonly, those who develop a lumbar strain or sprain are doing an activity that places their back at risk. This may be a sudden forceful movement, lifting a heavy object or twisting the back in an unusual manner. Knowing how to properly lift can help to prevent many back injuries.

Some well known factors that contribute to low back pain include:

- Poor conditioning, being generally unfit
- Obesity. Being overweight will put extra strain on your spine
- Smoking, and a poor diet or too much alcohol may all reduce healing time if you are injured or unwell
- Improper use/lifting technique or lifting and handling unnecessarily
- Peer pressure, continuing to use poor lifting and handling methods due to pressure from colleagues
- Stress – it causes people to take short cuts. Some clinical staff still believe that it is quicker to manually lift

a patient than to use equipment such as a slide sheet. This is not true.

- Fatigue. If you are tired and have been working long hours, your muscles may not work effectively to protect you.

The various types of injury are summarised below.

Intervertebral disc – prolapsed, degenerative

A prolapse of a disc (often called a slipped disc) happens when so much pressure is put on the disc that the gelatinous centre bursts out of the coating. This protrusion may then press on one of the nerves leaving the spinal cord and running just behind the disc, causing the nerve to become numb or to send pain messages to the brain. The most common place for a prolapsed disc to occur is in the lumbar (lower back) region, although it may occur in the cervical region (neck) or, less commonly, in other places down the spine. Discs are most easily damaged by heavy lifting. The increasing availability of MRI in recent years has revealed many answers to the causes of back pain including disc prolapse. However, disc degeneration and prolapse can be seen in a moderately high proportion of people who have never suffered from significant back pain.

Muscle strain

Most back pain comes from the soft tissues in the back such as the muscles. Usually they hurt because they are not moving as they should. Feeling stiff and achy may not mean you have done any damage – just that you could be using muscles that have not been active for a while. When bent or stooped, the disc becomes distorted and the muscles and ligaments are in a lengthened and weak position and cannot protect the back properly. Muscle strains are often a 'warning sign' and with appropriate rest and exercise, enough sleep and a good diet, should heal within 6 weeks.

Ligamentous damage

The main causes of damage to the spinal ligaments are trauma or sudden and excessive movements. These movements can arise from twisting, incorrect lifting technique or an awkward bend. This is why the 'normal position' should be maintained during moving and handling. These actions can cause the ligaments to become overstretched causing a strain or sprain. In severe injury, the ligament can actually tear. Poor posture and not standing straight (favouring leaning on one leg more than the other), can also cause the lower spinal and pelvic ligaments to gradually become stretched, which results in spinal deformation.

Malalignment of facet joints

Degenerative changes begin with an annular tear, in either a normal disc, or in one that has already begun to dry out. In time, the facet joints will become affected. The facet joints will be subjected to increased wear-and-tear because the shock-absorbing function has been lost. In addition, as the disc continues to degenerate, disc space height will decrease. Since the facet is comprised from the vertebrae above and below the disc, as the disc collapses, the two bone ends will slide past each other, causing malalignment. This is called facet subluxation. Such malalignment will result in even greater wear-and-tear on the facets. The articular cartilage of the facets is the smooth covering of the bone ends that allows them to flow smoothly over each other trillions of times throughout our lifetime. Increased wear-and-tear and malalignment damages the articular cartilage until the facet joint is bone on bone. The loss of articular cartilage is, by definition, degenerative arthritis.

 Did you know …?

- Back pain is common but not normally serious. With rest, appropriate exercise and advice, most people get better within 6 weeks
- You may never find out the exact cause of your pain – 85% of back pain sufferers will *never* know the cause
- Non-steroidal anti-inflammatory drugs (NSAIDs) such as ibuprofen, can help to relieve back pain
- Exercises to strengthen your back and your 'core' can help people with back pain

LEGAL MATTERS

There are a number of pieces of legislation associated with manual handling. This section outlines the key regulations and the responsibilities laid down within them.

Health and Safety at Work Act, 1974

This act aims to ensure the health, safety and welfare of all employees by laying down three main areas of responsibility: for the employer, for equipment and for employees.

The *employer* has a responsibility to provide a safe and healthy working environment by considering the following points:

- What is the likelihood of an accident occurring?
- What is the severity of the risk?
- How might the risks be controlled (to the lowest level reasonably practicable)?
- What are the costs associated with these control measures?

In addition, every employer has to ensure that employees are provided with

* Information, instructions, training and supervision

Any *equipment* used at work must be maintained in good working order, safe to use and regularly checked.

The *employee* has a responsibility to report where he/she feels that they are working at risk by:

* Taking care of their own health and safety and that of others
* Cooperating to ensure their own safety and that of others
* Not damaging or disabling equipment
* Undertaking any necessary training.

Management of Health and Safety at Work Regulations, 1999

These regulations require appropriate control measures to be adopted to eliminate or reduce risks in the workplace. The regulations recommend that a written record giving appropriate details is kept of any assessments or checks made in the workplace. Furthermore, employees have a duty under the regulations to use equipment in accordance with training and instruction given by the employer.

Manual Handling Operations Regulations, 1992 (Revised 2004) (MHOR)

Manual Handling Operations Regulations came into force on 1 January 1993, to implement European Directive 90/269/EEC. The regulations add to the duties placed on employers by the Health and Safety at Work Act (1974). The regulations clearly establish a hierarchy of measures for dealing with risks from manual handling to be carried out if the weight being handled falls outside the recommended guidelines (lifting from the optimum position at waist height, which is 16 kg for females and 25 kg for males). These regulations cover Manual Handling Operations, including the handling of people, but generally the transportation or supporting of a load, i.e. lifting, lowering, pushing, pulling, carrying, or moving: by hand or bodily force.

The employer's risk assessment shall:

* So far as reasonably practicable, avoid the need for his/her employees to undertake any manual handling operations at work, which involve a risk of being injured
* Make a suitable and sufficient assessment of all such manual handling operations that cannot be avoided
* Take appropriate steps to reduce the risk of injury to those employees arising out of their undertaking any such manual handling operations to the lowest level reasonably practicable
* Review the situation as necessary
* Provide information on the loads being handled.

The employees shall:

* Follow appropriate systems of work laid down for their safety
* Make proper use of equipment provided for their safety
* Cooperate with their employer on health and safety matters
* Inform the employer if they identify hazardous handling activities
* Take care to ensure that their activities do not put others at risk.

Provision and Use of Work Equipment Regulations, 1998 (PUWER)

These regulations necessitate the prevention or control of risks to people's health and safety from equipment provided for use at work.

Employers must:

* Ensure that all equipment is suitable for the work, and is used for the purpose for which it was intended, e.g. bed sheets and pillow cases are not intended or safe for moving and handling use
* Maintain equipment in a safe condition so that health and safety is not at risk
* Regularly inspect equipment to ensure it continues to be safe for intended use.

Employees must:

* Only use equipment for the purpose for which it was intended
* Report any defects immediately
* Not use work equipment without first receiving adequate training and supervision.

Lifting Operations and Lifting Equipment Regulations, 1998 (LOLER)

The Lifting Operations and Lifting Equipment Regulations are concerned with the suitability of lifting devices, ensuring that equipment is of suitable strength and stability and that it is marked in a manner appropriate for reasons of health and safety.

Every employer shall ensure that:

* Lifting equipment is of adequate strength and stability for each load/person
* That machinery and accessories for lifting loads/people are clearly marked to indicate their Safe Working Load (SWL)
* Equipment that could be used in error to lift people is clearly marked 'Do not use to lift people'
* Lifting operations are planned by a competent person, appropriately supervised and carried out in a safe manner

- Equipment used to lift people should be examined by competent people every 6 months and other lifting equipment every 12 months
- All maintenance and inspection work carried out on equipment should be logged.

The Human Rights Act, 1998

Article 3 of the Human Rights Act states that: 'no one shall be subjected to torture or degrading treatment or punishment'. Although not specifically related to moving and handling, it brings to question the concept of consent and the rights of both the handler and the patient, which may in some cases result in dilemmas. For example, a patient may refuse the use of a hoist which they might consider degrading but may also be deemed too heavy for staff to manually lift, as it would put their own health and safety at risk. The act in this case protects both parties. The patient's right to dignity and humane treatment and the staff's right to not put themselves unnecessarily at risk.

The Reporting of Injuries, Diseases and Dangerous Occurrences Regulations 1995 (RIDDOR)

This final piece of legislation is only concerned with the legal requirements for reporting injuries. The regulation details the types of reportable injuries and the use of accident books and reporting mechanisms. In the event of an injury, the responsibility of reporting it lies with both the employee and employer.

MANUAL HANDLING RISK ASSESSMENT

The decisions made associated with moving or handling a patient should encourage and enforce safer handling.

What is safer handling?

The aim is to eliminate hazardous manual handling in all but exceptional or life-threatening situations. Patients should be encouraged to assist in their own transfers and appropriate handling aids should be used whenever they can to reduce the risk of injury. The objective is to emphasise the importance of enabling the patient to help themselves as much as possible. This permits the patient to be as independent as they can be within the constraints of their condition and individual capabilities. This concept is not only safer for the handler but also for the patient. In the case of a deteriorating condition, it may preserve what little ability the patient has for as long as possible and for a recovering patient, it provides the exercise and strength required for their mobility to increase over time.

All manual handling tasks carry a certain amount of risk, particularly the potential of a musculoskeletal injury. Risk assessments aim to identify potential areas of risk by gathering information relating to the task which may impact on the way it is carried out, e.g. is it likely to cause a major injury; would you have to perform the task regularly. This principle of gathering information in order to make a sound judgement applies to all manual handling tasks. Risk assessment may be formal and recorded on specific documents and kept with patient's notes; this is often the case for inpatients or those likely to be having repeat care over a period of time. Furthermore, they can be generic relating to a clinical room or space and the type of work that can be practically and safely carried out there. Risk assessment may also be more informal in nature and assimilated during a brief contact with a patient, as is often the case for radiotherapy practitioner–patient contact, although some radiotherapy patients with complex needs are likely to have a more formal arrangement if they are going to be receiving a regular treatment regime.

In accordance to the Manual Handling Operations Regulations, 1992/2004, if the employer cannot avoid the need for manual handling, a risk assessment should be carried out by a competent person. The risk assessment should be suitable and sufficient to adequately reduce or control risks within the workplace. The risk assessment considers the likelihood that harm or injury may occur to staff and others and a document should be produced, which details what these risks are, identifies who may be at risk and how the risks could be reduced or controlled.

The Manual Handling Operations Regulations, 1992/2004 requires employers to look at four specific things when undertaking a risk assessment:

- Load
- Individual capability
- Task
- Environment

And when the handling of people is being carried out the following should be taken into account:

- Environment
- Load
- Individual capability
- Task
- Equipment.

Table 14.1 provides further explanation of each of the elements considered when carrying out a risk assessment.

The purpose of undertaking a risk assessment is to identify where any hazards may be and what the level of risk may be. The next step is to decide how the risks may be eliminated or controlled and to relay this information on to those affected. All inpatients will have been risk assessed on admission to a hospital and this would be repeated as a patient's condition/ability changes. Documentation associated with this risk assessment is called a Patient Handling Plan and can be found in the Patient

Table 14.1 Factors considered during moving and handling risk assessment

Environment	*Is there enough room to carry out the task without putting staff in a poor posture, such as bending, reaching away from the body, twisting and/or stooping?* If not, the layout of the area may need to be altered by moving or removing furniture. *Is the floor in good condition?* Slippery, wet or uneven floors maintained poorly all pose a risk to the handler. Floors should be well maintained and alternative routes considered if loads or patients need to be moved up steep narrow steps or slopes. *Lighting conditions* are important especially when working in light or darkened rooms in order to permit the visualisation of positioning beams. Light switches could be positioned close to point of need in order to facilitate efficient and safe transfers.
Load	Objects are considered with regards to weight, bulk and coupling when being handled. Some loads can be broken down into smaller loads, e.g. a bale of blue rolls for use on examination surfaces can be easily broken down into individual rolls for distribution to their point of use or storage. Alternatively, loads could be stabilised by the use of a trolley for transportation. This may be helpful in receiving and distributing deliveries of bulk medical supplies such as disposable syringes or laser film. When handling people, consideration must be given to the characteristics of that person which might influence safe manual handling practice: weight; size; height; age; cognitive function; ability to communicate; physical condition; how to promote independence; prognosis; patient motivation; pain and medication received; behaviour and predictability; ability to mobilise; infection control issues; skin condition; level of help required; dignity; lines; drains monitors and prosthetics. The above list is by no means exhaustive and what might apply to a patient at one time may be different on a future visit to your department as a patient's ability and characteristics can fluctuate with progression of a condition and treatment regimes.
Individual capability	Refers to the handler's capabilities. Staff need to be fit and well trained and motivated. Additional considerations need to be given to staff who are pregnant, suffering ill health or recovering from a previous injury. Staff who are particularly tall or short are likely to be at more risk of injury, as they may have to adapt to the limits of equipment or working with a member of staff with a greatly different height. Where a task may require specific training it will not be considered suitable for all members of the team to contribute without additional training or experience, e.g. a log roll.
Task	Loads and people are capable of behaving unexpectedly. The task should be reviewed to assess its association with bending; reaching; twisting; stopping or holding at a distance from the trunk; in addition excessive lifting, lowering or carrying over a distance needs to be taken into account. Can any of these actions be reduced or controlled by a change in practice?
Equipment	The equipment used for manual handling purposes should be both appropriate for the people it is being used with/for and the task being carried out. The assessment of equipment should also take into account its maintenance in order to keep it in functional and safe working order and the servicing requirements as stipulated by the law.

Care Plan. This may be particularly useful to radiotherapy teams seeing a patient regularly. Radiotherapy practitioners will commonly draw on their experience within the clinical environment in order to perform dynamic informal risk assessments of the situations and patients they meet during their time at work.

MANUAL HANDLING PRINCIPLES

This chapter highlights the fact that every manual handling situation is unique, with its own special set of circumstances. As a result, rather than trying to exactly follow a prescribed way of doing things, the most effective way to approach and manage a manual handling situation is to follow a core set of manual handling principles. This section summarises the three areas covered, incorporating the load or patient, the individual/s performing the procedure and the environment or equipment with which you have to work.

The load or patient

The load or patient is probably your first consideration and this should be a decision as to whether manual handling is required at all. A load can be broken down into smaller portions – e.g. a large box often contains a number of lighter modules within it which can be moved one at a time. Additionally, if a patient is able to undertake all or part of the movement themselves you should take time to provide instruction and encouragement and allow them to do so independently.

The assessment of risk covered earlier in this chapter forms part of the judgement decision you make regarding the management of the load or patient. Time should be taken to think through the movement, identifying and reducing potential risk to the load/patient and yourself. By thinking through the potential options of managing a load, you will also be able to select the most suitable technique. Your choice of technique can often be dictated by protocols and the patient may have a manual handling assessment in existence providing guidance on how he or she is currently handled. However, it should be acknowledged that some clinical areas will not always accommodate the equipment that your patient may be used to using. For example, restrictions on hoist use may be presented by an X-ray or radiotherapy couch being at a fixed height. Some equipment may be contraindicated in an MRI scan room.

The individual/s performing the procedure

Being aware of your limitations and capabilities as a manual handler is important if you are going to avoid future injury or risk to your patient. Consider your size, strength and build in relation to the task ahead. Bear in mind your current level of fitness and how you are feeling relative to the procedure you wish to perform, e.g. if you are currently in pain from an existing injury or have a disability you may need to reconsider or adapt your approach to the task ahead to suit your abilities. Clothing and footwear could also impact on your ability. If it is restrictive or impractical, you are likely to risk injury to yourself. Ideally, footwear should not be too high, the toes should be enclosed, the foot should be supported and the sole of the shoe non-slip.

Your level of experience is also worth taking into account, e.g. a practitioner who has never used a hoist should not attempt to do so without advice and support from someone who has knowledge and experience of that specific piece of equipment. Selecting an appropriate technique for the task will take into account your level of training, assessment of the situation and your prior knowledge and experience with the type of load given. A number of procedures should not be attempted single-handed and if you feel that alone you are not able, then another colleague or even a team of people should perform the manual handling task together. If this is the case, then a person should be selected to lead the procedure in order to avoid confusion and ensure a coordinated approach is achieved.

If working alone with a patient, it is still vital to ensure you take a lead role in order to gain the successful cooperation of the patient. It is the lead person's responsibility to provide clear and simple communication to members of the team and the patient. Ideally, prior to starting the movement it should be explained, including the instructions which will be used; understanding should be check and then the instructions carried out as described.

Once a procedure is underway, the individual should have an awareness of the position and action of their body in association to the task. In order to facilitate the safest movement, the following should be achieved where possible:

- As the head leads in natural body movement, lead any movement with your head
- To improve stability, a stable base should be adopted; with your feet shoulder width apart
- To keep your spine in line, maintain a natural posture. Avoid twisting by making sure you position your feet and move your body when moving from one position to another and avoid bending your back by keeping your knees flexed. Over-reaching and stooping should also be minimised
- To reduce the strains on your musculoskeletal system, keep the load as close to your centre of gravity as possible
- In order to maintain a good grip on your load or patient, consider the use of handles or handling belts and test the achievable grip prior to beginning a movement
- In order to improve efficiency, where possible, use momentum by facilitating small rhythmic rocking movements in unison towards the direction of the travel.

Environment and equipment

In order to avoid trips, falls and hazards, the environment should be cleared of clutter and suitable space should be made in order for the manual handling task to be carried out without compromising anyone's safety. Where possible, lighting should permit a clear view of where you are going and your field of view should not be obstructed by the environment, object or patient you are moving.

You should be familiar and trained in any equipment you have selected to utilise from a manual handling procedure. Furthermore that piece of equipment should be suitable for the task and in good working order. It is good practice to visually inspect equipment for damage or signs of wear and tear and also take into account size or weight restrictions, which may prohibit its use for a particular task.

'COMMON SENSE' ERGONOMICS

Eliminating all manual lifting may not be possible in all areas of work but it is still important to reduce the risk of injury and this can be achieved by looking at ergonomic issues. Ergonomics simply means fitting the task to the person. It is about designing and arranging the workplace to fit the task.

Imagine sitting at a workstation in a medical imaging or radiotherapy department; lots of people will be using this computer, screen and keyboard every day, so it is important to consider its design and how it can be safely used.

> **!** As an ergonomic example you might like to ask yourself the following questions:
>
> - How long do I spend at a computer each day?
> - Should I stand or sit?
> - Does the monitor and keyboard pivot and tilt to avoid glare on the screen?
> - Are the characters on the screen clear and readable?
> - Is the style and size of the mouse comfortable to use?
> - Is the desk free from clutter/big enough for the mouse/keyboard/monitor?
> - If there is a chair, is it adjustable and in good condition?

There are four key areas where changes can make a big difference to the way you work:

1. *Environment.* There must be sufficient space to arrange furniture and equipment appropriately for the patient handling task to be done and to be able to manoeuvre equipment easily.
2. *Equipment.* All furnishings and equipment must be suitable for their purpose, easy to move, easy to use and where applicable, adjustable in height to allow good working postures and positions. In your everyday working life, you should consider taking care of your back during all your tasks.
3. *Work organisation.* It is really important that staffing levels are appropriate for the demands of the work, and the dependency of the patients.
4. *Training.* Staff and students normally attend manual handling training at induction and are annually updated. Many clinical areas have Manual Handling Advisors who provide training, advice and information on local manual handling issues.

If new equipment is provided in your department, ensure you are trained and competent in using it. It is really important that you are familiar with the hoist which is used in your department if you have one. Training on use of the hoist must take in the clinical department because of the differing hoists available. Some hospital trusts have a 'hoist team' who will come and move a patient if required, as the hoist may be shared between many clinical areas.

Some examples of ergonomic issues facing practitioners include:

- Lifting, supporting, pushing and pulling patients
- Working in an awkward, unstable or crouched position, including bending forwards, sideways and twisting the body when positioning patients

- Lifting loads at arm's length
- Lifting with a starting (or finishing) position near the floor, overhead or at arm's length
- Handling uncooperative or falling patients.

SAFE HANDLING PRACTICE

Selecting the most suitable technique to use for the patient and practitioner is a fundamental moving and handling principle, which should be considered in advance. The following section provides a quick reference guide for some of the most common procedures needing to be performed along with a technique profile.

Remember: Wear suitable clothing and footwear. One of the reasons you have a uniform is so that your natural body movement is not restricted by clothing, and your shoes should be comfortable, non-slip, supportive, flat and with a closed toe. Maintain a natural upright posture, keeping the spine with its natural curves in a 'normal' position. This is when the spine is at its strongest. Ensure you can get and maintain a good grip when handling patients and loads and adopt a stable base. By separating your feet (about shoulder width apart) you improve your stability and reduce spinal rotation.

The handhold is one of the most useful methods of obtaining a grip on your patient if they have the ability to stand by themselves with limited support. A palm to palm handhold should be utilised and it important that thumbs and finger are not linked in any way as this may cause a risk of injury if your patient becomes unstable. A basic handhold is shown Figure 14.1.

Standing up from a sit

Prior to standing a patient up from a chair or examination table, he or she should be encouraged to adjust their position so that they have the most chance of standing successfully. In all cases where the stand is being performed from a chair with wheels, the brakes should be securely on and any floating table tops should be locked. Here, we will consider a stand from a chair but the

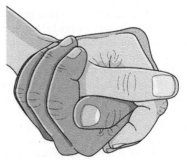

Figure 14.1 The basic handhold.

principle is the same for a stand from an examination table.

The patient's feet should be shoulder width apart with one foot in line below the knee and the other slightly back nearer the chair. The patient should move towards the front of the chair with their weight forward over their knees. If present, hands should be placed on the arms of the chair. Where possible, momentum can also aid getting the patient into the standing position with well instructed and synchronised rocking just prior to the stand. A suitable instruction for the patient is: *'ready, steady, stand'*. This instruction should be clearly communicated to the patient before attempting the stand to ensure the patient is aware of the commands and when to act upon them.

Caution: The stand should only be attempted if you are confident of the patient's strength and ability to weight-bear. If there is any doubt, test the patient's leg strength as part of your risk assessment by asking them to raise their leg against your hand.

Ideally, our role in the stand is to provide confidence through being present and providing clear instruction. This will encourage the patient to maintain their own independence and mobilisation capacity. If arms are not present on the side of the chair we could also incorporate the handhold mentioned previously, in order to give some stability to the movement.

For the less steady patient, further support can be provided with either one or two practitioners aiding the movement. The single practitioner should position themselves to the side of the patient facing the direction of travel with their feet in a stable base position. With the far hand being placed on the front of the patient's shoulder and the near hand spread low across the patient's back the movement can be made smoothly together. If a second person is utilised in this situation, then the second person mirrors that of the first with arms crossed behind the patient's back. To enhance this technique further, a handling belt could be utilised to improve grip. In the case of a two person stand, it is important that just one practitioner gives the instructions and leads the movement in order to minimise any confusion (Fig. 14.2).

> **!** *Note on walking frames:* If your patient has a walking frame this should not be used for standing, as it may tip towards the patient. Walking frames should be held onto only once the patient is in the upright position and can then be used to enable unaided walking.

Sitting from a stand

Prior to sitting down, the surface of any floating table should be locked and brakes on wheelchairs should be on. Where a height adjustable table is being used, the level should be brought to a level to suit the patient's stature and be positioned just above the backs of the patient's knees. The patient should be positioned so that they can feel the front of the table or chair with the backs of their legs. Weight should be distributed evenly through both feet and if armrests are present, these should be used to control the sit as the patient bends their knees and hips

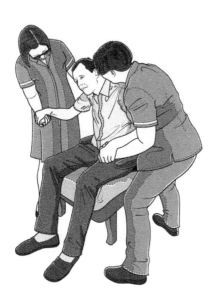
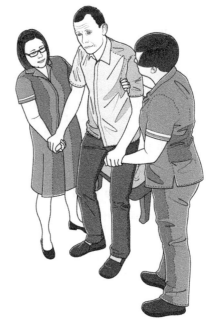

Figure 14.2 The two person stand.

and sits towards the front of the chair or table. The patient has two options for moving backwards into a secure and suitable position, either by shuffling from side to side or lifting using their upper body strength and pushing with their feet. If being supported by the practitioner, the command *'ready, steady, sit'* should be communicated to the patient and used in order to signal the change in weight distribution.

Sitting a patient forward

As with other movements, when a patient is moving or being assisted on a mobile surface, the brakes should be on and secure. As with standing up, a semi-independent patient should be encouraged to propel themselves into a sitting position in bed unaided using their arms and hands against the bed or secured cot sides.

The addition of a bed ladder can further support the patient with reasonable upper body strength. Bed ladders can be attached to the end of the patient's bed and also used on an examination table providing a suitably strong anchorage point can be identified. The ladder should be adjusted to reach the patient's groin area to ensure maximum effectiveness. To use this equipment, the patient is asked to cross their legs and walk their hands along the ladder, bringing them into a sitting position. For postoperative patients, the action of crossing their legs relaxes the abdominal muscles, so that moving into the sitting position is less painful.

Where a bed ladder is not suitable, two practitioners can perform a sit using an elbow to elbow hold. The handlers should face the patient, placing their feet into a stable position with their knee at the level of the patient's hip. The handlers should offer their nearside arms to the patient using an elbow to elbow grip, holding one another just above the elbow and not on the joint itself. The patient is brought forward by the handlers as they transfer their weight backwards through their legs following a *'ready, steady, sit'* command. In this case, to limit the possibility of injury, explanation and familiarisation of commands and the movement should be given to the patient prior to beginning. Due to the need of the patient to use their upper body strength, this technique is not suitable for patients with prohibitive arm or shoulder conditions.

Moving a patient up the bed

In the past, many staff may have resorted to using bed sheets to move a patient up the bed. This is, however, not recommended due to the risk of sheets tearing and the potential of friction burns being inflicted on the patient's skin. Positively encouraging an able patient to move up the bed can be achieved by suggesting that they bend their knees while pushing their heels into the bed and coordinate this by placing their hands flat on the bed behind them and lifting themselves backward towards the head of the bed. Equally, it may be more comfortable for them to slowly shuffle backwards by transferring their weight from one side to the other, supporting themselves on each side with their hands.

For the less able patient in need of assistance, a slide sheet enables a patient to be moved around their bed with a much reduced risk of damage to their skin and a greatly reduced amount of pushing and pulling required by staff using alternative methods. Today, there is a huge range of slide sheets available on the market, which may be either disposable or intended for repeated use, with or without handling straps. They all effectively provide a low friction surface on which the patient can easily glide on the surface they are lying on.

When being used it is essential that the bed brakes are on or the tabletop is locked. The optimal working height for the staff required to carry out the manoeuvre should be their median height in respect of their waists and pelvises. Slide sheets can easily be inserted under the patient by rolling them slightly in either direction, placing the first half under after the first roll and then unfolding the other half as the patient rolls in the other direction. Once on top of the slide sheet, staff should check that the patient's head, trunk, legs and feet are all on the slide sheet.

The patient being moved by slide sheet should be asked wherever possible to raise their head, placing their chin on their chest, and folding their arms in front of them. Staff should be positioned on either side of the bed near to the patients' pillow with one leg forward ready to transfer their weight backwards onto their other leg. A grip should be made on the upper part of the slide sheet or using an appropriate handle. The lead practitioner should give the instruction *'ready, steady, slide'*. Working together, the practitioners should gradually slide the patient up the bed. It is important not to lift with the slide sheet and if the patient is challenging, it may be necessary to undertake the procedure in stages.

> **!** *Slide sheet safety:* Slide sheets by their very nature are slippery and can therefore be a hazard. Sheets should never be left on the floor or under an unattended patient, in order to limit the possibility of accidents occurring. Always check slide sheets for signs of wear and tear prior to use.

Once the patient is in a suitable position, the slide sheet can be removed by pulling it towards the head of the bed from under the patient. It is important not to leave the patient on the slide sheet or pull it out towards the lower end of the bed, as this can cause the patient to slide back down the bed.

Lateral transfer

The lateral transfer should only be considered if no means of imaging or treating the patient is possible with them remaining *in situ* on their trolley or bed. Approximately 90% of all the assisted transfers undertaken are lateral transfers. A board device most commonly known as a 'Patslide' is probably the most recognised tool to aid a lateral transfer and is widely used in both imaging and radiotherapy departments. It is designed to act as a bridge spanning any gaps that occur between beds, trolleys and tables. The smooth upper surface provides low resistance, allowing for easy transfer and it can be used in conjunction with a sliding sheet. The underside has non-skid inserts permitting it to grip to the surface. It is ideally suited for use in the clinical area, as it is easy to clean, quick to use and permits a lateral transfer of vulnerable or immobile patients safely and with minimal risk of injury to staff.

For this illustration, the patient will be transferred from a bed to a table but this description can easily be applied to other surfaces. With the bed brakes securely applied, a Patslide can easily be inserted under part of the patient using a half roll, leaving the other half of the slide available to cover any gap remaining between the bed and the table. The bed and table should both be adjusted to appropriate heights for the staff performing the transfer – they should be adjacent to one another and closely aligned, giving a slight inclination in the direction of travel from the bed to the table to aid the movement with gravity. On the command of '*ready steady slide*' the patient can be gently pushed by the staff on the bed side and pulled towards the table by the staff opposite. While the movement is taking place, it is helpful if the patient can raise their head towards their chin and keep their hands on their chest. Once completed, the Patslide can be pulled out and the bed moved away.

The motion of the lateral transfer can be scary for patients who often cannot visualise how high they are and where the edge of the surfaces are. A clear explanation and some reassurance of how far and in which direction they will be moving should prevent the patient from panicking when the movement begins.

Other products which can support the lateral transfer are available and can be of benefit where workflow is particularly high or patients are commonly bariatric. These are generally more expensive, such as air-assisted tools, which support some of the weight of the patient by allowing them to hover as the lateral transfer is performed.

DANGEROUS OR PROBLEMATIC SITUATIONS

It is not always the movement itself that causes the potential danger, but rather the situation itself. This section will consider some of the common problems a practitioner may be faced with in their daily working environment.

Hoists

One useful piece of equipment which has yet to be mentioned is the hoist. This may have a role to play in manoeuvring the patient from the floor onto a surface or from a chair to a bed/table or vice versa. In the imaging or radiotherapy department, the hoist can become useful in complex cases where other methods may not be suitable, e.g. if a table is of a fixed height and cannot be adjusted to a suitable position for a patient to safely sit onto.

Hoists are not however commonly used on an everyday basis and this can create unfamiliarity with the required procedures. Each hoist is very individual in design. Patients also place themselves in a very vulnerable position when being hoisted and must trust the skill and experience of the staff operating the hoist. Errors can easily be made if brakes are left on during an ascent or descent, which could lead to the equipment becoming unbalanced. Furthermore, the use of an incorrectly sized sling can result in the patient's safety being seriously compromised once they are raised. As such, the use of a hoist should be limited to a hoist team which has received adequate training and has regular practice in its use.

Log rolls

Log rolls are performed when there is a need to support and maintain the alignment of the patient's spine. This can be due to a chronic condition or as a result of a recent injury where the extent of damage is not yet known. In either case, the procedure requires careful handling and control with teamwork being paramount.

The procedure requires a team of 4–5 people, all of whom should be skilled in the movement. The lead person will take responsibility for the head and neck; this is likely to be a doctor. They will ensure that all team members are clear about individual roles and ready before proceeding to give any instructions. The principle is to perform a smooth and coordinated patient roll from their back to their side and commands are given as the patient moves both onto their side and back into a resting position again. The movement can be used in conjunction with physical examinations of the patient's back and during lateral transfers using a Patslide. This movement should not be attempted unless you feel confident to take part and have a good understanding of the procedure.

Bariatric patients

Epidemiological studies in the Western world indicate that the number of bariatric patients is increasing. Extremely heavy patients can present a number of manual handling challenges with regard to their treatment and management. Failure to address these situations may lead to patients and staff requiring increased medical or healthcare intervention, following incidents in the workplace. Handling risks can be minimised by ensuring that appropriate and specialist manual handling equipment is available as soon as is reasonably practicable without compromising patient dignity.

Every piece of equipment used to support patients, such as beds, trolleys, chairs, hoists and slings, has a Safe Working Load (SWL). The specialist equipment we use, including the MRI, CT and radiotherapy treatment couches is no exception. It is imperative that the SWL is not exceeded, as it will affect the stability and function of the equipment. For much of this equipment, both the patient weight and width should be taken into account.

Bariatric patients can mobilise either using mobile walking devices or lifts. A device needs to be operated within the correct weight limit and a risk assessment should always precede any procedure. Slings need to be the right size and have the right safe working load. If they do not fit properly, they can cause pain and discomfort for the patient.

Equipment suggestions for bariatric transfers include:

- Crutches that take up to 25 stones (159 kg)
- Walking frames that take up to 50 stones (317 kg)
- Gait trainers (taking up to 300 kg) can be an invaluable aid to rehabilitation of the bariatric patient
- Gantry systems can take up to 500 kg and be easily moved
- Specialised bariatric slings, not just an ordinary sling in larger sizes
- Sliding sheets for sling application.

The falling patient

Falling patients present a risk not only to themselves but to those who care for and handle them. Most falls can be successfully managed by preventing their occurrence in the first place and risk assessment lies at the heart of this process. For example, when mobilising a patient, the correct handling techniques and walking aids should be used, and the environment should be prepared to minimise distractions or possible hazards. If the patient is falling and cannot be instructed to stand, they must be lowered to the ground or allowed to fall without putting the handler at risk of injury. The patient must not be held or supported in any way which prevents the handler from releasing them. The handler must avoid any method of support that allows the patient to grab hold of them. The handler must not rush to rescue or attempt to catch a patient. This is very dangerous and can result in serious injury to the handler.

UNSAFE HANDLING PRACTICES TO AVOID

The following types of patient transfer or lift are unsafe and using them could not only result in disciplinary action for those involved but could cause serious harm to both the patient and handler. They are mentioned here so that you may be aware of *don'ts* in the workplace, which unfortunately are sometimes still encountered.

UNSAFE! – The *'drag lift'* is any way of handling a patient where the handler places a hand or arm under the patient's axilla (armpit). Common situations where a drag lift has been used includes moving the patient up a bed; sitting the patient up from a supine position; bringing the patient from sitting to standing and moving the patient from one seating position to another, e.g. from a wheelchair onto a treatment or imaging table. So why has this lift been banned in the workplace? Despite it being quick and at first sight easy to perform for the handler, it is not without its risk to them. The weight of the patient is carried a distance away from the handler's body and involves a twisting action. This creates a shearing force across the handler's shoulders, which could result in ligament and muscle damage. Practitioners using this lift will find that the patient relies upon them for all of their support as they have moved their arm into a position where they are powerless to help. For the patient, it is both uncomfortable and painful. The patient's shoulder is at risk of joint dislocation, brachial plexus and soft tissue damage. The friction from the dragging motion contributes to the formation of pressure sores and there is a risk of dropping the patient, causing injuries. This lift is often resorted to as a time-saving measure by rushed staff who are unwilling to wait for the patient to perform the task independently.

UNSAFE! – The *orthodox or 'cradle' lift* is dangerous as it requires the practitioner to lift and twist while leaning forward, multiplying the effect of any load. The orthodox lift involves two carers placing their hands beneath the arms or behind the back and underneath the client's leg. This manoeuvre involves the carer lifting at arm's length, while twisting at the trunk and holding the load away from the carer's centre of gravity causing a great risk of injury to the carer. This is likely to cause injury to the client's shoulder's and knees.

UNSAFE! – The *shoulder or 'Australian' slide/lift* is a manoeuvre whereby a client can be moved onto a bed by two carers working together. When using this technique, both carers face in the opposite direction to the client. The carers have their inner knee on the bed and their outer foot on the floor. They then bend forward to place their inside shoulders under the client's upper arm, prior to carrying out the slide/lift. This technique results in danger to the carers due to an uneven loading, with force being applied to one shoulder only. Clients can also find the manoeuvre invasive of their personal space. Injury can occur to the client due to the carer's shoulder being placed beneath their underarm, resulting in soft tissue damage and possibly injury to ribs. Shearing and friction can occur to the client's sacral area and heels.

UNSAFE! – The *front assisted one carer pivot transfer ('bearhug')*. This technique involves transferring a client from one seated position to another by holding and lifting the client by a transfer belt, bear hug or otherwise. It is a manoeuvre which involves a high risk of twisting for the carer. There are risks of unstable postures for both client and carer. The carer has difficulty in controlling the amount of effort required to carry out this technique, and there is a risk of patient collapse which may injure both the client and carer; this technique should therefore be avoided.

 Other dangerous practices:

- The use of poles with a canvas is also no longer considered to be acceptable as it is a whole body lift
- Lifts involving the patient putting their arms around the practitioner's neck bring a high risk of neck injuries to the hander should the patient collapse

SOME TIPS FOR EVERYDAY BACK CARE

Vary your posture and aim to stand for some of the day. Remember to do exercises whenever you have the opportunity. Exercise is the most important thing you can do to reduce your risk of developing a back problem or to manage an existing problem. Regular exercise will:

- Develop strong muscles
- Increase flexibility in the joints
- Keep you fit
- Make you feel good
- Release your body's natural pain killers – endorphins

Avoid lifting and sustained head-down work when using a computer for extended lengths of time.

Common causes of back problems include:

- Poor workplace design and inadequate/infrequent training
- Extended periods in fixed positions
- Lifestyle: lack of exercise, sagging mattresses, poorly supported armchairs and sofas, poor lifting and carrying methods
- Repetition of poor posture

Common effects of back problems include:

- Loss of ability to walk, sit, bend or lift
- Incontinence
- Intractable pain
- Depressions
- Sciatic pain
- Loss of sensation/numbness in limbs and feet.

Advice for back pain used to be to rest and not do anything until the pain had gone. This is not helpful as muscles become weak and joints become stiff. Recovery becomes prolonged as it is harder to get moving and then the mood is affected due to inactivity.

The following are some suggested exercises to strengthen the spine to improve or maintain fitness for manual handling tasks.

Do not continue these exercises if there is any discomfort whatsoever!

Sitting exercises

Try and do these exercises as often as possible through the day, and repeat each 10 times. These exercises are designed to relieve the tension on your upper back and neck.

Leg lifts

Put both feet on the floor. Make sure your lower back is supported against the back of the chair. Lift your leg until the knee is fully extended, flex your foot, and point your toes towards the ceiling. Hold for a count of 5. Lower the left leg and repeat with the right leg. Repeat each exercise 5 times.

Shoulder shrugs

Slowly rotate your shoulders in a circular motion, first forward, up towards your ears, backward and down. After 10 forward circles, reverse and circle back, up, forward and down.

Head turns

Tuck your chin down, trying to make a double chin. Turn your head slowly to the right, hold for 5 seconds then turn back to the start position and then turn slowly to the left.

On your feet

These are designed to stretch and strengthen your back. Try and do each 10 times.

Pelvic tilts

Tighten your abdominal muscles and tuck your buttocks under while tilting the pelvis up and forward. Hold for a count of 10 then relax.

Arm stretches

Gently stretch your left arm above your head as far as you can without straining. Hold for a count of five and repeat with the right arm.

Wall slides

Place both heels 20 centimetres from the wall, facing away from the wall. Let your arms rest across your chest and slide down the wall until you are in a semi-sitting position, keeping your heels on the ground and maintaining the normal curves of the spine. Hold this position for as long as you can (the length of a nursery rhyme is a good guide).

At home

Stretching and flexibility exercises at home will help you reduce the risk of injury at work. Try and hold each for a count of 10, and repeat 10 times.

Pelvic tilts

Lie on your back, knees flexed, feet flat on the floor. Tighten your abdominal muscles, squeeze your buttocks together, and flatten your back against the floor.

Trunk flexion

Lying on your back, put the foot of your left leg flat on the floor and pull the right knee up to your chest. Keep your lower back on the floor and pull your right knee on to your chest. Repeat with the left.

Modified sit-ups

Raise your head and reach your fingers towards the knees, simultaneously tightening the abdominal muscles.

Back bends

In the press-up position, lying face down, try to straighten your elbows while keeping your hips in contact with the floor.

Back extensions

Lie face down with arms by your side. Raise your head and shoulders off the floor.

Back extension and flexion

Kneeling on all fours, shoulders and knees at a comfortable width apart, arch and hollow the back slowly.

Want to know more?

Core stability and strength is now recognised as one of the best ways to work your body and improve back, joint and postural problems. Why not join a Pilates or yoga class, or a core stability class in your local gym? These use controlled movements that re-educate the whole body. The body is healthy when the muscles working around the spine are long and strong. Finding a qualified instructor is crucial, but these classes will help you to keep your back healthy for a long career in healthcare. So why not give it a try?

KEY POINTS

The golden rules of handling

1. ASSESS the situation
2. PLAN your move
3. PREPARE
4. Keep your spine in normal position line and bend at the hips and knees
5. Transfer your body weight to move any load and always move a load within your base of support.
6. Keep as close to the load as possible and have a firm hold
7. Have a firm and stable base; move within your base; check footwear and clothing allow movement
8. Brace your abdominals but don't hold your breath
9. Avoid twisting and jerky movements
10. Coordinate any techniques and only when ready carry out the move

Section | 5 |

Infection control

Chapter | 15 |

Immunology and infectious diseases

Suzanne Easton

INTRODUCTION

The immune system provides internal and external mechanisms that the body utilises to prevent the 'invasion' of pathogens. These pathogens range from the smallest virus surviving within the hosts cells through to large parasitic worms living in the large intestine. The first-line of defence is through physical barriers in the form of the skin and mucous membranes. If this barrier is breached then the immune system takes over in an attempt to destroy the pathogens. This can be generalised or cell-specific. Pathogens are evolving and the immune system adapts and develops to address this evolution. The immune system can be diminished by illness and can also react in an inappropriate manner giving the individual allergies and conditions specific to the immune response.

PARTS OF THE IMMUNE SYSTEM

The majority of cells involved in immunity are derived from components within the bone marrow. Direct contact with epithelial cells, fibroblasts and macrophages will allow differentiation of the cells into different types of blood cells. These cells circulate in the blood and have the ability to enter tissues as required. The formation of these cells is termed *haematopoiesis* and occurs from specialised haemopoietic stem cells in adult bone marrow and the liver and spleen in the fetus and neonate.

Cells and molecules of the innate immune system

Phagocytes make up the majority of white blood cells and are known as *neutrophils*. Other phagocytes include *monocytes* and *macrophages*. Monocytes circulate in the blood and settle in the tissues as macrophages. Through a process known as *chemotaxis*, the phagocytes are attracted to the site of the microbe. The phagocytes adhere to the cell and then ingest it to cause its destruction. This is known as *phagocytosis* (Fig. 15.1). A coating of antibody will improve the ability of a phagocyte to destroy the microbe.

Natural killer cells (large granular lymphocytes) are found in all tissues of the body, but primarily the blood, and provide protection against viruses and some tumours. As the virus alters the surface of the outer molecules of the cells, the natural killer cells are able to attach and bind to the cell and then release perforins to destroy the cell. The natural killer cells also release interferon gamma which protects adjacent cells from infection.

Mast cells are found in connective tissues and similarly formed, and functioning basophils are found in the blood. Mast cells are usually closely associated with blood vessels and are found in the subepithelial areas of the gastrointestinal, genitourinary and respiratory tracts. In the cytoplasm of both these cell types, there are large electron dense granules which are released when the mast cells or basophils bind with certain substances. This results in the release of histamine and cytokines. The release of histamine results in vasodilation and, in severe cases, can lead to a severe anaphylactic response.

Langerhans cells, follicular dendritic cells and interdigitating cells provide the link between the innate and

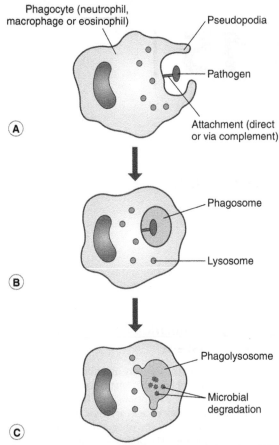

Phagocyte (neutrophil, macrophage or eosinophil)

Pseudopodia

Pathogen

Attachment (direct or via complement)

(A)

Phagosome

Lysosome

(B)

Phagolysosome

Microbial degradation

(C)

Figure 15.1 Phagocytosis. *(Reprinted from Kitchen G, Griffin J. Crash course: immunology and haematology, 3rd edn. 2007. Mosby, with permission from Elsevier.)*

adaptive immune systems. They are similar in appearance to the dendrites of the nervous system. These cells identify antigens in the innate immune response and initiate the adaptive immune response.

Eosinophils, platelets and erythrocytes also have a role in the innate immune system. Eosinophils are primarily used for the extracellular killing of parasites which cannot be phagocytised. They also contain histamines to balance the effects of the histamine released by mast cells. Erythrocytes are important for the removal of immune complexes in long-term infections and some autoimmune diseases.

Protection and control against infection is provided by proteins known as the *complement system*. These proteins can be activated by the microbes or through the adaptive immune system. The complement system can cause acute inflammation, assist in the attachment of a microbe to the phagocyte, kill the microbe or attract neutrophils to the site of infection.

Acute phase proteins are a group of plasma proteins and limit the damage to tissues caused by trauma, infection or malignancy. They are usually produced in the liver in response to certain cytokines or microbial stimulus. These proteins ensure the optimal functioning of the complement system.

Cytokines are small molecules and, depending on their source, will be called *interleukins*, *monokines*, *lymphokines* or *chemokines*.

Cells and molecules of the adaptive immune system

Lymphocytes are key to the function of the adaptive immune system, providing specificity and memory. There are two types of lymphocytes involved in the response: *B cells* and *T cells*. These have similar structures, but have different antigen receptors and molecules on the surface to enable interaction with other cells. T lymphocytes are produced in the thymus and each cell has receptors specific to just one antigen. Mature T cells migrate to secondary lymphoid tissues (spleen, mucosa-associated lymphoid tissue or lymph nodes) and mediate protection. B cells are formed in the bone marrow and are also found in secondary lymphoid tissues. With the support of the T cells, the B cells will react to antigens, producing either memory cells or plasma cells, which produce and secrete antibodies.

Antibodies are sometimes known as *immunoglobulins*. They are specific to certain antigens and fall into five categories (IgM, IgG, IgA, IgE and IgD). The antibodies have a high affinity for the antigen, binding tightly to the antigen. The affinity is higher in antibodies produced in a memory response when compared with those produced in a primary response. The classification of the antibodies determines their function and their response to other cells:

IgM – Immunoglobulin produced as the primary immune response or first exposure

IgG – Main circulating immunoglobulin for secondary immune response

IgA – Secreted immunoglobulin in bodily fluids at mucosal surfaces

IgE – Response to parasites and inappropriate response causing allergy

IgD – Antigen expressed on B-cells, however its role in not known.

IMMUNE DEFENCE

The innate immune system provides the first-line of defence and occurs rapidly after the introduction of a

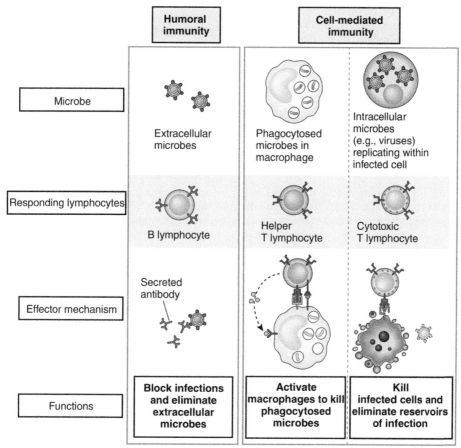

Figure 15.2 Types of adaptive immunity. *(Reprinted from Abbas A, Lichtman A. Basic immunology, 3rd edn. 2006. W.B. Saunders with permission from Elsevier.)*

pathogen. This system provides the acute inflammatory response taking place between hours and minutes. There is some specificity for certain microbes, but there is no 'memory' of previous encounters with a specific microbe. In contrast, the adaptive immune system is very specific, with memory, but takes time to develop and react. The innate system utilises natural barriers such as the skin and mucous membranes, phagocytes and natural killer cells, soluble mediators and pattern recognition molecules.

In contrast, the adaptive (or acquired) immune system uses lymphocytes, B- and T-cell receptors and secreted molecules such as antibodies (Fig. 15.2).

The two systems work together through cell contact and the interaction of cytokines and chemokines. There is also sharing of some cells and molecules from one system to the other. The 'memory' involved in the adaptive immune response is caused by the presence of a large number of antigen-specific cells. These are formed through the response of lymphocytes with receptors to the presence of an antigen. The lymphocytes bind to the antigen which triggers the production of clone cells specific to the antigen. These cells react with the antigen, eliminating or neutralising it.

KEY PRINCIPLES OF INFECTIVE MECHANISMS

Infective agents

Infection may be autogenous (self-infection) or exogenous where the source is external. Autogenous spread involves infection from one part of the body to another. Examples include *Escherichia coli* (*E. coli*), which can be spread from the anus to the urinary tract or the spread of infection through the blood from one area to another.

Exogenous spread can be subdivided into direct and indirect transmission. Direct transmission involves direct contact between individuals spreading the infection; indirect spread does not require contact between individuals. Methods of indirect spread include:

- Air-borne infection
- Inanimate objects
- Ingestion of infected materials
- Contaminated surgical instruments or needles.

Bacteria

Most bacteria are unicellular organisms, although some may be clusters or chains (Table 15.1). The majority do not require a host to survive and are known as *saprophytes*. Some do require a host and may be commensal, where they co-exist with the host; pathogens where they invade and damage the host; anaerobic which do not require oxygen to survive and aerobic which require oxygen to survive. Identification of bacteria is made on their reaction to different types of stains. Bacteria cause damage to their host in two ways:

1. The breakdown of the host's defence mechanisms, usually through the release of enzymes that disrupt the cell membrane
2. The release of toxins as the bacteria dies or the release of endotoxins as the bacteria multiplies.

Viruses

Viruses are small infectious agents (Table 15.1). They measure between 20 and 400 nm. They have a central core of nucleic acid which is surrounded by a capsid. This is known as a *virion*. The nucleic acid will determine the classification of the virus. Ribonucleic acid (RNA) viruses include rhinoviruses responsible for the common cold and deoxyribonucleic acid (DNA) viruses, which include the herpes virus responsible for cold sores.

Fungi

These are usually in the form of spores and require specific conditions to survive on the host (Table 15.1). The most common fungi are *Candida albicans* which depends on warm moist conditions to survive, resulting in thrush.

Protozoa

Protozoa are organisms which have a complex life cycle which ensures transmission and survival (Table 15.1). Infection with protozoa is intracellular and can become chronic due to their ability to escape into the cytoplasm after phagocytosis.

BARRIERS AGAINST INFECTION

There are three key barriers to infection: physical or mechanical, chemical and biological in the form of normal flora. These barriers are part of the body's innate defences.

Physical

Physical barriers are usually in the form of mucosal membranes and the skin. Close fitting cells prevent most pathogens from entering the body. This is assisted further by the rinsing action of tears, saliva and urine, preventing colonisation of epithelial tissues. Within the respiratory tract, mucous secretions trap microorganisms which are then expelled through coughing, sneezing and the movement of cilia. This is known as the *mucociliary escalator* (Fig. 15.3). Epithelial cells in the gastrointestinal and genitourinary tracts also provide a barrier against infection.

Chemical

Within the stomach and vagina, the growth of microorganisms are reduced by the acidic pH of secretions. The pH of the skin is maintained by the lactic acid in sebum and lysozyme, an enzyme found in saliva, sweat and tears, which can destroy microorganisms in the area of the secretion. Small peptides called *defensins*, fatty acids and antibodies will also provide chemical protection against pathogens.

Biological

Non-pathogenic bacteria are found on the surfaces of epithelial cells. These do not cause illness in the individual. They protect the body by fighting pathogenic bacteria for nutrients and sites for attachment and also through their ability to produce antibacterial substances. The biological protection can be disrupted by antibiotics and can lead to infection.

Active immunity

The process of active immunity requires the individual to be infected or vaccinated with a specific pathogen. This involves the combination of adaptive and innate immunity. The active response to the infection results in resistance to later exposure and infection.

Passive immunity

Passive immunity is immunity acquired from another source that stimulates the adaptive response mechanism.

Table 15.1 Some important human pathogens

Organism	Disease	Organism	Disease
Bacteria		Mumps virus	Mumps
Staphylococcus spp.	Boils, septicaemia, food poisoning	Respiratory syncytial virus	Bronchiolitis
Streptococcus spp.	Tonsillitis, erysipelas, scarlet fever, pneumonia	Orthomyxoviruses	Influenza
		Rhinoviruses, coronaviruses	Common cold
Bacillus anthracis	Anthrax	Rhabdovirus	Rabies
Corynebacterium diphtheriae	Diphtheria	Papillomavirus	Warts
Clostridium spp.	Tetanus, gas gangrene, botulism	Herpes simplex virus	Herpes
		Varicella-zoster virus	Chickenpox, shingles
Neisseria spp.	Meningitis, gonorrhoea	Epstein–Barr virus	Infectious mononucleosis
Escherichia coli	Urinary tract infection, gastroenteritis	Human immunodeficiency virus	AIDS
Salmonella spp.	Enteric fever, food poisoning	Flavivirus	Yellow fever, dengue
Shigella spp.	Dysentery	Rotavirus	Gastroenteritis
Vibrio cholerae	Cholera	**Fungi**	
Proteus spp.	Urinary tract and would infection	*Candida albicans*	Thrush, dermatitis
Haemophilus influenzae	Meningitis, pneumonia	Dermatophytes (e.g. *Trichophyton* spp.)	Ringworm
Bordetella pertussis	Whooping cough	*Cryptococcus neoformans*	Meningitis
Yersinia pestis	Plague	**Protozoa**	
Brucella spp.	Undulant fever	*Plasmodia* spp.	Malaria
Mycobacterium spp.	Tuberculosis, leprosy	*Leishmania* spp.	Leishmaniasis
Legionella spp.	Legionnaire's disease	*Toxoplasma gondii*	Toxoplasmosis
Treponema pallidum	Syphilis	*Trypanosoma* spp.	Trypanosomiasis
Chlamydia spp.	Trachoma, pneumonia, genital tract infection	**Helminths**	
Viruses		Cestodes (e.g. *Taenia* and *Echinococcus* spp.)	Cysticercosis, hydatid disease
Polioviruses	Poliomyelitis	Trematodes (e.g. *Schistosoma* spp.)	Schistosomiasis (bilharzia)
Hepatitis viruses (e.g. A, B and C)	Hepatitis	Nematodes (e.g. *Ascaris, Necator, Wucheria, Onchocerca, Dracunculus* and *Toxocara* spp.)	Ascariasis, hookworm disease, filariasis, river blindness, guinea worm disease, toxocariasis (larva migrans)
Rubivirus	Rubella		
Measles virus	Measles		

Spp. indicates that multiple species cause disease. (Reprinted with permission from Todd I, Spickett G. Lecture Notes: Immunology, 5th edn. 2005. Published by Wiley-Blackwell.)

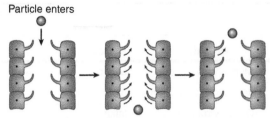

Particle enters

Figure 15.3 The mucociliary escalator. *(Reprinted from Immunology, 2nd edn. Lydyard P, Whelan A, Fanger M. ©2004, Cengage Publishers, reproduced by permission of Taylor & Francis Books UK.)*

This can be naturally from the mother while nursing, or artificially from another source such as the injection of immune serum. Immunity will be achieved for the lifespan of the antibodies, but it does not produce life-long immunity, which is achieved with active immunity.

SPECIFIC IMMUNE MECHANISMS

Vaccination

Vaccination is a form of active immunisation. This will provide rapid immunity to a specific pathogen. The individual will demonstrate a primary immune response with clonal expansion of B and T cells. This in turn leads to the formation of memory cells. Subsequent exposure to the pathogen will result in a secondary immune response.

Vaccines fall into six categories determined by a number of key features:

1. Live attenuated (oral polio, rubella, measles, mumps)
2. Killed (influenza)
3. Subunit (non-conjugated pneumococcal)
4. Recombinant (hepatitis B surface antigen)
5. Toxoids (diphtheria, tetanus)
6. Conjugates (meningococcal, *Haemophilus influenzae* type B (Hib))

The type of vaccine will be determined by: the level of immunity required; the response by the body to the introduction of the pathogen; the cost; the stability of the vaccine during storage and introduction; length of immunity period and finally, the side-effects caused by the vaccination itself. Not all vaccines are 100% effective and some individuals will not react adequately. This is not always a problem, as the risk of contact with the infection source is reduced if a large proportion of the population is immunised. Some vaccinations are given in combination to ensure an adequate immune response. Vaccines from the subunit group will not invoke an immune response in

isolation and are given in combination to ensure a reaction. Vaccinations usually require more than one does to ensure an immune response occurs. The first dose results in the production of IgM, with the second booster resulting in the rapid production of IgG. Between the initial and booster injections the production of antibodies is maintained ensuring the production of B and T cells.

Unfortunately, a number of infectious diseases have not had vaccines successfully developed yet. This is due to the fact that the key antigen does not provide a protective immune response. The development of antigens in combination with other substances (conjugates) has recently resulted in the successful introduction of the Hib vaccination. Infectious diseases with no satisfactory vaccines include human immunodeficiency virus, herpes simplex virus, tuberculosis, cholera, leprosy, the common cold and all parasitic infections.

HYPERSENSITIVITY REACTIONS

Hypersensitivity is the occurrence of an excessive and inappropriate inflammatory response to an antigen. This is a normal immunological process, it just occurs at the wrong time or place. Hypersensitivity occurs in response to a normally harmless substance such as pollen or peanuts, an infection that is not being cleared or an autoantigen. Reactions are classified into four types: I, II, III and IV (see below).

Type I

This reaction causes immediate degranulation of mast cells and basophils. It is caused by an overproduction of IgE to an environmental substance, but initial exposure must occur prior to the reaction to initiate sensitivity (Fig. 15.4). Type I reactions include:

- Pollens causing hay fever
- Reaction to house dust mites giving allergic asthma
- Systemic reaction to penicillin or peanuts resulting in anaphylaxis.

Type II

This is sometimes called *antibody mediated hypersensitivity*. This occurs when antibodies target the cell surface resulting in cell destruction. This is seen in incompatible blood transfusions, autoimmune haemolytic anaemia and haemolytic disease in the newborn.

Type III

This physiological reaction results in the production of lattices composed of antibodies and antigens known as an *immune complex*. The immune complex is broken up and transported by red blood cells to the spleen where they are

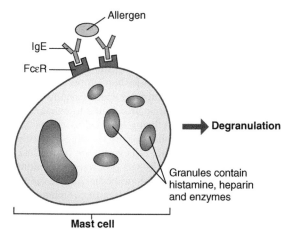

Figure 15.4 The immune mechanism of type I hypersensitivity. *(Reprinted from Kitchen G, Griffin J. Crash course: immunology and haematology, 3rd edn. 2007. Mosby, with permission from Elsevier.)*

phagocytised. Examples of this reaction are seen following intradermal or subcutaneous vaccination in individuals who have appropriate levels of circulating antibodies, resulting in reddening and inflammation of the injection site.

Type IV

This is a delayed response and is important for the removal of intracellular pathogens. This type of reaction is most commonly seen in the form of contact dermatitis to metals. Skin patch testing is used to determine the antigen causing the reaction.

ANAPHYLAXIS

Anaphylaxis is a severe type I hypersensitivity reaction affecting the respiratory and circulatory systems. During a reaction, the body mistakes the proteins within the substance causing the reaction with harmful antigens and releases a large number of antibodies. This triggers the release of histamines resulting in a number of physiological changes including vasodilation, reduction in blood pressure, increased fluid production and the relaxation of muscles. The key triggers for a reaction are medications, certain foods and radiographic contrast medium. Adrenaline (epinephrine) is required to halt the reaction with antihistamines and corticosteroids required in most cases. Individuals who have had an anaphylactic reaction should take extreme care and avoid known triggers. They should carry an EpiPen or similar adrenaline auto-injector to treat further severe reactions if there is accidental exposure to a trigger.

AUTOIMMUNE RESPONSES

An autoimmune response is an immune response against self antigens. It occurs when an autoimmune response leads to tissue damage. Contributing factors include: age, gender, infection and genetics. Autoantibodies are seen more often in older people, and women are at a greater risk. The key factor in the development of autoimmune disease is an environmental trigger or the inheritance of susceptible genes. Clusters of antigen-specific autoimmune disease are seen in some families and infections such as *streptococci* and malaria have been linked to specific autoimmune diseases. Certain drugs are also believed to trigger an autoimmune response, which resolves when the drugs are discontinued. Individuals with a reduced immune system are also more likely to develop autoimmune disease. It may be organ-specific or systemic. Systemic autoimmune disease is seen in systemic lupus erythematosus. It is also seen in rheumatoid arthritis, vitiligo, multiple sclerosis and type I diabetes. Organ-specific diseases include myasthenia gravis and Graves' disease. The main aim of the treatment for an autoimmune disease is to suppress the autoimmune response. This is achieved using non-steroidal anti-inflammatory drugs or corticosteroids. Cytotoxic drugs, ciclosporin or steroid sparing agents may also be used to remove lymphocytes. Some self-antigens may not be able to function properly and in these cases, replacement may be required. One example is the use of insulin in insulin-dependent diabetes.

The mechanisms involved in an autoimmune response fall into a number of distinct categories:

- Tissue damage caused in the same way as a 'normal' protective response through phagocytosis, interference with the cell function or the activation of complement
- Cell destruction caused by the antibodies binding to self-cells causing damage or destruction
- Antibodies can interfere with or enhance the function of a self-cell. One example is overstimulation of the thyroid in Graves' disease.

IMMUNOLOGY RELEVANT TO CANCER PATIENTS

The body's response to tumour cells is very similar but the inverse of the reaction to a transplanted cell. The body reacts to the non-microbial cells as the immune system identifies them as foreign. This is due to the presence of antigens on the surface of the tumour. Tumour-associated antigens are found on normal cells and less commonly tumour-specific antigens are found. These antigens can be used to differentiate between normal cells and tumour cells. They can also be used to identify the origin of the tumour as they demonstrate the same characteristics as the normal cells or origin. This information can be used to assist in the planning of any treatments. Tumour cells can be produced as a result of mutated cellular proteins, products of an oncogenic virus, incorrectly formed molecules or from oncogenes or tumour suppressor genes. A tumour is differentiated from a normal cell by a number of properties. These include:

- A lack of response to regulation
- Invasiveness
- Changes in antigens.

It is believed that normal killer cells will identify and destroy tumour cells as they develop, however this reaction is decreased in individuals with a reduced immunity. A response to tumour cells occurs in a similar way to a normal infection from antigens; however, this response is not enough to prevent the rapid development of the tumour even in immunocompetent individuals. Some tumours are able to evade detection by the immune system (immunosuppressive). These tumours are known as *antigen loss variants*, as they stop expressing the antigens that are causing the immune response. This allows the tumour to continue growing and spreading. Vaccinations against tumours associated with viruses are now becoming available. Some 70% of cases of cervical carcinoma are caused by the human papillomavirus (HPV) and all females are now offered vaccination in the UK at the age of 12 years. While the vaccination will not treat cervical cancer or treat an existing infection, it will prevent the initial infection from the virus.

Immunosuppression

Immunodeficiency can be caused by tumours, particularly those originating in the immune system. Examples of these are myeloma, leukaemia or lymphoma. The tumour can affect molecules regulating the immune response or alter the release of immunosuppressive molecules. Chemotherapy treatment and radiotherapy can destroy stem cells, lymphocytes and other cells important in the immune response resulting in immunodeficiency. Patients with immunosuppression/immunodeficiency will present with a non-classical presentation of illness as there is a subdued or lacking immune response.

Immunotherapy

Immunotherapy aims to provide a direct attack on tumour cells by modulating the immune system and directing it to tumour specific antigens. This in effect provides the patient with immunity against their own tumour. Immunotherapy provides treatment in some types of tumour

and is less demanding on the patient as a whole and results in less injury to the patient when compared with the effects of radiotherapy or chemotherapy. Treatment focuses on the stimulation of the immune system, vaccinating the patient with their own tumour cells or antigens. Cytokines are used to develop immunity and are used in conjunction with tumour specific regimes. Lymphocytes from a patient may be cultured to enhance the natural killer cells before being returned to the patient. Monocytes may also be cultured with cytokines, activating macrophage-activated killer cells which are reintroduced to the patient. Tumours may also be treated with monoclonal antibodies (mAbs). The antibodies kill the tumour cells through phagocytosis, activation of complement or apoptosis. This is a rapidly developing area of oncology and immunology with new drugs becoming available. Immunotherapy is not just limited to treatment of malignancy. A drug called Denosumab is used in the treatment of osteoporosis and a range of treatments for rheumatoid arthritis are available.

INFECTIOUS DISEASES ENCOUNTERED IN RADIOGRAPHIC PRACTICE

Pneumonia

Pneumonia is the acute inflammation of the lungs caused most commonly by *Streptococcus pneumonia*. Other causes of pneumonia are virus, *Haemophilus influenzae*, *Staphylococcus pyogenes*, *Escherichia coli* and *Legionella pneumophila* (Legionnaire's disease). It is transmitted by droplet infection and gains entry through the lower respiratory tract. The organism finds this easier if the mucociliary escalator or other defences are weak. This is especially the case if the individual has had a viral infection, poor cough reflex or has excess alcohol intake. Patients seen within the hospital setting often have underlying lowered immunity and then develop secondary pneumonia. Once the organism is in the lungs, it will induce an acute inflammatory response and this results in the production of fluid (exudate) and pus, which will fill the alveoli. This results in reduced gas exchange and a lowered PO_2. The collection of exudate and pus in the alveoli is known as *consolidation* and results in dullness to percussion. The consolidation may be either spread diffusely, known as *bronchopneumonia* or limited to specific lobes, known as *lobar pneumonia.*

Lobar pneumonia is most commonly seen in otherwise healthy young adults and is caused by *pneumococci* or *streptococci*-type bacteria with a sudden onset. Radiographically, the infection is localised to individual lobes. Infected lobes appear dense and opaque due to the consolidation. Treatment is usually effective with antibiotics with exudate being absorbed by the alveoli walls.

Bronchopneumonia is more common and seen primarily in the elderly. It takes advantage of the body's already lowered immunity and will infect the lungs bilaterally, usually in the lower portion. The alveoli become filled with exudate and pus will build up in infected areas. This results in the destruction of lung tissue. The patient will present with a raised temperature, productive cough and green, purulent sputum. This can cause chronic damage to the lungs and can be a cause of death in many patients with other terminal illnesses.

Tuberculosis

Tuberculosis (TB) is a bacterial infection, spread by the inhalation of droplets of saliva from an infected individual. The bacteria responsible are *Mycobacterium tuberculosis*. While it is spread through droplets from coughs and sneezes, extended exposure is necessary to become infected. It is usually transmitted between members of the same family or home or those who have a lowered immunity. There are a number of factors which will increase the risk of infection. These are:

- Family member who is already infected
- Travel to areas of the world where TB is common
- Being part of a community with origins in an area of the world where TB is common
- Lowered immunity
- Elderly or very young
- Extended, close contact with an infected individual
- Poor health/lifestyle

Once the bacteria have entered the body it will take time to develop symptoms. Symptoms are usually related to the development of the infection within the lungs. Symptoms of pulmonary tuberculosis include:

- Worsening cough and breathlessness
- Productive cough with phlegm which becomes bloody
- Weight loss
- High temperature
- Tiredness.

Less commonly, TB is seen outside of the lung region. This is due to the spread of the bacteria. TB can be found in bones and joints, lymph nodes, gastrointestinal tract, urogenital tract and the nervous system.

The diagnosis of pulmonary tuberculosis is through phlegm and sputum samples and the use of chest X-rays to support the results. Active pulmonary TB will be seen as areas of consolidation or cavities in the upper lobes. There may also be mediastinal or hilar lymphadenopathy. Old inactive TB will be seen as pulmonary nodules in the hilar or upper lobe regions of the lungs. TB in other regions of the body can be diagnosed through the use of other imaging techniques, depending on the region and the selection of the most suitable technique.

Latent TB can be identified using the Mantoux test. This involves injecting PPD tuberculin into the skin. If sensitivity occurs, then there is latent TB within the body. A severe reaction would suggest active TB. A mild skin reaction may occur if the individual has had the Bacillus Calmette–Guérin (BCG) vaccination. A newer screening test called the 'interferon gamma release assay' (IGRA) is now being introduced to identify latent TB in individuals who have had a positive Mantoux test; those being screened on entry to the UK; those who are starting treatment that will reduce immunity and healthcare workers.

Treatment for pulmonary TB utilises a combination of antibiotics for 6 months. This will destroy both the active bacteria and any dormant bacteria that may become active in the future. It may take several weeks for symptoms to decrease. The antibiotics used for uncomplicated TB are isoniazid and rifampicin for 6 months supported by pyrazinamide and ethambutol for the first 2 months. Latent TB is not always treated as the individual does not have symptoms and in older patients, the treatment may cause liver damage. Extrapulmonary TB can be treated with the same antibiotic combination, but treatment will be continued for a year to ensure the bacteria are destroyed. Individuals with TB in the heart or brain may be prescribed prednisolone, a corticosteroid for 2 weeks. Drug resistant TB is an increasing problem.

Hepatitis

Hepatitis can be caused by alcohol, drugs, other chemicals and viruses. There are a number of forms of hepatitis caused by viral infection. Symptoms are initially very non-descriptive with flu-like symptoms, lack of appetite and a rash. The individual will develop jaundice and at this stage, the initial symptoms may reduce. The jaundice is caused by inflammation and disruption of normal liver cell function and may result in liver necrosis and impaired bile drainage. Care should be taken to prevent infection from needle stick injuries in the workplace and the correct procedures should be followed if an injury is sustained. Prior to commencing work, practitioners should ensure they receive the required vaccinations against hepatitis infection. The most commonly seen types are hepatitis A, B and C, although there are other less common subtypes.

Hepatitis A (HAV) is primarily spread by poor hygiene and is the form seen when contamination has occurred from raw sewage in drinking water. It is an acute condition and once infection has occurred the body produces antibodies to prevent future infection. Initial infection can be prevented through strict personal hygiene and the avoidance of unpeeled or raw foods. Individuals are infectious for 2 weeks before and 1 week after the onset of jaundice and may incubate the virus for up to 28 days. A vaccination against HAV is available that lasts for 10 years.

Hepatitis B is spread by blood-to-blood transfer and is commonly seen through the use of shared needles, tattoos, sexual intercourse and breast-feeding, although the source is not always identified. Previously it had been contracted through blood transfusions, but this has now been eliminated through careful screening. Hepatitis B presents in both a chronic and acute form. The chronic form is seen in individuals who are unable to clear the virus from their bodies. Antibodies are produced but these are not in large enough quantities to clear the virus from the cells. This usually progresses to cirrhosis and may also lead to hepatocellular carcinoma. A lifetime vaccination is available and treatment using a number of regimes is also available, which is effective for some individuals.

Hepatitis C (HCV) is also transmitted through blood-to-blood contamination and can also pass across the placenta. It remains undetected for many years in some individuals and can be asymptomatic. Ultimately, it leads to chronic hepatitis, cirrhosis and individuals are more susceptible to infection from hepatitis A and B. HCV levels can be reduced through the use of a combination of interferon and ribavirin but there is currently no vaccination available.

Clostridium difficile

Clostridium difficile (C-diff) is a Gram-positive bacteria that causes diarrhoea, blood stained stools, fever, abdominal cramps and in severe cases, pseudomembranous colitis. Symptoms are caused by the inflammation of the lining of the large bowel. It is not normally seen in children under the age of 2 years, but is more common in adults over the age of 65 years. C-diff is found normally in the intestine of 2–5% of the adult population and two-thirds of all children, but over-colonisation can occur in individuals who have had the normal balance of flora in the intestine upset by long-term antibiotics. This can occur up to 10 weeks after the end of the antibiotics course. It can also be seen in patients being treated with chemotherapy.

Individuals most vulnerable to C. diff are those who:

- have been treated with broad-spectrum antibiotics
- have had to stay for a long time in a healthcare setting, such as a hospital
- are over 65 years old
- have a serious underlying illness or condition
- have a weakened immune system
- have had many enemas
- have had surgery to the intestine.

C-diff is transmitted through the oral–faecal route with the transmission of spores between individuals and is most commonly transmitted in close social interactions such as those seen in hospitals and nursing homes. The spores are not affected by the acid within the stomach, but react with bile and multiply once they enter the colon. The spores are difficult to eradicate as they remain active on surfaces for long periods of time and are not destroyed with conventional alcohol-based handwashes. The use of gloves, aprons and effective hand-washing with soap and water is effective in preventing transmission. The use of bleach-based cleaning products is even more effective at reducing infection. Patients with suspected C-diff should be nursed on their own with separate toilet facilities. All inpatients in the NHS over the age of 65 years are now routinely screened for C-diff as it can be confused with Norovirus, each having similar symptoms but different treatments. Diagnosis is made through the identification of C-diff toxins within a stool sample from the individual. C-diff is treated with a course of antibiotics, either metronidazole or vancomycin, although this is dependent on the bacteria not developing resistance to the antibiotic regime. The spores also have a protective layer making antibiotic treatment difficult. A failure to treat C-diff with suitable antibiotics can lead to sepsis and perforation and it is for this reason that treatment is started before a positive diagnosis is confirmed. In mild cases, stopping the initial course of antibiotics is enough to allow the body to balance the levels of flora in the intestine and halt the symptoms.

MRSA

MRSA is meticillin-resistant Staphylococcus aureus, a common bacterium found on the skin, which is resistant to antibiotics including meticillin. The infection enters the body through a break in the skin, multiplying causing symptoms. The symptoms will vary depending on the site of infection but usually involves reddening of the skin and discomfort. Staphylococcus aureus (SA) is a common bacteria found on the skin surface of approximately one-third of the population. This level of colonisation increases in the population of a hospital due to an increase in contact with infected individuals. It is most commonly found in folds of skin around the groin and armpit and in the nose but does not cause problems for the majority of people who are colonised by the bacteria. MRSA will not infect a healthy person, but those in hospital are more susceptible for a number of reasons. The key reasons are:

- There is a route of entry for the bacteria in the form of a surgical wound or a catheter
- They are more vulnerable individuals with a decreased immunity
- They are in contact with a large number of individuals increasing the rate of spread.

The rate of spread can be halted by effective screening of all planned hospital admissions to ensure any MRSA infection is identified and precautions can be put into place.

Infection can occur when a break in the skin such as a wound or bed sore becomes colonised with MRSA. A healthy individual will be able to resist the infection, however a lower immunity or individuals outlined above will not be able to fight the infection. This will be seen as redness, swelling and tenderness in the area. There may also be pus within the wound. If the infection enters the blood stream, it will cause septicaemia, meningitis, pneumonia, endocarditis or septic arthritis.

Treatment is with antibiotics, but due to the resilience of the SA to antibiotics, the choice of effective treatments is limited. Treatment regimens include intravenous vancomycin or linezolid. The patient should be nursed in a side room with suitable protocols implemented, but visitors are not prohibited. Visitors should, however, be encouraged to employ effective hand-washing techniques before and after visiting.

Human immunodeficiency virus (HIV)

The human immunodeficiency virus (HIV) reduces the human immune system. An individual who has HIV has a reduced immune system, making the individual more susceptible to serious infections and certain types of cancer. HIV infects CD4 cells, which are responsible for fighting infection. HIV is a retrovirus, reproducing itself within the cells of the individual, releasing copies of itself into the blood stream. Once infected the cells are destroyed. The body will attempt to regenerate the cells which have been destroyed but this is not effective and will eventually lead to a decline in the number of CD4 cells, leading to a reduction in immunity. HIV is spread through the exchange of bodily fluids, including semen and blood, usually associated with sexual contact or the sharing of needles. The virus can also be transmitted from mother to child through the placenta, although drugs are now available to prevent this happening. In the early days of the presence of the virus it was possible to be infected through blood transfusions. Since 1985, all blood donations in the UK have been screened prior to transfusion to eliminate infection. This is not the case in all countries and infection during a transfusion is still possible in areas where screening is not carried out.

The initial stage of HIV infection is called *primary HIV* or *seroconversion*. Many individuals develop symptoms but are not always aware of the cause, as they are common to a number of illnesses. These include fever, tiredness, sore throat, joint and muscle pain and a blotchy rash. Diagnosis is only possible through a blood test to identify the presence of the virus. This can be detected with in a week of infection, but a negative result usually requires a re-test at 3 months. After this initial phase, the symptoms recede and the individual is in the asymptomatic phase. They may go for a number of years with no symptoms; however, the virus is still active within the body. The final, late stage infection is commonly known as *AIDS* and can take up to 10 years to develop from initial infection.

Individuals with HIV will require regular blood tests. These identify the CD4 count and the viral load of the blood. A CD4 count above 500 indicates a low risk of HIV-related infection; below 200 the risk is very high. The viral load will be used to determine the effect of a medication on the presence of the virus. Medication can reduce the viral load to an undetectable level. Treatment for HIV uses combination therapy with a range of drugs. The virus is able to mutate effectively and so combinations are used which can be changed. Treatment starts when the CD4 drops below 350 or an HIV-related illness such as Kaposi's sarcoma is diagnosed. Treatment is also started in individuals with hepatitis B or C, those at risk from heart disease or stroke and during pregnancy to protect the unborn child. There are a large range of drugs which are effective in the treatment of HIV, but are specific to the individual and this will change as the disease progresses.

Protozoa

A number of protozoa can cause illness in individuals. These include, but are not limited to, toxoplasmosis from *Toxoplasma gondii*, malaria from a parasite transmitted by the anopheles mosquito and giardiasis caused by *Giardia intestinalis*.

Toxoplasmosis is caused by the parasite *Toxoplasma gondii*. This is found in undercooked or raw meat, raw cured meat, cat faeces and unpasteurised goat's milk. Toxoplasmosis can also be contracted by individuals working with sheep during the lambing season. *Toxoplasma gondii* cannot be transferred from one individual to another, except for transmission from a pregnant mother to her child. This is known as *congenital toxoplasmosis* and occurs when a mother becomes infected during pregnancy or up to 3 months prior to becoming pregnant. The risk of infection in the child increases as the pregnancy progresses. In the majority of individuals, infection does not cause any symptoms. In some cases, the individual will develop enlarged lymph nodes and symptoms similar to flu. In the developing fetus, effects can range in severity from stillbirth through to no symptoms at birth, but symptoms may develop later in life. Toxoplasmosis can be fatal in individuals with reduced immunity. Most individuals do not require treatment but in severe cases, pyrimethamine and sulfadiazine will be prescribed.

Malaria is caused by four parasites, spread by the female *Anopheles* mosquito. The most prevalent and potentially most serious is *Plasmodium falciparum*, but others include *Plasmodium vivax*, *Plasmodium ovale* and *Plasmodium malariae*. Inherited immunity to *P. vivax* is seen in many West African individuals and resistance can be acquired by repeated infection to any of the four types. This takes between 5 and 20 years to develop and withdrawal of exposure may result in the loss of this immunity. The initial stage of infection which affects the liver is usually symptomless and it is not until the infection enters the blood and causes the rupture that the classic symptoms of chills, fever and sweats known as 'a crisis' are seen. This is caused by the induction of inflammatory cytokines. The main complication of malaria is anaemia. An additional complication with *P. falciparum* is cerebral malaria which can lead to coma and death. Other organs can be affected and complications including pulmonary oedema in the lungs, hypoglycaemia, lactic acidosis or adult respiratory distress syndrome may be seen. Malaria can cause severe immunosuppression. Treatment is primarily through prevention or anti-malarials, but these vary depending on the malaria strain and sensitivity. Supportive measures for complications may be required in addition to the anti-malarials.

Giardiasis is caused by the transmission of the parasite *Giardia intestinalis* through the faecal–oral route. The parasite develops a protective shell called a *Giardia cyst* while in the intestine. The cysts are passed with stools and can survive for months outside of the body. They are spread in drinking water that is contaminated with faeces, primarily in areas with poor sanitation and limited clean water. Giardiasis can also be spread with poor personal hygiene through contamination during food preparation. Transmission is also seen in childcare workers who change nappies with poor hand-washing before and after each child. Diarrhoea is the most common symptom of giardiasis. Other symptoms can include vomiting, abdominal cramps, bloating, nausea or weight loss. Symptoms take between 4 and 10 days to develop after infection and left untreated, can last for up to 2 months. Some untreated individuals suffer from chronic giardiasis where symptoms persist for a number of years. Treatment is effective with a course of metronidazole.

KEY POINTS

The prevention of cross-infection between patients and practitioners is possible if a number of key procedures are followed. Depending on the patient history and the protocols in place within the individual hospital trust, the precautions and measures may vary. The areas highlighted below are a guide, but practitioners should take time to become acquainted with their own Trust's protocols and procedures. (See also Chapter 16, Methods of infection prevention.)

- Hand-washing is essential to prevent the spread of infection. Depending on the infection type, soap and water or alcohol gel is needed to remove infection. This should be carried out between patients regardless of known infection. A large number of the conditions described in this chapter may not be known about by the patient and so precautions should be taken at all times

- Masks are needed to prevent air-borne transmission to patients who may have lowered immunity. They are also required where a patient has active tuberculosis
- Physical barriers are necessary to prevent infection of the patient or the healthcare professional. These are usually in the form of aprons and gloves and masks when needed as outlined above
- The timing of a patient's examination or treatment should be planned to reduce the risk to other patients in the waiting room and their time away from the ward should be minimised. Timing should also be considered to ensure there is time to clean the room and equipment before and after the patient's visit to reduce cross-contamination
- Barrier nursing may be in place and special care should be taken during imaging and treating these patients to ensure the protocols in place are maintained
- Some patients with highly infectious conditions or severely reduced immunity may be in isolation. Treatment and imaging of these patients should be carefully planned utilising the skills of the whole multidisciplinary team involved in the management and care of the patient
- Infections such as *Norovirus* and *C. diff* will pass between patients very easily and if an outbreak is suspected then the ward will be closed to visitors and new admissions. In these circumstances, only examinations and treatments that are essential should be performed and strict adherence to protocols should be in place.

Chapter 16

Methods of infection prevention

Jenny Lorimer

This chapter will consider:

- Common infective organisms
- Virulence of those organisms
- Important factors that affect resistance in both the individual and the population

INTRODUCTION

It is important that we prevent our patients from infective organisms within the clinical environment. There are vast numbers of infections which can be caused by five main types of infecting agent: bacteria, viruses, fungi, prions and parasites. Particularly relevant to the clinical environment and our patients are bacteria, viruses and fungi and these will be the focus of this chapter. In addition, activity elements are included in this chapter for you to check your levels of knowledge and understanding.

Infection can be defined as the invasion of, and the increase in microorganisms in the normally sterile tissues of the body. A successful breach of the individual's barriers and immune defence mechanisms is required for an infective process to take place. It is a fact of everyday life, that infection is a common cause of morbidity and mortality throughout the world. This is true whether we consider our own domestic environment, the industrial

> **!** We need to consider a broader aspect than only the clinical environment as we ourselves, as healthcare professionals, may unwittingly act as a means of spread of infection.

workplace or the healthcare settings where we work. Gaining an understanding of the factors influencing infection is the first important step in preventing the spread of infection.

It is recognised that transmission of infection can be by four different mechanisms. Animal to human and environment to human are acknowledged but for the purposes of our work in healthcare, it is both human to human and medical institution to patient, *nosocomial*, that are most important to consider. Infections are caused by pathogens and these are microorganisms that are normally absent from the body. Pathogens have the important capacity to invade the body and then cause disease.

In considering the main infective organisms, the distinction between commensals and pathogens will be referred to. Commensals can be described as microorganisms that are normally present within the body. In health they do not cause disease and may be in some circumstances an advantage. The word pathogen is also used to describe a microorganism but the important distinction is that pathogens usually cause disease. Pathogens can be non-living, e.g. a chemical, but can occur more commonly as living microorganisms, e.g. bacteria.

MICROORGANISMS RESPONSIBLE FOR DISEASE COMMONLY ENCOUNTERED IN HEALTHCARE

Table 16.1 lists a number of microorganisms that are usually absent from the body, but which all have adaptations or mechanisms that allow them to invade the body and cause disease. Many of these are commonly encountered, and they all may be encountered in the healthcare environment. The method the organism uses to spread and the disease caused by the organism are included.

Table 16.1

Name of organism	Disease caused	Method of spread
Bacteria		
Staphylococcus (including MRSA)	Wound infections Respiratory infections Cardiac infections CNS infections Intestinal infections Bone and joint infections	Contaminated objects Skin to skin contact
Streptococcus	Upper respiratory tract infections Meningitis Bacterial pneumonia Endocarditis	Person-to-person contact Discharges from the nose or throat Infected wounds on the skin
Clostridium	Botulism Colitis Tetanus	Usually spread on the hands of people who come into contact with infected patients Environmental surfaces (e.g. floors, bedpans, toilets) contaminated with the bacteria or its spores Very hardy and can survive on clothes and environmental surfaces for long periods
Listeria	Influenza-like illness Meningoencephalitis/septicaemia Spontaneous abortion	Most cases are food-borne (meat, processed foods, soft cheeses and meat-based pates). Mother to fetus *in utero* or during birth
Escherichia coli	Food poisoning Urinary tract infections (UTIs) Bacteraemia	Food contamination or person to person spread
Mycobacterium tuberculosis	Tuberculosis (TB)	Only the pulmonary form of TB disease is infectious. Transmission occurs through coughing of infectious droplets
Viruses		
Adenovirus	Upper respiratory tract infection Acute diarrhoea	Air-borne droplets or nasal secretions
Varicella-zoster	Chickenpox Shingles	Can be spread by direct contact (shingles is a reactivation)
Epstein–Barr	Infectious mononucleosis	Saliva-droplet spread
Coryza	Common cold	Air-borne droplets or nasal secretions
Rhinovirus	Mild upper respiratory tract infection	Air-borne droplets or nasal secretions
Rotavirus	Gastroenteritis	Person-to-person spread (especially healthcare workers)
Rubella	German measles	Air-borne droplets

Take time to study the table so that you are familiar with the organism, its method of spread and the disease caused when you come across them on clinical placement.

Activities

- List all of the organisms that may be spread by hands (person to person).
- List all those spread by air-borne droplets.

POSSIBLE MECHANISMS OF INFECTIVE TRAVEL

As healthcare professionals we all have a legal, professional and moral duty to prevent and control the spread of microorganisms within our working environment.

Three different and distinct routes of movement of micro-organisms must be considered. These are from patient to patient, patient to staff member and staff member to patient. All of these routes can be considered in terms of a single model. It is helpful to use a model to understand the complex nature of the interaction between pathogens, human beings and the environment (Fig. 16.1).

Organism

After the invasion of the body by a microorganism, there are normally no initial indications that anything has happened. A period of incubation follows, and length of this time interval will depend on the microorganism. The incubation period can be defined as the time between the invasion of microorganism into body and appearance of clinical signs of disease. During this time, the micro-organisms reproduce until there are sufficient pathogens to cause adverse effects. The individual may experience a prodromal period. This will vary both with the invading pathogen and the individual. The affected person may feel a loss of appetite and be suffering from fatigue. Other signs include a headache, or a feeling that 'something is wrong'.

When the affected individual is a patient, the practitioner needs to consider how to interrupt any potential

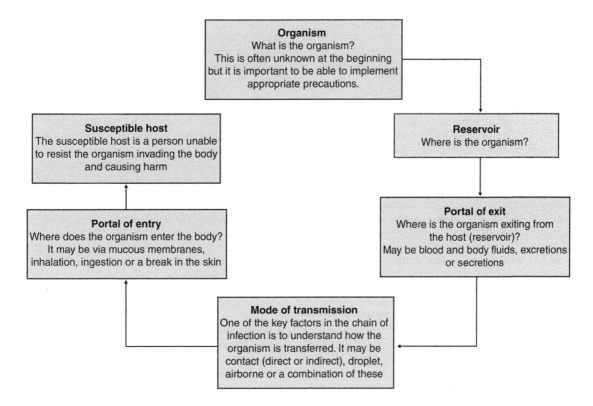

Figure 16.1 A model showing the complex nature of interactions between pathogens, human beings and the environment.

spread of disease. This will vary depending on the specific clinical setting. At this stage, the type of infection, and therefore how it is likely to be spread are probably not going to be known. The healthcare professional needs to think about all the following methods of disease transmission to prevent the spread of disease. Methods of transmission to consider include the spread by air-borne particles or droplets, by direct skin contact or by contact with body fluids.

Activities

- What would you do if a patient sitting in the crowded waiting room was obviously suffering from a heavy cold?
- What preventative measures would you consider if you are asked to perform an examination or treatment on a patient suffering from TB?
- You are asked to perform a procedure on a patient who is known to be suffering from *Clostridium difficile* (*C. diff*). What precautions may be required?

Reservoir

> **!** In the clinical environment the reservoir is any person, substance or piece of equipment in which an infectious agent normally lives and multiplies. It is common for the reservoir to harbour the infectious agent without injury to itself.

The reservoir serves solely as a source from which other individuals can be infected. It is from the reservoir that the infectious substance is transmitted to a susceptible individual. Any object can become a reservoir, and in a hospital the range and number of objects is almost endless. Common reservoirs have been found to be moving and handling equipment, nurses' scissors, stethoscopes, mattresses, pillows, call bells, cassettes, keyboards, lead aprons and anatomical markers.

The potential for the medical imaging department to be involved in the transmission of infective disease cannot be questioned because of its central role in a hospital. A large number of patients, from the very young to the elderly, use medical imaging services and they will have a wide cross-section of illnesses and diseases. These same patients are likely to be susceptible to infection. Many will have suffered trauma, have had operations or have a compromised immune system because of disease. Similarly, the radiotherapy department has to be equally concerned with the transmission of infection. While not normally as central as a medical imaging department, the challenges faced by the radiotherapy department are

of a similar magnitude. Both departments have a high workload with a large number of patients visiting each day. The radiotherapy department will have to consider that the majority of the patients are likely to be immunocompromised, and any risk of infection needs to be considered very carefully.

For many of these patients imaging examinations will involve direct contact between their skin and computed radiography (CR) imaging cassettes or treatment equipment during examinations. Research in medical imaging has suggested that up to one-third of cassettes are contaminated with potential pathogens such as *Staphylococcus aureus* and so the potential for cross-infection has to be very real. Radiotherapy departments can consider the risks to be of an equal magnitude. In medical imaging, the potential becomes even greater when mobile radiography is considered when the patients being imaged are even more likely to be vulnerable to cross-infection. Impermeable, disposable cassette covers should be used for cassettes in imaging patients who are 'inpatients' or who have been admitted to the hospital as they are most likely to be at an increased risk. Additionally, since cassettes act as reservoirs for potential pathogens, there can be little argument against medical imaging departments having effective methods for both monitoring and maintaining the cleanliness of cassettes. The argument for equipment in radiotherapy departments must be equally persuasive.

Another known possible reservoir within the medical imaging department is lead rubber aprons. While lead rubber aprons are not likely to come into direct contact with patients' skin, they are worn in environments where the risk of transmission of infection must be minimised, e.g. operating theatres, intensive care units and suites for interventional radiology. Since lead rubber aprons have been proven to be reservoirs for potential pathogens departments should maintain and monitor their cleanliness to protect patients from the risk of cross-infection.

A very mundane possible vector within the imaging department is radiographic anatomical markers. As they are an essential, they can be regarded as one of the most frequently handled pieces of imaging equipment. Yet, because each individual responsible for imaging will have their own personal anatomical markers, which are returned to their uniform pocket at the end of the examination, they are likely to be overlooked as important imaging equipment. These anatomical markers can become highly contaminated and they need to be regularly cleaned with a suitable disinfectant wipe or alcohol gel to decrease the risk of contamination.

One complication of decreasing the risks of cross-infection within a medical imaging department can be the specialist nature of some of the equipment. For example, ultrasound equipment has been demonstrated as a reservoir for potential pathogens, but the ultrasound probes cannot be cleaned with standard alcohol wipes because of the delicate construction. It is also relevant to mention that there have been proven cases of nosocomial infections from ultrasound gel. The specialist nature of an ultrasound department means that cleaning and decontamination guidelines need to be specific to the imaging methods and equipment used.

Moving away from the specialist nature of the medical imaging department, one area that affects all healthcare workers is that of uniforms and their contribution to the risk of cross-infection. There is no evidence that contaminated uniforms have caused a nosocomial infection.

> **!** The perception of uniforms posing an infection risk seems to be held by the general public and media. It is possible that wearing uniforms outside of the clinical environment may damage the public's confidence in the healthcare professions.

It is inevitable that a uniform will become contaminated during normal working, but the contamination can be limited by the proper wearing of personal protective equipment.

Activities

- Is it acceptable to wear your uniform on your way to and from work when you travel by car?
- You have just finished a busy day at work. List the ways in which you could potentially transmit pathogens to another person from normal day-to-day contact.
- Identify one item of healthcare equipment that is repeatedly in use in your working environment, e.g. immobilisation aid, tourniquet. Track how many times the piece of equipment is used during 1 day. What would this equate to over 1 year? How is the equipment cleaned? How often does cleaning occur?

Portal of exit

The portal of exit refers to how and where the microorganism leaves the reservoir or host. Breaking the cycle of infection at the exit portal gives us fewer, more specific opportunities to think about. At this stage, knowing the type of microorganism means that specific measures can be taken. When considering the patients presenting to a radiotherapy or medical imaging department it is highly likely that the presence and the type of microorganism is going to be unknown. The most important method of preventing the spread of infection at this stage is by reducing the risks as far as possible. Both practitioners and patients should always minimise the effects of coughing and sneezing. It is important to remember that contaminated

secretions are a greater threat on hands or on tissues than in air. These can easily be transferred to other equipment which will then act as a reservoir. As a practitioner, if you are in the clinical environment while having a minor infection involving coughing and sneezing, you should cover your nose and mouth with a mask.

> **!** Being a practitioner, part of your daily routine in getting ready for work should include covering any break in the skin or mucous membranes with a suitable barrier.

For patients, specific routes should be considered as a potential mechanism for a possible pathogen to be passed on. Commonly this will include blood and body fluids, excretions or secretions. The likely paths of escape of the pathogen will include faeces, urine, wound discharge, mucus, blood and vomit.

Activities

Compile a list of the possible reservoirs of infection that are likely to be found in a medical imaging or radiotherapy department. If you are a radiotherapy student discuss your list with a colleague from medical imaging and vice versa. What pieces of equipment are common between the two disciplines? How is each of pieces of equipment kept clean? Is there any knowledge and areas of good practice that can be transferred from a radiotherapy department to a medical imaging department and vice versa?

Mode of transmission

Preventing the transmission of infection within the clinical environment has been a hot topic for a number of years as many studies have demonstrated a clear link between personal and environmental hygiene and the rates of infection. The impact of the spread of infection will often affect both patients and healthcare workers. A useful illustration of this is the number of deaths of healthcare workers during the Severe Acute Respiratory Syndrome (SARS) epidemic during 2003. There is a wealth of evidence that demonstrates links between a lack of training and education and the level of non-compliance with infection prevention processes with an increase in the number and incidence of healthcare associated infections. Such is the strength of the evidence base that prevention of infection is a very high priority within the National Health Service (NHS). Since 2000 over £68 million has been invested across the UK in preventing healthcare associated infections.

There have been several government policies to combat the widespread incidences of infection spread in clinical environments. Procedures that you are likely to be aware of in the clinical environment include specific objectives such as the inclusion of infection prevention policies in the induction of all new members of staff, or the requirement that all staff have education and training on prevention and control of infection in their personal development plans. More recent evaluations of transmission on infections within the clinical environment show that rates are significantly decreased from rates detected 10 years ago. While this is excellent news, the continued decrease will not be sustained without increased and persistent vigilance, monitoring and assessment.

Within the healthcare environment, the ways in which a pathogen may travel from the reservoir to a new host is well evidenced and understood. The four ways of transmission that are relevant within the healthcare setting are contact, both direct and indirect; air-borne; consumption and exposure to blood. Direct contact is where the new host has actual contact with an infected person. While this is hopefully unlikely it becomes more of a risk if the infection has not been diagnosed so that proper precautions can be taken. Indirect contact is when the new host is in contact with surfaces that have been touched, and so contaminated, by the infected person, or where droplets of fluid from the infected person have landed. The most important category of indirect contact is through spread on unwashed hands. Air-borne transmission occurs most commonly when tiny infected particles from an infected person are released when they cough or sneeze. These can be inhaled by the unwitting new host. Although it may seem that consuming or swallowing food or water that has been contaminated with microorganisms may be unlikely within a healthcare setting, it becomes a significant reality when unwashed hands are considered. The last category of transmission, and perhaps the one that is most readily associated with the healthcare environment is exposure to blood through needlestick injuries.

There are three important steps that should form part of our everyday working lives to prevent the spread of infection. These should be so second nature that they are performed automatically, every time, almost without conscious thought.

1. Any piece of equipment that is used in caring for patients and has become soiled with blood, body fluids, secretions and excretions should be handled so that the risk of contamination of clothing, skin or mucous membranes is prevented. This prevents the transfer of microorganisms to ourselves, other patients or the environment.
2. All re-usable equipment is always cleaned appropriately after use.
3. All single use items are always disposed of properly immediately after use.

Portal of entry

Preventing the spread of infection is most concerned with reducing the risk of contamination in everyday clinical practice so that everyone is able to play a part in ensuring that the healthcare environment minimises the risk of possible infection for patients, practitioners, clients and visitors. Considering the possible portals of entry of the pathogen forms the cornerstone of preventing contamination. It is important to consider inhalation; ingestion; breaks in the protective skin barrier, e.g. surgery, intravenous lines, injury; and mucous membranes, e.g. mouth, eyes and nose. The four most important measures to be taken are:

1. Hand hygiene
2. Wearing personal protective equipment
3. Practising aseptic technique
4. Safe disposal of sharps.

These will now be considered in turn.

Hand hygiene

It is vital that all healthcare workers understand that effective and careful hand-washing minimises the number of microorganisms on the hands. In the clinical environment, the microorganisms often come from contact with body fluids and contaminated surfaces. Careful hand-washing will often break the chain of infection transmission and therefore reduce person-to-person transmission.

While all healthcare workers will understand the importance of hand-washing it cannot be ignored that compliance is often less than it should be. Possible reasons for this may include a lack of appropriate equipment; low numbers of staff meaning an increased pressure on staff time; allergies to hand-washing products; a poor level of knowledge among staff about risks and procedures; the time taken for proper hand-washing; and careless attitudes among staff towards infection prevention. Another possible reason is the drying effects of regular hand decontamination. If this is found to be a problem, then an emollient hand cream should be regularly applied to protect the skin.

Hand-washing with soap and water will kill many transient microorganisms and the rinsing with running water allows them to be physically removed from the hands and disposed of safely. An alternative is the decontamination of hands with waterless, alcohol-based hand gel. This will either kill or inhibit the growth of microorganisms in deep layers of the skin. Decontaminating hands is not appropriate when hands are soiled.

How to wash your hands

The following steps assume that the healthcare worker is wearing essential jewellery only, has short, clipped natural nails and is wearing sleeves that end above the elbow.

The first step should be removal of any jewellery being worn (rings, watches).

1. Wet your hands and wrists, making sure you keep your hands and wrists lower than your elbows (this makes the water flow down the forearm and hands to the fingertips and so avoids arm contamination).
2. Apply soap to both your hands and create a thorough lather.
3. Using firm, circular motions wash your hands and arms up as far as the wrists. Ensure you cover all areas including palms, back of the hands, fingers, between fingers, knuckles and wrists.
4. You should continue to rub the lather for a minimum of 10–15 seconds.
5. Rinse your hands thoroughly, again keeping the hands lower than the forearms.
6. This process can be repeated if your hands are very soiled.
7. Dry both your hands thoroughly with disposable paper towels, a clean dry towel or air-dry them.

Hand disinfection

During clinical work, waterless, alcohol-based hand rubs can be used as hand-washing is not always necessary. The alcohol hand-rubs are suitable for quickly decontaminating your hands between patients. It is important that hands are clean if only an alcohol gel is to be used. If hands are soiled then you should wash your hands as detailed in the process above. Dispensers should be placed within each examination room and outside each patient room, when considering mobile examinations.

Three key learning points on the effectiveness of hand disinfection and compliance by healthcare workers depend on the following:

1. The type of alcohol gel available. This will vary in different clinical environments
2. The volume of hand rub to be used. This varies between products
3. The reading and adhering to instructions for use.

The product should be put into the palm of one of your hands. You should then rub your hands together, covering all surfaces of hands and fingers, until your hands are dry. You should make sure that the alcohol gel covers all of both hands and that areas of skin are not missed. There are many recommended methods for doing this and practitioners must adopt a responsible method of application.

This procedure should not be rushed and may take up to 30 seconds. This is the time taken for the alcohol gel to evaporate, leaving clean, dry hands.

 You should not rinse your hands after the gel is applied.

Personal protective equipment

There will be occasions when you will need to wear personal protective equipment. The equipment is designed to interrupt the cycle of infection. Infection may either be a known condition, e.g. in the barrier nursed patient; or may be a possibility, e.g. in the road traffic accident; or may be required for the cleanliness of the environment, e.g. in the operating theatre. As with hand-washing, it is important the practitioner knows and understands the precautions being taken. Compliance with the precautions is equally important for the health of patients and staff alike. When implemented and adhered to, barrier methods, e.g. gloves, gowns and masks, together with effective hand-washing and antisepsis, are very effective methods in reducing the transmission of disease.

Full personal protective equipment

Although in the past there has been much discussion on the order in which protective clothing is worn, it is now believed that the order is not important and the following sequence is given merely as a suggestion.

1. Wash your hands
2. Put on protective clothes, e.g. scrubs, in the designated changing room
3. Change your shoes to the provided boots or clogs. An alternative to this is to use shoe covers
4. Put on cap and mask (see below)
5. An impermeable apron should be worn if splashes of blood or body fluids are anticipated
6. Protective eye goggles may be required.

Caps

Caps should be worn when it is possible that splashes of blood or body fluids are to be expected. They are also appropriate when it is necessary to protect the patient from microorganisms that are present in the hair. The cap worn should be disposable and waterproof. It is usual for caps to be available in a range of sizes so that hair can be completely covered.

> **!** When you remove your cap you should hold the inside of the cap and lift it straight off your head. While removing it you should turn the cap inside out and fold it so that the inside is not exposed to the environment.

Caps should always be disposed of in the proper container. After removing your cap you should wash your hands straight away.

Masks

Surgical masks are used by healthcare workers to help to protect them from inhaling respiratory pathogens such as TB. They assist in preventing the spread of infectious diseases that are spread by the droplet pattern such as meningococcal meningitis. In particular environments such as theatre, they are used to protect the patient from the risk of infection from the healthcare workers.

Masks may also be worn by patients who are known, or suspected to be, a risk of transmitting a communicable disease such as TB. They are important when the patient is transferred from one place to another or visiting a hospital department, e.g. medical imaging, radiotherapy or physiotherapy.

Surgical masks are disposable and designed to be worn once for a maximum period of 4–6 hours. They should be disposed of immediately after use and should not be left to hang around the neck. If the mask you are wearing has been soiled you should immediately change it and wash your hands to prevent contamination.

You should always wear a mask when there is a risk of 'splashing' of blood or body fluids, secretions or excretions. Wearing a mask is essential if you know or suspect that a patient has an infectious disease that is spread by the droplet route.

Before taking a mask from the container, your hands should be clean and dry. All practitioners should know how to properly wear a mask and should consult the instructions if they are not sure, as there will be some variation in the type of mask available in different departments and hospitals. Special consideration is needed if you wear glasses. The lower edge of the glasses should press over the top edge of the mask. This will make the mask fit more securely and help to prevent fogging of the lenses of the glasses.

> **!** While wearing a surgical mask you should avoid talking, sneezing or coughing.

When removing your mask you should hold it only by the strings. Masks must be disposed of in the appropriate container and after removing your mask you should wash your hands.

Gowns

Disposable gowns are designed to protect the healthcare worker's clothing or uniform from contamination. You should wear a gown when there is a risk of contamination with microorganisms from blood, body fluids, secretions and excretions. Gowns are normally disposable and each should be worn only once. As soon as you have completed the examination or episode of care, the gown should be disposed of. Gowns should be clean and are not sterile.

They are made of a material that is resistant to fluids. When putting on a gown you should make sure that the neck is high, and that the gown is long enough to cover your clothing. Where disposable gowns are not available, reusable cotton gowns are worn with a plastic apron over.

When you put on a gown you need to make sure it covers as much of your clothing as possible, particularly at the back, and you will need help to fasten the waist tapes. When removing your gown it is important to touch as little of the outside of the gown as possible. The waist tapes should be undone while still wearing gloves. When you have done this remove and dispose of your gloves and continue removing the gown by touching only the inside as far as possible. As you remove it you should turn it inside out (as with the cap), roll it into a ball and dispose of it in the correct container. After removing the gown you should wash your hands thoroughly.

Aprons

The most important function of an apron is to protect the healthcare worker from contact with contaminated body fluids. Plastic aprons worn either over clothes or over a gown are used when caring for patients where the possibility of splashes with blood or body fluids is likely. If a gown is of impermeable material an apron is not necessary. Aprons are usually plastic and disposable. The apron should be long enough to cover the healthcare worker's uniform but should not touch the floor. The apron should be wide enough so that the ties can be secured at the back. Aprons should always be worn tied at the back to make sure they protect the wearer. Hands should always be washed before putting an apron on and after it has been removed. When removing an apron it should be removed by touching the inside surface only, as the inside can be thought of as 'clean' and the outside contaminated. The apron should then be folded so that the outside surface is folded into the inside and disposed of in the correct container.

Protective eyewear

During extreme circumstances, such as major trauma, there may be a risk that blood or body fluids may splash on to the healthcare worker's face and/or eyes. The risk of contamination can be reduced by the use of face shields or protective goggles. These should be worn in addition to ordinary spectacles where used. Disposable face shields or goggles are preferable but some may be reusable, and will need to be cleaned thoroughly after each use.

Gloves

All healthcare workers must be familiar with wearing gloves as they are commonly used throughout all aspects of healthcare. Gloves must always be worn when there is a potential for exposure to blood, body fluids, secretions or excretions. Gloves should be changed when they become soiled; between different procedures of care on one patient; and between patients. It is important that gloves are removed immediately after completing a procedure and hands are always washed immediately. Healthcare workers should make sure that they do not contaminate their environment before removing used gloves. You should take care not to touch any equipment, controls or other objects such as door handles, telephones, or items belonging to the patient. At times when this is going to be difficult, e.g. replacing the covers over a patient, ask for the assistance of another member of staff, who has not had potential contamination.

There are different types of gloves available within the clinical environment and the correct type should be selected for the task to be performed. Disposable, clean gloves can be used for all aspects of patient care where there is a potential for contamination. In order to decrease the potential for contamination, sterile gloves must be used for any invasive procedure. More heavy duty gloves are needed for cleaning the environment, handling soiled linen or clothing, and for cleaning spills of blood or body fluids. These gloves can usually be cleaned and reused.

Before putting on any types of gloves, the healthcare worker should be sure that the gloves are not damaged and that they will fit properly. You should first wash and dry your hands. Gloves should be picked up by the cuff and pulled onto the hand. The second glove should be put on in the same way.

When removing protective clothing, gloves should be the first items to be removed as they are most likely to be contaminated. The first glove should be removed by taking the outside of the cuff and then pulling the glove off so that it turns inside out as it is removed. The second glove is then taken off by taking the inside of the cuff and pulling it off, again so it turns inside out as it is being removed. When the gloves have been removed they should be rolled up and disposed of in the correct container. Hands should then be washed thoroughly.

Many studies have been conducted on the use of gloves within the clinical environment. Results of these studies often conflict with each other which has the potential of leaving the healthcare worker confused about what is the correct procedure to be used. Healthcare workers generally use gloves correctly, although some professions are thought to be more compliant with correct glove use than others. Some studies have found that healthcare workers often use gloves when they were not required. While this is not a detriment to spread of infection, it does have a disadvantage if gloves are worn in preference to hand-washing once gloves have been removed.

It is important to remember that wearing gloves does not remove the need for hand-washing. Some authors suggest that healthcare workers consider gloves to be used for their own protection rather than protection of both staff and patients. This can be illustrated by healthcare workers failing to change their gloves between different procedures on the same patient. One key learning point for all healthcare workers is that gloves should be worn only once for only one aspect of care on a single patient. This important point can be thought of as an example of the directive from the Medical Devices Agency (MDA). The MDA regard gloves as single-use medical devices (MDA 2000). The second key point is to remember that hand-washing is still required after an episode of care, whether gloves have been worn or not.

Activities

- When you are next on placement find time to practise putting on and taking off personal protective equipment. With permission, work in pairs with one person observing the other. Offer each other hints and tips on when areas of possible contamination might occur.
- Choose three organisms from Table 16.1. Explain and justify which items of personal protective equipment would be effective in preventing the spread of infection for each organism.

Aseptic technique

Aseptic technique is the term commonly used to describe a variety of methods used to prevent contamination of wounds and other susceptible sites by pathogens that could cause infection. The purposes of aseptic technique are to:

- Prevent the introduction of pathogens to a site
- Prevent the transfer of pathogens from the patient to staff or other patients.

It is accepted that aseptic technique is an important method of preventing the spread of pathogens to patients from both clinical staff and the environment they work in. Since 2001, the Aseptic Non Touch Technique (ANTT) has been used across large parts of the NHS and aims to decrease the variables in practice across an enormous clinical workforce. The technique was introduced with the aim of improving the quality of practice and so decrease infection rates. Where measurable, audit of data from Trusts suggests that aseptic technique has become more standardised and that healthcare associated infection (HCAI) rates have been decreased.

The ANTT guidelines work on the basis that it is not possible for a technique performed on a patient, e.g. i.v. cannulation to be aseptic in a typical healthcare setting because the environment where the procedure is taking place contains microorganisms in the atmosphere. Aseptic technique becomes more focused when clinical staff are able to identify the most critical areas and sites and assess how they are to be protected during a procedure. Peer reviewed clinical guidelines, which use pictures with minimal instructions, give guidance to practitioners in a way that is both simple and visual. The guidelines have been developed using best practice and key guidance documents.

It is recognised that the ANTT clinical guidelines are not the only way for a healthcare worker to practise aseptic technique, but they do have the advantage of offering a standardised approach.

Techniques that require aseptic technique in a radiotherapy or an imaging department are numerous and varied. In accordance with guidance all healthcare professionals performing an aseptic technique should be properly educated and trained in the procedure to be undertaken. If the two key points (given above) are remembered and applied to the clinical setting, the procedures needed for asepsis can be determined. The first point was to: *prevent the introduction of pathogens to a site.* Any procedure where a piece of equipment is introduced into a site that is sterile asepsis should be used, e.g. intravenous cannulation or injection, arterial injection, catheterisation of the urinary bladder. Asepsis is not essential if the site is not sterile, e.g. the upper or lower GI tract. Although it is important to add that a high standard of cleanliness should always be used. Most aseptic procedures in the radiotherapy or medical imaging are performed with sterile, gloved hands. A clean area is created around the site of the procedure using a sterile towel. The person carrying out the procedure will be wearing appropriate personal protective equipment, e.g. a clean, disposable apron and sterile gloves. For many imaging procedures, much of the equipment will be in a pre-packed sterile equipment tray. Additional items, such as catheters will need to be added to the tray. These will be individually enclosed in sterile packing and will be carefully added to the equipment required.

The second key point was to: *prevent the transfer of pathogens from the patient to staff or other patients.* In an imaging or radiotherapy department, this needs to be considered as anything that is removed from a patient, e.g. biopsy specimen, body fluids, etc. and these need to be considered as potential sources of infection.

> ! Specimens must be sealed and enclosed in appropriate containers. Body fluids, secretions or excretions need to be disposed of according to protocol.

Outside of the radiotherapy and imaging departments the process for aseptic technique may be achieved differently, e.g. in an operating theatre, but the two basic principles remain the same.

Activity

Discuss with a colleague the infection prevention measures that are used in different areas of the hospital.

Safe use and disposal of sharps

During many aseptic techniques 'sharps' will form an essential piece of equipment. A 'sharp' can be thought of as any item that has corners, edges or projections capable of cutting or piercing the skin. These will be varied but include needles, cannulas, scalpels and biopsy guns. Whatever the procedure or the piece of equipment being used, the Medical Devices Agency has issued guidelines which should always be followed. These include:

- A sharp should never be passed directly from hand-to-hand. Handling should be kept to a minimum
- Whoever uses the sharp must dispose of it themselves
- Needles should never be recapped or re-sheathed, broken or disassembled before use or before disposal
- Used sharps should be disposed of into a sharps container by the user at the point of use
- Sharps containers should not be overfilled.

Susceptible and contagious groups of staff and patients

Nosocomial infections are thought to occur in up to 10% of all patients admitted to hospital in the UK. The possible consequences of these infections are delayed recovery, increased complications and may ultimately result in the death of a patient.

> ! As healthcare professionals we have to recognise that many of the patients we care for are at a high risk of developing an infection despite all of the preventative measures that are taken.

Factors that can increase the susceptibility to infection include: age, e.g. the elderly and very young; underlying diseases such as diabetes mellitus; HIV positive patients; patients with extensive burns; treatment with drugs that suppress the immune system. Other patients will have had procedures that disturb the ability of the skin to act as a physical barrier to infection such as surgical operations and indwelling catheters or lines. In hospitals we are likely to be in contact with patients who have had transplant surgery, either of tissue or a whole organ. These patients require immunosuppressive drugs as part of their postoperative care to help prevent transplant rejection. This suppression of the immune system puts the patients at increased risk of nosocomial infections.

Whatever the pathological cause of the threat to the immune system, as a general rule if a patient has a decreased number or activity of B cells, they will be susceptible to bacterial infections. A deficiency of T cells will have the consequence of making the patient increasingly vulnerable to viruses and parasites.

In order to protect patients, it is important that all healthcare workers take responsibility for their own health and recognise that their health may have an impact on those that they are caring for. This may be as fundamental as covering a break in skin with a suitable dressing. A more difficult judgement to make is that of taking time off sick when we ourselves are unwell. We are not able to spread infections to patients when we take time off sick appropriately and with good judgement. Against this, all healthcare workers will recognise the pressure to keep working in areas where there are shortages of staff or increased workloads.

THE CLINICAL ENVIRONMENT

As in our own homes, the hospital environment becomes contaminated with dust, debris and chemical residues.

> **!** The large number of people living and working in and passing through the hospital means that the level of organic material and potentially pathogenic microorganisms accumulates at a rate that needs constant attention.

The only way to keep the environment safe for patients, staff and visitors is to remove and/or destroy all of the contaminating material regularly and at appropriate intervals through both cleaning and disinfection. This decontamination means that the environment remains safe, as any debris, dust or potential pathogens are not allowed to accumulate in volumes that would pose a risk.

Cleaning involves the physical removal of dust, debris and chemical residue, as it would in our homes. This cleaning does not destroy microorganisms but reduces the quantity of possible pathogens present. Any possible pathogens cannot be quantified, either before or after cleaning, and the process is very dependent on the efficiency and regularity of the cleaning.

Disinfection is the process that reduces the number of viable microorganisms, both those that are pathogenic and those that are not. Some pathogenic organisms such as some viruses and spores are not destroyed by disinfection. These have to be physically removed from the environment by efficient and effective cleaning.

It is imperative therefore that any facility built for healthcare needs to be both well designed and well maintained. Properly designed cleaning regimes need to be applied to both clinical and non-clinical areas since people move between the two. The level of cleanliness needs to be sufficient in order to prevent the likelihood of spread of HCAIs. Unfortunately for us as practitioners, there is little evidence as to what is sufficient or acceptable as a perfectly sterile environment is not achievable. The design and layout needs to be one that does not allow microorganisms

to collect in sufficient quantities to become an infection reservoir. Areas that need particular attention are any horizontal surfaces and fabrics. Perhaps particularly relevant to medical imaging and radiotherapy departments are the existence of narrow, inaccessible areas that are hard to clean. Also, there should be sufficient storage space that allows a good layout for both working and cleaning. Equally as important as the buildings are the fittings such as basins, taps and hand-drying facilities.

Activities

Draw a plan of an imaging or treatment room that you are familiar with. Imagine you are responsible for the decontamination of that room for a period of 1 week. Design a schedule that would allow you to keep the level of cleanliness of the area at an acceptable level. Make a particular note of areas that could likely become reservoirs for microorganisms.

CLEANING, DISINFECTION AND STERILISATION OF MEDICAL EQUIPMENT

All healthcare workers need to be aware of and be able to comply with all infection prevention and control measure. Regular audits will monitor practice and identify any inappropriate actions. It is important for all practitioners to have a basic level of understanding of the key points so that they may take appropriate action when required in caring for their patients. Decontamination is the process of making a piece of equipment safe for re-use and the next section will explain key terms and practices to enable you to comply with infection control policies.

In medical imaging and radiotherapy departments, many items are re-usable and therefore can transmit pathogens. Almost all pathogens are within visible soiling and so a number of steps may be necessary to make a piece of equipment suitably clean.

Microorganisms have differing levels of resistance to disinfection or sterilisation and the selection below indicates the level of virulence of some pathogens.

Viruses	Susceptible
Some bacteria, e.g. *Staphylococcus aureus*	
Fungi	
Some bacteria, e.g. *Mycobacterium tuberculosis*	
Bacterium spores, e.g. *Clostridium difficile*	
Prions	Resistant

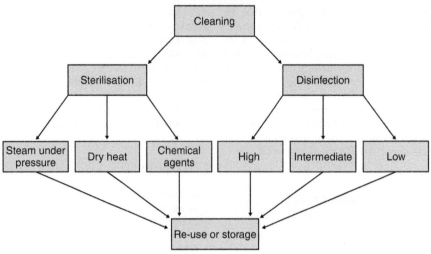

Figure 16.2 The decontamination process.

The decontamination process involves a number of processes and steps which can be employed depending on the nature of the object and how it is used. Figure 16.2 indicates how these processes may be used to achieve objects that are clean and ready for re-use or storage.

KEY POINTS

- In the clinical environment, it is common for infective agents to harbour in certain places, known as reservoirs, e.g. lead aprons used in fluoroscopy, uniforms, etc. As practitioners you need to find out which reservoirs apply to your practice, and ensure that they are disinfected regularly
- The four main means of transmission of a pathogen from a reservoir to a new host are: air-borne, through contact, through consumption and exposure to blood

- The four most important measures of preventing the spread of infection are: maintain good hand hygiene, wear protective clothing, use an aseptic technique and safe disposal of sharps
- In order to protect patients, all healthcare workers must take responsibility for their own health and recognise that their health may have an impact on those they are caring for

Section | 6 |

Medical imaging procedures

Fluoroscopy

Saminah Yunis

FLUOROSCOPY IMAGING EQUIPMENT AND DOSE

Fluoroscopy is an imaging technique commonly used to obtain real-time moving images of the internal structures of a patient through the use of a fluoroscope. In its simplest form, a fluoroscope consists of an X-ray source and fluorescent screen between which a patient is placed. However, modern fluoroscopes couple the screen to an X-ray image intensifier and video camera allowing the images to be recorded and played on a monitor. This immediate imaging is invaluable during interventional procedures such as cardiac catheterisation, thin needle biopsies of tumours and localisation of foreign bodies.

Fluoroscopy examinations require the potential risks from a procedure to be carefully balanced with the benefits of the procedure to the patient. While those performing the procedure always try to use low dose rates, the length of a typical procedure often results in a relatively high absorbed dose to the patient. Recent advances include the capturing of digital images and flat panel detector systems, which reduce the radiation dose to the patient still further.

Since the year 2000, flat panel detectors have begun to be installed in the UK. They are either amorphous silicon or amorphous selenium, together with a thin film transistor array to produce an electronic signal.[1]

National reference doses have been derived for those medical X-ray examinations and interventional procedures where dose measurements on adult patients are available from a sufficiently large sample size to be representative of national practice.

Table 17.1 demonstrates data compiled by the Health Protection Agency[1] (HPA) that analysed the doses to patients from radiographic and fluoroscopic X-ray imaging procedures in the UK.

The operator's training in performing fluoroscopic investigations and completing a diagnostic examination combined with experience of working with fluoroscopic equipment can greatly influence patient radiation dose during fluoroscopy. Care should be taken in ensuring only suitably qualified and competent staff use this equipment. All radiation reduction techniques should be applied, e.g. removal of grids for paediatric patient examinations. Use the equipment to its full potential, e.g. use of collimators and filters and any dose reduction devices and programmes set by the manufacturers.

Modern fluoroscopy equipment has the capability of pulsed fluoroscopy, where the X-ray beam is emitted as a series of short pulses rather than continuously. Due to the reduced frame rates, pulsed fluoroscopy can provide substantial dose savings. This technique is valuable when performing paediatric examinations.

> **!** Management of patient radiation dose involves the combination of both the fluoroscopic equipment design, which determines the amount of radiation required to produce an image, and the control of the image by the operator, who ultimately determines the total number of images acquired during the procedure (Fig. 17.1).

Table 17.1 Recommended national reference doses for diagnostic fluoroscopic examinations on adult patients

Fluoroscopy procedures	DAP per exam (Gy/cm²)	Fluoroscopy time per exam (min)
Barium or water soluble enema	24	2.8
Barium follow through	12	2.2
Barium meal	14	2.7
Barium meal and swallow	11	2.2
Barium or water soluble swallow	9	2.3
Fistulogram	13	3.8
Hysterosalpingogram	3	1
Micturating cystourethrogram (MCU)	12	1.9
Sialography	2	1.7
Small bowel enema	48	9.2

Modern fluoroscopy systems based on image intensifiers are extremely flexible devices and permit operation in a wide range of modes for dynamic and static imaging. Accompanying this flexibility is the fact that different imaging modes have different dose characteristics, which can make dosimetry a difficult task. Fluoroscopes typically have the capability of operation in a number of dynamic imaging modes: normal fluoroscopy, high-dose fluoroscopy and conventional and digital cine fluoroscopy. In addition, these systems may record analogue or digital static images (e.g. conventional photospot images, digital photospot images). The operator should have knowledge of the relative dose characteristics of the different imaging modes, and it is important that these modes be properly configured and maintained during the life of the system.[3]

The most significant things to help reduce paediatric and adult patient dose during fluoroscopic examinations are the following:

- Position the patient as close as possible to the image intensifier
- To avoid excessive skin dose the X-ray tube should be as far away as possible from the patient table
- The lowest acceptable frame rate, last-image-hold and fluoroscopy loop facility should be used. However, this will be dependent on the equipment
- Some centres prefer to set a 'floor' (a kVp) below which the system will not go, such as 70 kVp for paediatric patients and 80 kVp for adults
- Using additional copper filtration also reduces patient dose.

When referring to fluoroscopic examinations, most departments associate barium studies and gynae/urological contrast studies as the majority of the work performed within this modality. Interventional radiology tends to be classed

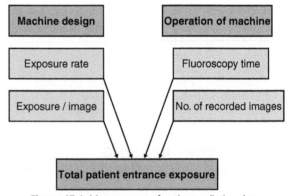

Figure 17.1 Management of patient radiation dose.

separately despite the majority of interventions performed using the same imaging technique and equipment.

FLUOROSCOPY AND THE PATIENT

Performing fluoroscopic procedures involves teamwork. A combination of professions including nurses, practitioners and doctors may be required to perform the procedure. Team work plays a role to ensure the workflow and wellbeing of the patient.

In general radiography, the turnaround of examinations are quick and contact with the patient is for a short time, as opposed to fluoroscopy where the examination times are longer and therefore there is time to possibly forge a greater relationship with the patient. Successful relationships between patients and healthcare professionals depend upon trust.

Ideally, it is important for this process to begin before the patient even attends the department. Some fluoroscopic procedures will require patients to have prepared by fasting, following diets and having taken bowel preparation. This is the point where the relationship begins with the patient.

> **!** Clear concise instructions as well as a good patient information leaflet[4] will allow the patient to gain confidence in the capabilities of the professionals delivering their care. Once a patient attends the department, prior knowledge about the procedure can alleviate some of the anxiety a patient feels.

FLUOROSCOPY AND SKILLS MIX

Performing fluoroscopic examinations was one of the first areas in which radiographers have been able to expand their role. Many procedures including barium studies, sialography, hysterosalpingograms (HSGs) and cystography are performed and reported by advanced medical imaging practitioners rather than radiotherapy practitioners. This role development has enabled some of the first 'consultant radiographers' to be appointed within this modality.

Skills mix has also seen the development of the assistant practitioner role within this modality. Nurses have also been replaced by the development of the healthcare assistant during simple fluoroscopic examinations allowing radiology nurses to also extend their role in other areas e.g. inserting Hickman lines.

FLUOROSCOPY EXAMINATIONS

Barium studies

Nationally, there has been a decline in the number of barium studies being performed. This has been mainly due to the availability of endoscopy, which is seen as the 'gold standard' in investigating the gastrointestinal (GI) tract.

Examinations of the GI tract account for the majority of work performed in this modality on both adults and paediatrics.

The examination of both the upper and lower GI tract include the features in Table 17.2.

Examinations of the lower GI tract

Fluoroscopic examinations of the lower GI tract, i.e. small bowel, large bowel and rectum are performed for a variety of reasons ranging from altered bowel habits to constipation or diarrhoea, bleeding per rectum, abdominal pain, anaemia and evacuation difficulties.

Table 17.2 Studies of the gastrointestinal tract by anatomical locality

Upper GI	Lower GI
Barium swallow	Barium enema
Barium meal	Water soluble enema
Barium small bowel meal	Small bowel follow through
Small bowel enema-enteroclysis	Small bowel enteroclysis
Barium follow through	Defecating proctogram
Video fluoroscopy	Herniogram
Nasogastric tube insertion	Loopogram/fistulogram

Although the number of examinations has been declining nationally with the availability of endoscopic procedures, sigmoidoscopy and colonoscopy, CT colonography barium and water soluble enemas are still being performed at a varying rate. With an ageing population who are not fit for colonoscopy and with a limited CT colonography service, numbers may begin to increase.

Some examinations of the lower GI tract come with specific issues and need to be addressed to ensure the patient is compliant with the examination. For example, good preparation is vital in a barium enema; all patients should receive detailed information and instructions on the reasons and requirements for the bowel cleansing treatment. The practitioner must explain the procedure in detail before starting the examination.

> **!** Practitioners must not rely on the patient having read the patient information leaflet and therefore should inform the patient that the barium enema can sometimes cause abdominal cramps and that it is completely normal to have the urge to have a bowel movement.

Some patients may not be able to retain the barium and it is not uncommon for some leakage of the barium to occur, especially in elderly patients. If this does happen the patient should not feel embarrassed and care should be taken to help clean the patient quickly at the same time preserving the patient's dignity. If patients are not provided with this information during the examination they may become distressed and may feel humiliated.

Due to the patient having multiple bowel movements during the preparation the rectum may be sore and irritated, therefore care should be taken when inserting the enema tip. The practitioner must take note of any history of acute angle glaucoma and tachycardia in case an injection of Buscopan is needed. Patients should be completely covered by a blanket or sheet at all times.

> **!** Care must be taken when placing the patient in the upright position as many patients may feel weak after the lack of food and undergoing the bowel preparation.

Also due to the antispasmodic the patient may experience a dry mouth and have blurry vision. The patient should be informed of the need to drink plenty of fluids after the barium enema and that having white stools following a barium enema is normal.

Bowel preparation

To minimise faecal contamination, it is common to use oral bowel cleansing preparations before radiological assessment of the large and small intestine. They should be well tolerated by the patient, easy to administer and effective in cleansing the bowel.

A number of oral bowel cleansing agents are available currently within the UK, including:[6]

- Citrafleet® (DeWitt); sodium picosulphate and magnesium citrate
- Citramag® (Sanochemia); magnesium carbonate and citric acid
- Fleet Phospho–Soda® (DeWitt); sodium dihydrogen phosphate dehydrate and disodium phosphate dodecahydrate
- Klean Prep® (Norgine); polyethylene glycol
- Moviprep® (Norgine) polyethylene glycol
- Picolax® (Ferring) sodium picosulphate and magnesium citrate.

Although in general these preparations are safe and well tolerated, in 2009, the National Patient Safety Agency[7] (NPSA) issued a Rapid Response Report alerting clinicians and other healthcare practitioners referring patients for investigation that required oral bowel preparation to the potential risk of harm associated with their use.

The risks include:

- Renal failure as a result of phosphate nephropathy
- Complications of hypovolaemia
- Electrolyte disturbances
- Harm where there is a definite contraindication, e.g. bowel obstruction, ileostomy.

A significant amount of watery residue can be left by some types of bowel preparation within the gut lumen. However, this may result in undiagnostic views of the bowel mucosa during barium enema and CT colonography examinations.

These types of laxatives are therefore avoided for radiological imaging of the colon.

According to the Consensus guidelines for the prescription and administration of oral bowel cleansing agents, Picolax® produces the 'driest' bowel; Citramag® is intermediate; and polyethylene glycol preparations leave the highest amount of watery residue.[8]

PROCTOGRAM

This examination can be referred to as either an evacuating proctogram or defecating proctogram. The test only takes about 5 minutes, however prior to the examination, the patient is required to drink one or two cups of barium liquid, the purpose of which is to demonstrate the small bowel on the proctogram images. After waiting 1 hour following the drink of barium, the rectum is filled with barium paste by passing a rectal catheter through the anal opening. The patient will be asked to rest, squeeze and strain certain muscles and then defecate the rectal paste. If the examination is also required to evaluate the bladder a catheter will be inserted into the urinary bladder and filled with iodinated contrast medium. The patient will be asked to defecate under X-ray control so that the mechanism of rectal emptying can be evaluated.

> **!** It is important during this examination to maintain the patient's dignity by first ensuring only a minimum number of staff are present during the procedure. Second, try and keep the patient covered and third, use a screen around the patient to allow them privacy while they are defecating. The patient may be extremely embarrassed and will require reassurance.

It is not unusual for the patient to feel the urge to urinate and defecate during the examination. Toilet facilities should be close by for the patient's use after the examination.

Other fluoroscopic procedures include:

- Sinography
- Urethrography
- Dynamic joint imaging and pain injections
- Sialography
- Hysterosalpingography.

INTIMATE FLUOROSCOPIC EXAMINATIONS

There are many intimate fluoroscopic investigations performed in radiology departments on a daily basis. These may seem routine to the healthcare professionals involved in the procedure but for the patient these can be a very traumatic experience.

Intimate examinations need appropriate attention and understanding to enable trust and mutual confidence between the patient and practitioner. The correct setting, the importance of privacy, preservation of the patient's dignity and respect will all influence this type of examination. Express consent, either verbally or in writing, should be obtained for intimate examinations and serious consideration should be given to the need to provide a chaperone.[9]

PAEDIATRIC FLUOROSCOPY

The majority of fluoroscopic examinations are performed by dedicated radiotherapy practitioners with a special interest in paediatrics.

There are special considerations that need to be made when examining these patients.

The age of the child will determine how cooperative the child may be. A baby or young infant will not be able to understand what is happening and may become distressed at being held down. Involve the parents, ask them to hold the child or allow them to give the barium during a barium swallow/meal or follow through examination.

Consider adding flavours to the drink to try and make the examination a more pleasant experience for the baby or child.

Using child play specialists may be considered to help distract the child during the examination and to help put the child at ease.

PREPARATION OF THE PATIENT BEFORE AND AFTER FLUOROSCOPIC EXAMINATIONS

The majority of patients attending for a procedure under fluoroscopy will require some form of preparation. Due to individual preferences and availability, preparations may differ from department to department. Examples are given in Table 17.3.

PATIENT INFORMATION LEAFLETS

Improving information for patients was a commitment in the NHS Plan. When writing patient information leaflets, it is good practice to write from the patient's point of view and assume they have little knowledge of the subject. The exception to this is the 'expert patient' who has a long-term medical condition.

Tips for writing patient information leaflets[4]

Use everyday language. Avoid jargon and acronyms. Use plain language but be aware that childish language can be patronising

Use patient-friendly text. Use personal pronouns such as 'we' and 'you'. If it is difficult to avoid using medical terminology, such as 'nuclear medicine', explain what it means

Information should be in context with other information, i.e. letters and leaflets

Reinforce the information that patients have been told at the clinic

Explain instructions, e.g. the importance of taking bowel prep and diet restrictions

Help people make decisions by giving facts about risks, side-effects and benefits. Give alternatives to the examination

Do not confuse people by covering several treatments and conditions in the same leaflet

Tell people what other information, support and resources are available

Be up-to-date. Give the most recent practice and latest phone numbers

Let people know if information is available in other formats.

RESPECT, PRIVACY AND DIGNITY DURING FLUOROSCOPY EXAMINATIONS

In recent NHS Benchmark publications,[10] the importance of the patients' rights to being treated with respect, dignity and privacy is highlighted. *Respect* is defined as having due regard for the feelings and rights of others. *Privacy* is defined as freedom from unauthorised intrusion. *Dignity* is defined as quality of being worthy of respect.

The majority of patients in fluoroscopy are required to undress and wear a hospital gown. They may feel exposed due to the procedure they are about to undergo especially examinations of their bowel, which requires rectal intubation. A correct sized gown as well as a dressing gown may help to preserve a patient's dignity. Many hospitals advise patients to bring their own dressing gowns and this is often indicated in patient information leaflets and appointment letters.

> **!** Allow patients to get undressed close to the room so they are not walking through busy waiting areas. Good practice is to have separate waiting areas for patients who are in gowns and a separate area for males and females. However, space and workflow often make this difficult to achieve.

Table 17.3 Specific patient preparations and aftercare for fluoroscopic examinations

Procedure	Definition	Preparation required prior to procedure	Aftercare
Barium swallow	Investigation of the upper GI tract with barium	Nil by mouth 4–6 hours before procedure	
Barium meal	Investigation of the upper GI tract mainly stomach	Nil by mouth 8 hours before procedure	If Buscopan administered, warn patient of blurred vision; constipation
Barium swallow/meal	Investigation of the oesophagus and stomach after ingestion of barium liquid	As for barium meal	As for barium meal
Barium small bowel meal/enema/enteroclysis	Examination of the small bowel after injection of barium liquid or via a nasogastric feeding tube	For enteroclysis, no food or drink 8 hours prior	Warn of constipation
Barium enema	Examination of the large bowel by introduction of barium via a rectal catheter	Bowel preparation and fasting required	Use of toilet and washing facilities. Possible diarrhoea. Inform patient stools will be white in appearance. After affects of antispasmodic. Advice to drink plenty of fluids to reduce constipation
Proctogram	Examination of the rectum to determine the cause of evacuatory difficulty, pelvic floor pain and faecal incontinence	No food for 8 hours prior. Approx. 1 hour before procedure, patient to drink barium liquid. Change into gown	Use of toilet facilities
Water soluble contrast swallow	Examination of upper GI tract with a water soluble contrast[a]	None required	None required
Water soluble contrast enema	Examination of the large bowel by introduction of water soluble contrast[a] via colostomy or a rectal catheter	None required	Use of toilet and washing facilities
Sialogram	Investigation of the salivary glands following injection of contrast[a]	Removal of false teeth. Control images taken	Mouthwash provided
Dacryocystogram	Investigation of the lacrimal system following an injection of contrast[a]		Eye covered until patient is able to 'blink'
Urethrogram	Examination of the urethra after administration of contrast[a]	Micturate prior to procedure. Local anaesthetic applied	Warn patients of the chance of haematuria. Use of toilet and washing facilities
Cystogram	Examination of the urinary bladder after introduction of contrast[a] via a catheter	Micturate prior to procedure. Some patients may require sedation	Use of toilet and washing facilities

Table 17.3 Specific patient preparations and aftercare for fluoroscopic examinations—cont'd

Procedure	Definition	Preparation required prior to procedure	Aftercare
Hysterosalpingo-gram	Examination of uterus and fallopian tubes following cannulation of the cervix and injection of contrast[a]	Examination to be performed within 10 days of start of menstruation and when menstruation has ceased Empty bladder prior	Recovery time Sanitary pad provided Use of toilet and washing facilities Explain possible abdominal pain and 'spotting' After affects of antispasmodic if administered

[a]Radiopaque iodine-based contrast agent.

Access to toilets as soon as leaving the examination room will also help maintain the patient's dignity, especially after a barium enema, proctogram or hysterosalpingogram examination. Many radiology departments now have en-suite and shower room facilities.

Only allow those that are required to be present in the fluoroscopy room during the procedure. Locking the door will prevent anyone from entering. Trust approved interpreters should be used rather than family members to allow for patient confidentiality and dignity.

CONSENT FOR FLUOROSCOPY EXAMINATIONS

Effective communication with patients is key in providing good quality care and is vital in gaining valid informed consent.

! Good practice in gaining consent is part of an ongoing process of communication that respects patient rights and takes into account a patient's capabilities, concerns and circumstances.

Patient's capabilities, concerns and circumstances include:

- Their temperament, attitude and level of understanding
- Influences that are non-medical but may impact on their choice
- Disabilities or impairment
- Their individual circumstances and cultural norms
- Information provided to the patient in a form and language they can understand
- Response to their questions and concerns.

! Consent is a process – it results from open dialogue, not from getting a signature on a form. Whenever it is possible, before providing treatment or investigating a patient's condition you must be satisfied that the patient has understood what is proposed and the reasons for it. In addition, the patient must be informed appropriately about the balance between risk and the benefit of undergoing the investigation.

In each case where care is provided, a judgement needs to be taken on the basis of the nature of the procedure, level of risk versus the potential benefit, and an understanding of the needs of the patient. According to the Royal College of Radiologists' Standards for Patient Consent Particular to Radiology (2005), the person making the judgement must ensure the following:

1. The patient has the right information to make the decision
2. The information has been presented in a way that the patient can understand
3. The patient has shared in the process of decision-making and agrees with the outcome.

Apart from interventional procedures, the majority of fluoroscopic examinations do not require written consent. However, consent must be gained for all investigations before they commence. The types of consent that patients may be asked to give will be dependent on the procedure or treatment the patient is to undergo. The three types of consent are described below.

Written consent

1. Written informed consent must be completed and included in the patient's clinical record for: medical, surgical, radiology, endoscopy and oncology treatments/

procedures requiring general, regional or local anaesthesia or intravenous sedation

2. Invasive procedures or treatment where there are known significant complications or risks, e.g. lung, liver biopsies, angiography
3. Administration of blood products or the administration of a blood transfusion
4. Administration of medications with known high-risk complications
5. Participation in clinical trials and medical research.

Verbal consent

Verbal consent is where a patient states their consent to a procedure verbally but does not complete a written consent form.

Verbal consent is adequate for fluoroscopic procedures or treatments including:

1. Barium studies, e.g. enemas, proctograms
2. Joint injections under fluoroscopy
3. Urological investigations, i.e. cystogram, urethogram
4. Video fluoroscopy.

Verbal consent must be documented in the patient record.

Implied consent

Implied consent refers to when a patient passively cooperates in a process (such as taking medication or giving blood) without discussion or formal consent.

The principles of good communication apply in these circumstances and health professionals need to provide the patient with enough information to understand the procedure and why it is being done.

Implied consent does not need to be documented in the clinical record.

Case scenario 1

A parent brings in her 7-month-old baby or a micturating cystogram procedure.

What considerations need to be made?

- Ensure the environment is child-friendly; consider the lighting and colours; use distraction techniques; use a play specialist to assist during examination if possible
- Examination may be traumatic for the patient and parents so ensure good communication is maintained throughout
- Immobilisation of the patient: consider what is required and ask parents to be involved
- Radiation dose and reduction: consider that paediatric examinations may be possible without using grid facilities
- Ensure clear explanation and communication to parents throughout the procedure

- Ensure presence of only necessary staff in room
- Extra time will be required to perform the examination.

Case scenario 2

A 28-year-old female is attending for a hysterosalpingogram procedure.

What considerations need to be made?

- Consent: Information leaflets must be provided before the patient attends for her appointment and this will alleviate some of the anxieties the patient will have before the procedure. Good communication before and during the procedure will also help the patient to relax.
- Privacy and dignity: This is an intimate examination, therefore due to the nature of the procedure, only 2–3 people may be present in the room. Explaining the role of each person to the patient may help them appreciate the need for the others to be present. If possible, consider only female members of staff.
- Limiting radiation dose: Remove grid if possible. Newer fluoroscopy equipment may have last image hold or fluoroscopy loop hold options. Ensure you use a small collimation field. Gonad protection will not be possible due to the nature of the examination. Be careful not to change from a large field of view to an increased magnification, as this increases the exposure required by the image intensifier tube and the absorbed dose to tissues within the radiation beam will also be increased.
- The patient may have psychological issues around fertility and may be anxious about the results following the procedure. Information regarding the next step in the patient's pathway, i.e. outpatient appointments with the referring clinician must be communicated to the patient. If the results of the procedure are discussed with the patient, ensure that they understand.
- Aftercare and recovery: explain to patient that they may have 'spotting' of blood after the procedure and may experience lower abdominal pain/discomfort. Give them information on who to contact should the need arise. This information may prevent the patient from being alarmed later and should complications arise, they will be aware of who to contact.

ROLES AND RESPONSIBILITY OF THE MEDICAL IMAGING PRACTITIONER WITHIN FLUOROSCOPY

Patient care

- Correctly identify the patient with the 3-point check: (1) Name; (2) Date of Birth; (3) Address
- Maintain the privacy and dignity of patients at all times

- Adequately explain each examination to the patient in order to ensure that the patient is at ease
- Be aware of the basic principles of radiation protection in order to reduce the radiation dose to the patient as much as possible
- Understand the indications for and contraindications against the use of intravenous radiographic contrast, and be able to monitor its administration
- Be able to recognise and treat idiosyncratic reactions to intravenous contrast
- Develop an understanding of the indications and contraindications to the different types of enteral contrast, and the differences and relative merits of single and double contrast studies
- Develop knowledge of the preparation and aftercare required for the common and more complex examinations
- Understand the physics of radiation protection and how to apply it to routine studies
- Be able to answer all questions required to obtain consent from patient.

Interpersonal and communication skills

- Communicate with the patient at all times during the examination in order to ensure that the patient remains at ease
- Communicate effectively with all members of the healthcare team
- Expedite abnormal results to the referring physician (NPSA)
- Appropriately obtain informed consent
- Radiotherapy practitioners and advanced medical imaging practitioners need to produce concise reports which include all relevant information.

Professionalism

- Introduce yourself to the patient so that they are aware of your name, role and title
- Demonstrate respect for patients and all members of the healthcare team
- Respect patient confidentiality
- Present oneself as a professional in appearance and communication
- Develop a responsible work ethic with regards to the task given.

KEY POINTS

- It is important to be familiar and competent with the fluoroscopy equipment the operator is working with. This will ensure low radiation doses are utilised for every procedure. Also be aware of any manufacturer radiation dose reduction devices, e.g. virtual collimation, care positioning, grids
- To ensure cooperation of the patient during the examination, the patient must receive appropriate explanations before, during and after the examination
- Respect the patients' privacy and dignity by having only essential staff during the examination. This is most important for intimate examinations
- Professionals administering contrast agents must be aware of their indications and contraindications. Appropriate patient group directives (PGDs) must be in place to allow non-medical practitioners to administer them
- Good communication between professionals and patient is paramount.

Chapter 18

Interventional radiology

Andrew England

CHAPTER OUTLINE

This chapter will consider:

- Commonly encountered interventional radiology procedures
- Detailed descriptions of the Seldinger technique
- Special considerations, e.g. analgesia and sedation

INTRODUCTION

Interventional radiology (IR) is now a well-established part of modern medicine. Using imaging guidance (fluoroscopy, ultrasound, CT and MRI), IR can provide minimally invasive treatment options for a continually expanding range of diseases. Recent developments in imaging technology and instrumentation have also helped fuel the worldwide adoption of IR. Today, IR procedures provide an attractive alternative to surgery, often with lower mortality and morbidity rates, faster recovery times and at lower cost. IR procedures are performed via direct skin punctures (percutaneously) or through direct introduction of catheters and guidewires through orifices such as the mouth and anus. In addition to lower mortality and morbidity rates, there are several other key advantages which can help explain the rapid growth of IR (Table 18.1). Disadvantages are also evident and include the associated radiation burden, service availability issues, set-up costs and a lack of evidence for some procedures.

GROWTH OF INTERVENTIONAL RADIOLOGY

The birth of IR is, for many, attributed to Charles Dotter. On 16 January 1964, Dotter successfully undertook a percutaneous balloon angioplasty procedure to treat a focal stenosis of the superficial femoral artery.[1] Since then, there has been a massive explosion in both the variety and number of IR procedures performed. Almost every hospital within the UK offers some form of IR procedures; large hospitals may offer a full range of services and these are usually performed by dedicated *interventional* radiologists, or in some instances, practitioners or nurses. IR procedures are generally undertaken using conscious sedation instead of more risky general anaesthesia. The absence of a general anaesthetic has undoubtedly assisted in reducing mortality and morbidity and allows many of these procedures to be undertaken as a day-case or with only a short hospital stay. Day-case or short-stay procedures are highly attractive too for commissioners and hospital managers as they can show considerable economic benefits when compared with surgical alternatives. Day-case procedures are however, not suitable for all patients, careful selection is paramount and should ideally involve discussion within the multidisciplinary team (MDT) and include a face-to-face consultation with a member of the IR team. Measures should also be in place to allow a day-case patient to be admitted at short notice; this may be if there are unexpected complications or if there is a sudden change to the physical condition or social circumstances of the patient.

THE HEART OF IR: THE SELDINGER TECHNIQUE

The Seldinger technique, named after the Swedish radiologist Dr Sven-Ivar Seldinger, is a medical procedure used to obtain safe access to blood vessels and hollow viscera (Fig. 18.1). The Seldinger technique has led to the development of many successful IR procedures, including angioplasty, percutaneous nephrostomy and percutaneous gastrostomy. This technique is not without its risks, particularly when

Table 18.1 Advantages and disadvantages of IR procedures

Advantages
Often avoids general anaesthesia and its associated risks
Risk, pain and recovery time are often significantly reduced
Less surgical scarring and fewer complications associated with open procedures, e.g. infection and haemorrhage
Most procedures are performed on an outpatient basis or with a short hospital stay
Only treatment option for some patients
Many IR procedures are less expensive than the surgical alternatives

Disadvantages
Patients are awake and aware of what is happening and need to remain still for often long periods of time
Lack of service availability in some areas
Lack of an evidence base for some IR procedures
Expensive capital costs and training issues when starting a service

acquiring arterial access. Published evidence[2] indicated complications when accessing the common femoral artery, the majority of which were minor puncture site haematomas.

INFORMED CONSENT

Patients must be informed and provide consent before being examined, receiving treatment or having a procedure. Invasive procedures, such as those within IR, require a written record of consent. If this is to be valid then the patient must be given an adequate explanation of the procedure, its intended outcomes as well as the risks involved and the alternatives available. Information must be up-to-date, suitably structured and provided in writing where possible and the patient must be allowed adequate opportunity to make a fully informed decision. For this reason, many interventional radiologists will aim to see patients in a dedicated radiology clinic or on the hospital ward; either way steps must be in place to allow a patient adequate time to decide whether they wish to undergo the procedure.

> **!** The responsibility for obtaining informed consent rests with the clinician who is to carrying out the IR procedure.

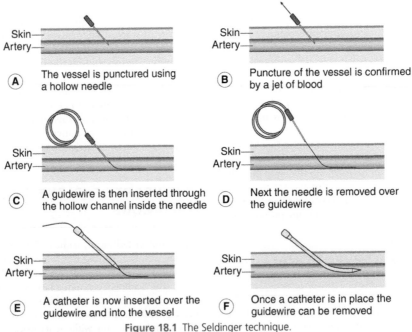

(A) The vessel is punctured using a hollow needle

(B) Puncture of the vessel is confirmed by a jet of blood

(C) A guidewire is then inserted through the hollow channel inside the needle

(D) Next the needle is removed over the guidewire

(E) A catheter is now inserted over the guidewire and into the vessel

(F) Once a catheter is in place the guidewire can be removed

Figure 18.1 The Seldinger technique.

In some instances, it is acceptable to delegate this responsibility to an appropriate healthcare professional (HCP). Some departments employ specialist nurse practitioners to admit, consent and discharge patients who are undergoing radiological interventions. Whoever is responsible for consent, this person must have the necessary knowledge and experience to provide adequate explanations to the patient. Within IR, consent can frequently involve more than one person. The referring clinician, who has requested the procedure, has a responsibility to explain the clinical need and the alternatives available to the patient. The interventional radiologist or HCP will then focus on obtaining consent for the requested procedure and explaining the intended benefits and risks. The provision of written information, e.g. patient information leaflets is encouraged, together with a complete assessment of the individual communication needs of each patient.

> **!** Consent is not only a legal and moral requirement but has been shown to provide further benefits. The provision of high-quality information prior to a procedure can reduce anxiety levels, improve compliance and help speed up recovery.

ANALGESIA AND SEDATION

Patients are often awake for their IR procedure, although this is advantageous in terms of a faster recovery and fewer risks, being awake may cause some distress for the patient. For most IR procedures it is also likely that a patient will experience some degree of pain. Inducing distress can affect patient cooperation and cause increased sympathetic activity. This can in turn lead to tachycardia and hypertension, both of which can lead to myocardial ischaemia or infarction in a susceptible patient.[3] To combat any distress and anxiety, a combination of sedatives and analgesic drugs are administered to enhance procedural safety, ensure maximal comfort and procedural success. Using sedation carries risks, especially when inappropriate techniques are used by inexperienced or untrained personnel. It is therefore crucial that IR practitioners have a thorough understanding of sedation and analgesia regimes. IR suites must be designed with sedation in mind, vital signs monitoring equipment, piped oxygen and suction must be available in the IR room, as well as any adjacent recovery areas. Nursing staff, who are familiar with the interventional department, should undertake preset pre-procedural patient checks and should be available to monitor patients both during and immediately after the procedure.

> **!** When the patient returns to the ward it is useful for a post-procedural information leaflet to accompany the patient. This can provide information on any sedation and analgesia administered and a brief summary of the procedure.

More importantly, it can provide information on the aftercare for the patient, e.g. mobilisation or additional observations required and the contact details for the IR department/interventionalist.

VASCULAR INTERVENTIONS

Peripheral artery disease (PAD) is caused by the narrowing of the arteries in the legs; this is commonly the result of atherosclerosis. Fatty deposits build up along the walls of the arteries causing stenosis and eventually vessel occlusion. Over half of the patients with peripheral artery disease (PAD) are asymptomatic. PAD is a progressive disease and in chronic cases, may progress into painful leg cramps, ischaemic rest pain and tissue loss. Best medical therapy is generally the first option for early PAD and includes smoking cessation and controlling any hypertension, hypercholestreolaemia and diabetes. Invasive interventions such as angioplasty, stenting or surgery also have a role but for more extensive/life-limiting PAD.

Angioplasty and stenting

The mechanical widening of a narrowed or occluded artery can be achieved using a balloon mounted on a catheter. The balloon is inflated across the lesion and can stretch the vessel returning it to its normal diameter. This procedure is given the term angioplasty or more precisely, percutaneous transluminal angioplasty (PTA). PTA has successfully been applied to almost all vascular territories, including the peripheral, carotid, renal, visceral and coronary arteries and can offer a much needed alternative to surgery. The implantation of a stent is another option for the treatment of a narrowed segment of artery. A stent is a tubular support device which when implanted inside a vessel, serves to restore luminal diameter and improve blood flow. Stents are indicated not only for the treatment of a stenosis but can be used to recanalise a chronic arterial occlusion, re-open an occlusive dissection following angioplasty and to treat fragile arterial plaques which have caused distal emboli.

The iliac arteries, because of their size, are well suited for radiological intervention. Initial technical success rates of >90% have been reported for angioplasty, together with

5-year primary patency rates of around 80%.[4] If the lesions are long and calcified, then the patency rates are generally lower. Angioplasty failure is also more likely in patients with chronically occluded vessels, symptoms of critical limb ischaemia or poor arterial flow within the calf-vessels and feet.[5] Stents are now routinely used within diseased iliac arteries and can deliver patency rates comparable with surgical bypass. Stents are not devoid of complications; stents can become occluded or re-stenosed from intimal hyperplasia. Additional interventional procedures may be needed, e.g. repeat angioplasty in order to maintain luminal patency. PAD is generally progressive and some patients, despite angioplasty and stenting, will require surgical bypass or even an amputation of the effected limb. Arterial angioplasty and stenting involve the administration of iodinated contrast media; this has nephrotoxic properties and it is recommended that pre-procedural renal function is checked.

Although angioplasty and stenting are widely used throughout the body, several reports have questioned its value. The ASTRAL (Angioplasty and Stenting for Renal Artery Lesions) trial suggested that there were no benefits from angioplasty and stenting when compared with best medical therapy for patients with renovascular disease.[6] Likewise, the implantation of a carotid artery stent (CAS) to prevent stroke has generated much debate. Randomised controlled trials (RCTs) comparing best medical therapy with surgery have shown a clear benefit for surgery in patients with a severe (>70%) stenosis.[7,8] When comparing surgical endarterectomy with stenting RCTs have generally failed to show any difference between the two treatments.[9] Others have reported an increased stroke risk from stenting[10] and this has led to many advocating surgery over stenting for the prevention of ischaemic stroke. As with all treatments, there are certain situations when a treatment may be substituted for a less favourable alternative. This may be at the request of the patient or if contraindications are present. Carotid stenting, although less favourable than surgical endarterectomy still has a place in the management of CAS. Centres may prefer CAS for cases of surgical re-stenosis or where a stenosis relates to previous radiotherapy of the neck. It is important to treat every patient as an individual; the pros and cons of each treatment must be carefully weighed up before deciding on management.

> **!** As with arterial disease there are also indications for stenting in the venous system. Chronic obstruction of deep veins may be treated by implantation of a stent. Extrinsic compression of veins resulting from malignancy, e.g. superior vena cava obstruction and recurrent fibrotic re-stenosis of veins can also be successfully treated by stenting.

Covered and drug eluting stents

Covered or fabric wrapped stents are often termed stent-grafts and are an essential component of any IR department. Vessel rupture occurs in a small number of patients following angioplasty[11] and this can be seen on angiography with the patient continuing to report pain at the angioplasy site following deflation of the angioplasty balloon. Vessel rupture can be quickly and successfully treated by implanting a covered stent. Other indications for a covered stent include the management of arterial trauma from either a blunt or penetrating injury, e.g. RTA or stabbing, the treatment of pseudoaneurysms and degenerative aneurysms of the aorta and peripheral vessels and for the treatment of recurrent intimal hyperplasia.

Drug eluting stents (DES) are specifically designed to deliver agents (e.g. sirolimus or paclitaxel) to the intima layer of an artery in order to prevent in-stent restenosis. DESs are predominantly used in the coronary arteries.[12,13,14]

Thrombolysis

Thrombolysis is the collective term for the breaking up and the dissolving of blood clots. Acute arterial obstruction can result from either an embolism or thrombus formation *in situ* and are emergency conditions. There are two IR-based thrombolytic treatment options available to treat an acute vascular occlusion, mechanical thrombectomy and chemical thrombolysis.

Mechanical thrombectomy involves the use of angioplasty balloons and large bore catheters to manually disrupt the thrombus and then remove it by aspiration. This is an entirely percutaneous procedure and is often followed by the infusion of thrombolytic drugs. There is also the possibility of using an AngioJet rheolytic system for mechanical thrombectomy. AngioJet (Medrad, Inc., Warrendale, PA) is a percutaneous catheter-based system that uses a high speed saline jet that produces a vacuum at the catheter tip allowing the removal of thrombus in acute occlusions of both the arterial and venous systems. Chemical thrombolysis uses drugs to enhance the body's own internal thrombolytic system. Commonly used thrombolytic agents include tissue plasminogen activator (alteplase, t-PA) and (reteplase, r-PA) and are delivered direct to the site of thrombosis by intra-arterial or intra-venously placed catheters positioned under fluoroscopic guidance. Chemical thrombolysis is a risky procedure and can cause haemorrhage at sites away from the initial blockage. Patients must be carefully screened before initiating treatment, those with a history of a previous spontaneous haemorrhage, e.g. cerebral or GI are usually excluded from treatment. Arterial access sheaths and catheters must be left in the occluded vessel while the treatment is delivered, usually >24 hours. In order to prevent migration of the thrombolytic catheter or serious puncture site complications, patients must remain on full bed rest. There is also the possibility of serious haemorrhagic complications from catheter thrombolysis. The intracranial haemorrhage risk is around 1% and consequently, patients must have regular neurological and cardiovascular observations. It is also likely that a patient will need to be managed in a high-dependency environment, which may form part of a dedicated vascular ward.

Embolisation

Clinically, there may be a need to reduce or stop the blood supply to an area, e.g. life-threatening GI haemorrhage. Embolisation is an IR procedure which can be used to cause temporary or permanent disruption to the blood supply to an area and help manage haemorrhage, tumours and abnormal blood vessels. A variety of embolic agents are available and selection is based on the indication for treatment and the anatomical region. Permanent embolic agents cause irreversible blood vessel occlusion; this can be achieved by internally blocking the vessel lumen using coils, glue or polyvinyl alcohol particles (PVA). Temporary embolisation can be achieved using autologous clot or gel foam and can maintain occlusion for a period of several days to a few weeks. Intravascular thrombin injections can also be used to cause immediate thrombosis, particularly useful when treating femoral artery false aneurysms resulting from incorrectly positioned arterial access. With any embolisation procedure there is the risk that the embolic agent can lodge in the wrong place and starve normal tissue of a blood supply. It is also possible that the catheter cannot be positioned in a blood vessel which feeds only the abnormal area. Infarction of normal tissue may be accepted as part of the embolisation procedure but if this is considered unsafe, then it will mean that the patient cannot undergo embolisation.

Venous access and filtration

Access to the central veins is often required for haemodialysis, parenteral nutrition and the long-term administration of antimicrobials and chemotherapy drugs. Access can be achieved using direct puncture into either the peripheral or central veins and provide long-term access via externally sited catheters or totally implantable ports. Venous access under imaging-guidance offers advantages over traditional anatomical landmark based methods. Higher technical success, fewer post-procedural complications, more accurate catheter placements, shortened procedural times, have all been reported when using imaging.[15]

Vena caval filters can be used to prevent pulmonary embolism from a venous thrombus. Debate exists regarding the precise indications for filter implantation and also the precise type of filter, timing of implantation and whether the filter should be eventually removed. Common indications generally include patients who have known deep vein thrombosis (DVT), who have absolute contraindications to anticoagulation or who cannot tolerate anticoagulation or where there is ineffective anticoagulation. Filters do not prevent venous clot formation but act as a trap within the vena cava to prevent clot moving into the pulmonary circulation. If a temporary filter is implanted, then there must be a robust system in place for arranging retrieval. Filters can incorporate into the caval wall with time; this can make delayed filter retrieval difficult and risky.

NON-VASCULAR INTERVENTIONS

Tumour ablation

Chemical ablation of a tumour is usually achieved by introducing a chemical agent, e.g. ethanol, directly into the lesion under imaging guidance, usually ultrasound and CT. Percutaneous ethanol injection (PEI) is performed by inserting a needle, usually under ultrasound guidance into the centre of the lesion. Absolute alcohol is then injected with the droplets appearing as an echogenic cloud moving away from the needle tip. PEI is particularly useful in treating hepatocellular carcinomas (HCC) in cirrhotic livers, however, multiple PEI sessions may be necessary in order to treat larger lesions.

Other ablative techniques use temperature extremes or radiofrequency (RF) energy to percutaneously treat solid tumours. Abnormal levels of temperature within tissues result in permanent cellular damage and coagulative necrosis. Tumour destruction can be achieved by cryoablation (freezing) tumour tissue. Tumours are cooled to at least $-35°C$ via injection of liquid nitrogen through cryoprobes. Common applications include the treatment of tumours within the skin, bone, larynx, prostate and liver. In reverse, cellular damage also occurs when tissues are exposed to temperatures over $60°C$; here coagulation and cell death occurs instantaneously. Radiofrequency (RF) ablation has emerged as the most predictable and safe technique for the percutaneous treatment of solid tumours.[16] An electrode is placed in the centre of the tumour and RF energy is applied which causes heating and tumour necrosis.

> **!** Generally, ablation can be painful and is either performed under general anaesthetic or with deep sedation with careful attention to ensuring adequate pain control.

Combined chemotherapeutic and embolic agents can also be instilled into vascular tumours via selective catheterisation of arterial feeder vessels (TACE). These embolic agents reduce the blood flow to a tumour and allow the chemotherapy drugs to remain within the malignant lesion for an extended period of time. Primary and secondary hepatic lesions are particularly amenable to TACE. Embolisation has a further role in the management of several other benign and malignant tumours. Embolic material delivered to the supplying artery can cause successful infarction of a tumour. The most common benign tumour to undergo embolisation is uterine fibroids. In uterine artery embolisation (UAE), PVA particles are injected until there is severely reduced flow into both uterine arteries. A recent RCT concluded that UAE for symptomatic fibroids provides a satisfactory alternative surgical hysterectomy.[17] UAE can be a painful procedure and it is essential that adequate post-procedural analgesia is prescribed. Pain management often includes a patient-controlled analgesia (PCA) infusion of an opiate, e.g. fentanyl, together with rectally administered diclofenac. Pain may continue for several days and discharge analgesic regimes must take this into account. Following discharge, it is usually recommended that the patient receives regular paracetamol and diclofenac (orally). UAE patients can also experience post-embolisation syndrome (PES), this includes fever, pelvic pain and a vaginal discharge. PES may also be accompanied by nausea and exhaustion and will usually pass with time. If the symptoms get worse then infection must be considered, if this is confirmed and found to be in the uterus, then hysterectomy may be considered. This is often essential in order to prevent the spread of infection and any life-threatening sepsis.

Image-guided percutaneous biopsy

Histological assessment of both liver and kidney tissue is a major diagnostic tool. Even with major developments in both biochemical and imaging techniques, biopsy still remains an important diagnostic tool. Biopsy can be used to sample general organ tissue or a specific abnormal anatomical part, e.g. a mass. Biopsy can usually be undertaken as a day-case procedure but careful consideration on the use of sedation and analgesia must be undertaken and include the assessment of pain in the post-biopsy period. The role of imaging is to help mark an entry site and advise on any 'no go' areas. More recently, image-guided biopsy techniques have evolved to include 'real-time' visualisation of the needle tracking into the biopsiable tissue. This method is generally considered to be associated with few complications and promotes a greater chance of successfully obtaining an appropriate sample.

Percutaneous abscess drainage

Image-guided percutaneous drainage of an abdominal or pelvic abscess is the primary treatment option for infected or symptomatic fluid collections when there is an absence of an indication for immediate surgery. Imaging is typically by ultrasound or CT and commonly utilises a transabdominal approach for drainage. For difficult to reach abscesses,

such as those deep in the pelvis, under the diaphragm or in the epigastric area, then access can be undertaken via the transrectal, transgluteal, intercostal or transhepatic routes. Treatment success is generally excellent, with primary success being reported in 86–96% of patients.[18,19]

There are two common methods for introducing a drainage catheter into an abscess. First, the trocar technique where a catheter mounted on a sharp trocar is inserted into the abscess under image guidance. This is the fastest technique but the trocar may be difficult to reposition if the track is suboptimal. Second, and the preferred option, is the Seldinger technique: a hollow needle is inserted into the abscess cavity; a guidewire is then placed into the cavity through the hollow bore of the needle. The drainage catheter is then placed over the guidewire after the needle has been withdrawn. In many instances, the needle track is dilated prior to the introduction of the drainage catheter. Catheters are retained in the abscess cavity, either by the formation of an internal coil or pig-tail at the end of the catheter. Other fixation devices include sutures or devices which adhere to the skin.

Percutaneous urinary interventions

Percutaneous nephrostomy (PCN) is the dominant urological IR procedure and is used to help treat renal stones and other causes of renal obstruction. PCN was first described over 50 years ago as a safe means of decompressing an obstructed kidney. Alternative indications include access for nephroureteral procedures and urinary diversion, e.g. in ureteric fistulae.

Most PCNs are carried out under conscious sedation together with antibiotics prophylaxis. Patients are commonly positioned prone with imaging by a combination of ultrasound and fluoroscopy. Access to the renal pelvis is achieved using a needle, guidewire and dilator. Once a track has been established, then a nephrostomy drainage catheter is placed over the guidewire into the renal pelvis and secured in place (seen as the internal 'pigtail'). Prior to the insertion of the guidewire, successful puncture of the renal collection system is confirmed by antegrade injection of iodinated contrast. For an obstructed system, this is usually preceded by a flow of urine up the needle immediately after puncture. In cases where infection is suspected, urine should be collected and sent for analysis. Occasionally, it is necessary to undertake a PCN in a non-dilated system, e.g. urinary leaks or non-dilated obstruction. This can be challenging,, especially when attempting to visualise the non-dilated renal pelvis using ultrasound. In patients with normal renal function, an intravenous injection of an iodinated contrast medium can be used to opacify the renal pelvis and allow puncture under fluoroscopic guidance. With PCN being a relatively traumatic procedure, patients should be advised to expect small amounts of blood in their urine for several days after the procedure.

Further urological interventions include the insertion of a nephroureteral stent via the nephrostomy tract. This can provide an option for providing internal drainage of the renal collection system directly into the bladder. These double-J internal ureteric stents are commonly used to provide drainage across a malignant ureteric obstruction, e.g. extrinsic compression from a prostate or gynaecological tumour.

Percutaneous radiological gastrostomy (PRG)

Gastrostomy is a procedure to insert a small tube directly through the skin and into the stomach. The primary indication for a gastrostomy is to provide nutrition in patients who are unable to swallow or take inadequate oral nutrition. Gastrostomy tubes are generally inserted under endoscopic guidance (PEG) but for some patients, oesophageal intubation with an endoscope may be unsafe. Radiologically inserted gastrostomy (RIG) provides an option for patients who have a moderate or severe respiratory impairment[20] and who are unsuitable for endoscopic intubation. The RIG procedure involves distension of the stomach with air via a nasogastric tube. Local anaesthesia is then applied to the anterior abdominal wall and gastropexy sutures are then placed between the anterior abdominal wall and stomach to provide immobilisation and prevent the gastrostomy tube being sited within the peritoneal cavity. The stomach is then percutaneously punctured, aspiration of air confirms successful cannulation and a guidewire inserted into the stomach and the tract dilated. Finally, a gastrostomy tube is tracked over the wire and into the stomach; fixation is by an internal pig-tail or inflated balloon. RIGs are totally percutaneous procedures and avoid any puncture site contamination risks, e.g. stoma metastasis from upper GI tumour seeding. There is a further IR gastrostomy procedure, which is a hybrid of a RIG and PEG and is called a per-oral image-guided gastrostomy (PIG). Again, the stomach is distended with air; Buscopan and local anaesthetic agents are administered. The stomach is then punctured through the anterior abdominal wall and a 4F haemostatic sheath is inserted into the stomach. A guidewire and catheter are then introduced through the sheath and manipulated under fluoroscopy in order to gain access to the lower oesophagus and exteriorised through the mouth. The wire is then exchanged for a stiff guidewire and a push–pull gastrostomy is inserted over the guidewire through the mouth and out of the anterior abdominal wall. PEG complications may be experienced either immediately after the tube placement or over subsequent years following implantation. Skin infections, tube blockages or the tube falling out are all possible and may potentially be avoided. It is essential that the patient and carers are taught how to care for the PEG tube. This information can be obtained from patient information leaflets, websites and nutrition nurses.

Stenting of the GI tract

Intubation of the GI tract for the treatment of strictures is a well-established practice. Certainly, the implantation of plastic prostheses into the oesophagus for the palliative treatment of malignant strictures has been practised for over 100 years.[21] Today, oesophageal stents can be placed under radiological or endoscopic guidance and there are many different stent designs available. These include both covered and uncovered self-expanding stents, some having the presence of an anti-reflux valve or the option for retrieval. Indications for oesophageal stenting now span beyond the palliative treatment of dysphagia and include the management of a trachea-oesophageal fistula, oesophageal perforation, extrinsic compression from mediastinal compression and in some situations, the treatment of benign disease. Regardless of the indication, oesophageal stenting involves conscious sedation with the patient positioned prone to avoid aspiration. Xylocaine spray is first administered in order to act as a throat anaesthetic and assist intubation. The oesophagus is then cannulated with a catheter and guidewire; this is then transversed beyond the tumour and into the stomach. Before the oesophageal stent can be delivered, the tumour must be delineated in order to define the location for the stent. One option is to inject an iodine-based contrast agent through the catheter while withdrawing back from the stomach. Radiopaque markers can then be temporarily stuck to the patient and provide a means to identify the full extent of the tumour. Once the location of the tumour is known, the stent delivery system can then be tracked over a stiff guidewire and deployed relative to the radio-opaque markers. Stent deployment can be painful; many operators will administer a small bolus of an intravenous analgesic agent, e.g. fentanyl prior to the start of stent delivery.

For benign disease, there is also the possibility of improving swallowing using balloon dilatation. Depending on the underlying aetiology, repeat procedures may be necessary in order to maintain adequate swallowing.

Stenting of the GI tract has expanded to include the treatment of strictures in the duodenum and more commonly the colon. For both areas, the primary indication is the non-surgical management of malignant obstruction. Stenting in both areas can be challenging, especially when presented with difficult anatomy resulting from the malignancy. Evidence from several RCTs comparing surgical gastrojejunostomy with duodenal stenting (DS) identifies that DS was associated with fewer complications, shorter hospital stays, lower post-procedural pain levels and a faster time to restoring oral intake than surgery.[22,23] Mortality rates were similar for both groups of patients. For colonic obstruction, the majority of patients are treated with emergency surgery which carries a significant risk of mortality and morbidity. Patients are often left with a permanent colostomy that diminishes their quality of life. The implantation of a colonic stent (CS) under fluoroscopy guidance is a potential alternative treatment option.[24] As with oesophageal stents, colonic stent, also have a role in treating benign disease. Benign colonic strictures, leaks and fistulae have all been successfully treated by colonic stenting under radiological guidance. Both duodenal and colonic stenting can induce the discharge of bodily fluids (vomit and faeces). This should be anticipated when preparing the room for the procedure and by having vomit bowls and inco-sheets readily available.

Colonic stenting requires prolonged rectal catheterisation; this is likely to induce some degree of anxiety and embarrassment.

> **!** It is essential that IR staff ensure good communication with the patient and perform steps to reduce any discomfort and anxiety, e.g. cleaning-up accidents and keeping the patient covered up where possible.

Percutaneous biliary procedures

Percutaneous biliary procedures involve the successful cannulation of the biliary tree using an aseptic technique. Following the initial needle puncture, catheters and guidewires can be manipulated within the biliary system under fluoroscopic guidance. Historically, percutaneous biliary procedures were undertaken purely for diagnostic purposes and involved passing a needle percutaneously through the liver and into a biliary duct. Iodinated contrast could then be injected into the bile ducts in order to delineate the anatomy. This technique called percutaneous transhepatic cholangiography (PTC) is only undertaken for purely therapeutic reasons today, most commonly in cases of biliary obstruction.

A total or partial biliary obstruction usually results from the presence of gallstones, inflammation or a tumour. IR treatment options include endoscopic retrograde cholangiopancreatography (ERCP) and percutaneous transhepatic biliary drainage (PTBD). PTBD is considered to be more invasive and risky and is therefore reserved for cases where ERCP has failed and there is a need to:

- Decompress an obstructed biliary tree
- Provide access for dilating biliary strictures and removing gallstones
- Divert bile away from bile leaks
- Allow the stenting of biliary defects
- Treat acute biliary sepsis.

Using PTBD, obstruction can be alleviated by placing a drain within the biliary ducts. These drains can be externally sited collecting bile into an external drainage bag or totally internal providing drainage directly into the duodenum. In some situations a combined internal/external drain can be implanted which will achieve dual drainage. If obstruction results from biliary stones then these can be removed percutaneously and allow a more definitive treatment option to be provided. If the source of obstruction is a malignant biliary stricture, e.g. compression from surrounding enlarged lymph nodes then a metallic stent can be placed in the biliary tree to restore patency removing the long-term need for a drain. As previously stated, percutaneous biliary procedures are not without risk. Cases of serious complications have been reported and these include sepsis, haemorrhage, localised infection and inflammation and death. Clinical teams must therefore carefully consider the age, condition of the patient, the underlying aetiology of the biliary obstruction and the degree of biliary dilatation before deciding on treatment.

Endoscopically guided biliary procedures are preferred and are undertaken alongside fluoroscopic guidance. This is either provided in the radiology department or using mobile imaging equipment within the endoscopy suite. Biliary interventional procedures are frequently undertaken on female patients of reproductive age. As with any procedure involving the use of ionising radiation, it is important that the practitioner excludes any possibility of pregnancy. This can be problematic in biliary procedures where the patient may be sedated outside of the radiology department. Good working relationships with the endoscopy/nursing staff will often lead to an accepted protocol for excluding pregnancy. Endoscopic procedures are preferred over percutaneous procedures because they avoid the risks associated with a needle. If the common bile duct (CBD) can be accessed via the duodenal ampulla, then this can be electrically cut open to improve drainage and allow biliary stones to pass. The CBD can then be easily swept with a balloon or basket to remove stones and if necessary, a stent can be placed to assist drainage and alleviate any remaining symptoms.

Vertebroplasty

Percutaneous vertebroplasty and kyphoplasty are valuable treatment options for providing pain relief to patients with painful osteoporosis with loss of vertebral body height or fractures and for patients with symptomatic vertebral haemangiomas and painful malignant tumours, e.g. metastases or myeloma.[25] For percutaneous vertebroplasty, an injection of acrylic bone cement directly into the vertebral body can relieve pain, stabilise vertebral fractures and in some cases, restore vertebral height. Kyphoplasty is similar to vertebroplasty but before the injection of acrylic cement, a balloon is inflated in the vertebral body in order to create a cavity. Using vertebroplasty, reports have suggested that pain relief will be experienced in around 58–97% of patients and that a decrease in analgesic requirements will be seen in 50–91% of patients.[25] Complications following vertebroplasty do exist and include damage to nerves and tissues following the introduction of the cement injection needle and from leakage of cement into the surrounding tissues.

NEW FRONTIERS

With the rapid development of IR, new treatments are rapidly becoming available and traditional management options are changing. For example ablative techniques used at one time to treat solid organ tumours and correct heart rhythm disturbances, are now being used inside blood vessels. Refractory hypertension (RH) can now be treated by renal denervation where catheter-based RF ablation is applied to the renal sympathetic nerves in the renal arteries. Also IR is emerging as an option for patients with multiple sclerosis (MS). There have been reports of a possible link between chronic cerebrospinal venous insufficiency (CCSVI) and MS. Venous angioplasty has been trialled as a potential treatment option, with several encouraging initial reports. High numbers of sufferers and the associated costs of managing these highly debilitating diseases are driving demand for alternative treatments. High quality research is still essential in order to determine the safety and efficacy of these new interventional therapies.

In future years, existing IR therapies are likely to play more of a dominant role in patient care. Catheter-directed embolisation is likely to play a more dominant role in the management of massive haemorrhage following a major trauma. UK major trauma centres are encouraged to have IR services available 24/7 and be located in close proximity to the Emergency Department. The potential of IR in controlling massive haemorrhage has also being widely publicised throughout the UK and a RCT has also been established to evaluate the efficacy and safety of embolisation in trauma. These factors are likely to contribute to significant changes in practice and are likely to be mirrored in many other disease areas, e.g. oncology.

KEY POINTS

- Interventional radiology (IR) is a subspecialty of radiology in which minimally invasive procedures are performed under image guidance
- IR procedures are attractive because they generally offer lower mortality and morbidity rates when compared with traditional surgical alternatives. For some situations, IR techniques may be the only treatment option available

- Over the past decade, IR has experienced rapid growth. Several limitations still exist, including a lack of research evidence for some procedures; initial set-up costs are high; expertise may not be readily available and there are risks from the use of ionising radiation and nephrotoxic contrast media
- The Seldinger technique is a fundamental component of IR; it provides access for guidewires and catheters into vascular and hollow/fluid containing structures
- Informed consent is a prerequisite for any IR procedure; patients must be provided with appropriate information on the procedure, intended benefits and possible risks
- Patient comfort and cooperation is paramount during IR procedures; this is often achieved using a combination of intravenous sedation and analgesia
- Vascular IR procedures are frequently used as a minimally invasive option for improving the blood supply to any area, e.g. angioplasty and stenting. More recent IR developments include the use of covered stents for treating arterial trauma and drug-eluting stents to prevent re-stenosis
- IR can provide a solution for reducing the blood supply to an area. Embolisation has evolved rapidly for the treatment of massive life-threatening haemorrhage, tumours and abnormal blood vessels
- Debate regarding the exact indications for IR procedures commonly exists, e.g. implantation of a vena cava filter. Many regulatory bodies are attempting to provide evidence and/or guidance on the safety and efficacy of various IR techniques. In the absence of an alternative, it is often difficult to limit the use of unproven IR techniques
- The range of non-vascular IR techniques is as wide as the available vascular procedures. Many solid and hollow visceral organ pathologies are now amenable to IR. In these situations, image guidance by ultrasound and CT has a much larger role
- In order to ensure acceptable patient comfort, an assessment of pain is recommended both before and at regular intervals during and after the procedure, appropriate mechanisms should also be in place for prompt pain management.

Chapter | 19 |

Ultrasound

Pauline Mitchell, Naomi Brown

INTRODUCTION

The aim of this chapter is not to duplicate what has already been discussed in Chapter 10 (see the section on Physical and biological effects of ultrasound) but to explore patient centred care that is essential to the efficient and effective delivery of ultrasound services. The qualities of interpersonal interactions, professional and organisational standards are essential to ensure the delivery and maintenance of a patient centred service and therefore it can be argued that professional standards concerning safety, training, communication, accessibility and evidence-based practice are fundamental to underpinning patient centred care.[1] The UK Association of Sonographers (UKAS) provide guidelines, as outlined in Box 19.1, for the conduct of sonographers to ensure that patient centred care is at the forefront of professional practice.

PHYSIOLOGICAL AND BIOLOGICAL RISKS

When discussing the safe provision of ultrasound services to the population it is necessary not only to consider the physical and biological risks of ultrasound to the patient but also the training of the practitioner to ensure that the equipment is being utilised appropriately. This section aims to outline practical steps which can be taken by the sonographer to reduce potential risks to patients when undertaking medical ultrasound examinations and are outlined in Table 19.1.

This section should be read in conjunction with Chapter 10, which details the physical aspects of radiation hazards and safety considerations associated with ultrasound.

Strategies and guidelines for best practice to minimise the risk to the patient have been well documented by several national and international ultrasound societies and governing bodies as listed below:[2]

- United Kingdom Association of Sonographers (UKAS)
- British Medical Ultrasound Society (BMUS)
- European Federation of Societies for Ultrasound in Medicine and Biology (EFSUMB)
- American Institute of Ultrasound in Medicine (AIUM)
- Australasian Society for Ultrasound in Medicine (ASUM)
- World Federation for Ultrasound in Medicine and Biology (WFUMB).

All the guidelines are basically centred around the concepts of the ALARA principle (risks should be 'As Low As Reasonably Achievable'), justification of the examination and the appropriate training of the operator. As mentioned in Chapter 10, at all times the operator must ensure that the Thermal and Mechanical indices displayed stay within the recommended range.

Ultrasound equipment is rapidly evolving, with new technologies providing more applications for the imaging modality. Some carry significant increases in dose to the patient and therefore, it is imperative that the operator is fully aware of the implications of their practice. The British Medical Ultrasound Society (BMUS)

Box 19.1 The Code of Practice for Sonographers

1. Sonographers have a duty of care to their patients and carers and to the minimisation of ultrasound exposure consistent with diagnostic needs.
2. Sonographers are ethically and legally obliged to hold in confidence any information acquired as a result of their professional and clinical duties, except where there is a legal obligation for disclosure.
3. Sonographers must be committed to the provision of a quality ultrasound service having due regard for the legislation and established codes of practice related to healthcare provision in order to minimise risk to patients, carers and other professionals.
4. Sonographers are legally and professionally accountable for their own practice and must not be influenced by any form of discrimination.
5. Sonographers must identify limitations in their practice and request training and support to meet their perceived needs.
6. Sonographers will take all reasonable opportunity to maintain and improve their knowledge and professional competency and that of their peers and students.
7. Sonographers must pay due regard to the way in which they are remunerated for their work.
8. Sonographers have a duty of care to work collaboratively and in cooperation with the multidisciplinary healthcare team in the interests of their patients.
9. Sonographers must act at all times in such a manner as to justify public trust and confidence, to uphold and enhance the reputation of sonography and serve the public interest.
10. Sonographers must ensure that unethical conduct and any circumstances where patients and others are at risk are reported to the appropriate authority.
11. Sonographers who are held accountable in another area of health care must relate this Code to others that govern their practice.
12. Student sonographers pursuing a qualification in medical ultrasound must adhere to their Universities' Codes of Conduct that relate to all elements of their ultrasound education and training.

(Reprinted with kind permission of the College of Radiographers/ United Kingdom Association of Sonographers.)

Table 19.1 Means of risk reduction in ultrasound

Decreases risk to patient	Increases risk to patient
Keep overall examination time to a minimum	Use of Doppler
Reduce dwell time (time spent in one spot)	Increased depth of imaging
Keep power to a minimum	Increased focusing
Use of freeze button	Use of harmonic imaging
Remove transducer from patient when not imaging	Scanning tissues with increased absorption co-efficient such as bone
Use of cine loop	Duplex imaging

Box 19.2 Practical means of risk reduction

The use of the cine loop function should be utilised wherever possible – not only does this reduce the ultrasound exposure to the patient but also if the operator ensures they rest their arm comfortably while reviewing the cine loop images, the potential for musculoskeletal injury to the sonographer is also reduced.

The operator should ensure that while the image is frozen, such as when undertaking measurements, they should not hold the transducer in the same position but instead rest it comfortably with the shoulder not extended and the wrist not being flexed unnecessarily.

The default output power level should be checked before starting each examination. Wherever possible, the output power should be reduced and not increased unless all other image optimisation techniques have been tried without success.

INTERVENTIONAL ULTRASOUND

When considering patient centred care, an understanding of what is important to the patient must be explored. Procedures that reduce the time a patient needs to spend at the hospital have a two-fold benefit in that the patient can remain in their own home and also the cost of care for the service provider is reduced. Ultrasound has rapidly become the modality of choice for the guidance of some interventional therapeutic and diagnostic procedures. Procedures including fluid drainage, biopsy, amniocentesis, chorionic villus sampling (CVS) in obstetric practice, fine needle aspirations (FNA), musculoskeletal (MSK) injections and gynaecological procedures are commonly undertaken within the ultrasound department. These less

produces guidelines[3] which outline the safe use of diagnostic ultrasound equipment. It is suggested that you should familiarise yourself with these guidelines in order to maximise benefit and minimise risk within the practical applications of ultrasound.

Musculoskeletal injuries are commonplace among sonographers[4] and by following the suggestions in Box 19.2, you will minimise not only the potential risks to the patient but also to yourself.

invasive ultrasound guided interventional procedures have resulted in reduced numbers of surgical procedures, thereby providing a more responsive delivery of treatment as well as reducing patient mortality and morbidity.[5]

Drainages, aspirations and biopsies are commonly undertaken with ultrasound guidance, sometimes in the ultrasound department and sometimes in other hospital locations. If the sonographer is working on the wards or in the intensive care unit then particularly high levels of infection control need to be adhered to. The ultrasound machine should be fully cleaned with effective products which will not damage it. It should be cleaned before and directly after use to minimise the potential spread of infection. More information about infection control can be found in Chapter 16.

An advantage of using ultrasound to guide needle placement is that the needle can be correctly positioned and that the required area sampled or drained as required. On some occasions, there may be a nurse or radiology assistant present to assist during the procedure. No matter whether working alone or with help, the equipment used during the procedure needs to be sterile in order to protect the patient from potentially introducing infections. Ensuring that sterility is maintained is part of caring for the patient.

When considering ultrasound guided interventional procedures, attention must be paid to the minimisation of mechanical trauma to the patient. The risks of mechanical trauma can be reduced by ensuring that the ultrasound practitioner has a good knowledge of the scientific principles of ultrasound, anatomy and practical ultrasound scanning.

Ultrasound guidance can be undertaken either directly or indirectly. Indirect guidance is more commonly undertaken for large uncomplicated fluid collections and is mainly undertaken by an ultrasound practitioner who will not undertake the interventional procedure such as the actual drainage of the fluid. It is suggested that when the ultrasound practitioner marks the puncture site for the drainage that the patient should be in the position that the interventional procedure will also be undertaken in order to avoid positional errors leading to mechanical errors or repeated attempts.[5]

Direct guidance is used for more complicated interventional procedures where the risk from mechanical trauma is much greater, e.g. in the case of procedures such as amniocentesis, CVS, core biopsy, FNA and MSK joint injections. The ultrasound guidance and the interventional procedure occur simultaneously, usually conducted by the same person and are in the main undertaken by a medical professional. However this situation is changing with the growth of advanced and consultant practice in the non-medical professions. It is suggested that all professionals undertaking direct guidance ultrasound interventional procedures should be appropriately trained in undertaking and interpreting ultrasound and that they should complete a minimum number of procedures each year in order to maintain competence.[6-8]

The use of contrast agents in ultrasound is increasing. The implication for the operator performing these examinations is that they need to be trained in intravenous cannulation techniques. Recognised courses are available which teach the theoretical knowledge, which can then be supported by practical skills development in the clinical setting, under the guidance of an experienced person. A sterile environment must be maintained while preparing the contrast agents for use. Additional technical ultrasound training might also be required to ensure that these procedures are undertaken safely and accurately. Sonographers are required to undertake continued professional development (CPD), to ensure they are up-to-date with their knowledge and techniques. Training in performing contrast examinations can be part of this CPD.

Gynaecological scanning accounts for a large quantity of a sonographer's workload. Examination of the female pelvis can be performed using transabdominal and/or transvaginal approaches. While technically, a transvaginal scan is not classified as an invasive procedure, a patient might regard it so and therefore it shall be mentioned here. Maintaining the patient's privacy and dignity during internal examinations is vitally important, alongside undertaking the procedure correctly and accurately. There are a variety of patient positions that this scan can be undertaken in and the sonographer needs to choose the position that is acceptable to the patient, while not compromising the technical requirements of the scan. There are also variations in how a patient is covered for the scan. Some are given a gown to wear; some are covered with a pillowcase, while others are given a piece of tissue couch roll to cover themselves with. Consideration should be given to any patient's cultural and religious needs regarding this. Although all the methods of covering the patient mentioned are acceptable from a sonographer's point of view – have we ever asked the women what they would prefer? Perhaps we should ask and have a variety of modesty covers available for patients to choose between.

ACCESSIBILITY AND PROVISION OF SERVICES

Ultrasound services have traditionally been offered as a Monday to Friday, '9 to 5' provision with little 'out of hours' expectation. The need to provide services at a place and time that is more convenient to the patient is becoming a major issue and it is here that ultrasound can have advantages over most other imaging and diagnostic practices. By increasing the availability and accessibility of certain ultrasound services, our patient provision can increase. Independent ultrasound service providers are currently leading the way in ultrasound provision by taking the examination to a place that is more convenient to the patient such as the GP surgery, therefore improving access and expediting the examination by providing most of the diagnostics in the primary care setting.

Historically, patient demographics have encouraged a 'postcode lottery' for the level of service a patient could expect. Waiting times for initial investigation and reports, diagnostic procedures provided and appointment times vary greatly across the country and it is these inconsistencies and inequalities in service provision that have a detrimental effect on patient centred care. Darzi's 2008 report 'High Quality care for All'[13] put the emphasis on service flexibility and responding to the needs of the service user providing them with real choices concerning their care and ultrasound services, are now beginning to answer this call, however there is still a long way to go. There is a move towards more evening and weekend working in some areas and patient choice has accelerated this process. In a competitive healthcare environment, Trusts which offer more limited hours of operation may find themselves at risk.[9]

Waiting times for diagnostic procedures have been targeted over the last 5 years in the UK as a direct result of the 18-week wait and the 2-week cancer plan. There is guidance available from the Healthcare Commission regarding the expected wait for an appointment when cancer is suspected[10] and ultrasound departments work towards meeting this. However, there are differences in the speed with which diagnostic test results are issued, not just for suspected cancer patients. The Royal College of Radiologists' guidelines indicate that a patient's examination results should be sent to the referring clinician within 14 days.[11] While many departments work within this time period, the delay of issue of results can delay patient treatment or reassurance.

Changes in working patterns and investment in training sonographers to undertake what was once predominantly a radiologist-led service has had a great impact on meeting the expectations of patients and the Department of Health (DoH). The increasing autonomy of sonographers, capable of both undertaking the scan and providing an accurate and diagnostic report, has had a major impact on reducing patient waiting times, alongside the development of innovations such as electronic reporting and voice recognition systems.

Although accessibility has been addressed with the common practice of extended working days and the advancement of patient electronic appointment booking systems, there are still issues surrounding inequalities in the quality of service delivery and 'out of hours' provision. Although it is common practice in computed tomography (CT) and plain X-ray radiography to provide an 'out of hours' sonographer-led service, this is not the case in ultrasound.

The issues of 'out of hours' ultrasound service provision are compounded when we consider the need to provide carotid artery ultrasound in a timely fashion for suspected stroke patients[12] (within 1 week of symptom onset). The provision of an 'out of hours' service in this area of ultrasound practice is essential for earlier diagnosis. Another area where an 'out of hours' service can benefit the patients, is in early pregnancies where complications are suspected. Decreasing the waiting time for these patients can have a profound effect on the patient's anxiety levels. Some research evidence suggests that anxiety levels can have an impact on pregnancy outcome and timely ultrasound can assist by revealing that a pregnancy is viable.

If the provision of ultrasound services is to be extended beyond '9 to 5', Monday to Friday, then this will have an impact of the staffing levels in an already short-staffed profession; it is nationally accepted in the UK that there has been a workforce deficit of sonographers for over a decade and this should be considered alongside service planning.

PATIENT CHOICE

Modern health service improvement emphasises providing a patient-led service and empowering the patient when considering the delivery of care has been at the forefront of all health service improvements.[13] However, empowering the patient means that we also need to provide them with information in order for them to make informed choice about their care. There are many issues to consider regarding informed choice and valid consent, one being that, in order to make an informed choice, a patient must have access to a good level of information concerning their health needs and care.

It is acknowledged that the patients of today generally have more access to information concerning their health and the care that can be provided via DoH and hospital information leaflets. However, widespread public access to the internet has proved to be problematic in areas such as obstetrics and oncology, since online information can be misleading and patients' expectations may be raised to unrealistic levels. The art of face-to-face communication with patients can be sidelined if over-reliance is placed on leaflets and posters and an assumed level of patient understanding by the professional can lead to patient dissatisfaction. Sonographers must be encouraged to ensure that the patient is fully compliant with the examination prior to commencement and that they understand the role and limitations of the scan; this is particularly important in the field of obstetric scanning.

It can be argued that patient choice has become the driver for most healthcare reform but patient choice must always be tempered with the benefit to the health of the patient. This beneficence is important when we consider ultrasound scanning as it is considered to be a relatively risk free examination and is therefore open to inappropriate use.

SOCIAL SCANNING

Pregnancy is an exciting time for a woman and her partner and the opportunity to see their baby on ultrasound is often greatly anticipated. There has been a growth in the independent sector of 'non-medical' obstetric scans which have sometimes been referred to as 'social scans'. The internet is full of offers of videos, pictures, 3D and 4D scans of babies during pregnancy. These are not all offered routinely as part of NHS scans. The medical justification for such things is not always evident and BMUS has provided guidelines for sonographers concerning 'social scanning', indicating that obstetric scanning should have medical justification.

One area of contention is that of sexing the baby. At the 20-week anomaly scan it can be possible to determine the sex of the baby, depending on the baby's position. Some parents do not wish to know the gender in advance of the birth, whereas for others finding out the sex of their unborn child before it is born is important. Accurate determination of the gender of a baby on ultrasound is not always possible and false information may be given. Taking into account these and other reasons, some hospitals have a policy not to disclose the gender during pregnancy. This can sometimes cause distress to the parents and the sonographer. Some parents question whether the hospital has the right to choose whether to disclose the sex of their unborn baby.

Antenatal ultrasound requires a high level of concentration by the sonographer. Having lots of people present in the ultrasound room during the scan can be an unwelcome distraction and may affect the sonographer's ability to successfully carry out the scan. Due to this, there is often a limit set to the number of people that can accompany a woman for her pregnancy scan. However, this can lead to a conflict of purpose between the sonographer and the patient and requires excellent interpersonal skills to ensure this situation is managed appropriately.

PSYCHOLOGICAL CONSIDERATIONS

Patients attending for an ultrasound examination may be anxious and worried about the implications of their results and this can manifest itself in different behavioural patterns. It is the responsibility of the sonographer to identify these anxiety patterns and address them accordingly; no two patients react or respond in the same way and everyone must be treated as an individual. Some patients may present in an agitated aggressive manner, while others may appear withdrawn and uncommunicative. The sonographer will need to be able to calm and reassure the patient in order to put them at ease.

It is normal practice in the majority of ultrasound departments not to provide the patient with a verbal report at the time of general and abdominal non-obstetric ultrasound examinations. The dynamic nature of the ultrasound scan can place the sonographer in a difficult position when approached by an anxious patient asking questions concerning the scan results. It could be argued that withholding information from the patient at this time can increase anxiety levels and that if the scan appears normal, divulging this to the patient could potentially alleviate some of the psychological pressure. However, difficulties arise when findings are unequivocal, as is often the case with ultrasound, since it has a high sensitivity but much lower specificity when providing diagnosis. Patients may place unrealistic expectations on the accuracy of ultrasound scanning, since they may not fully understand its limitations.

Antenatal ultrasound screening examinations pose dilemmas when considering the psychological impact on the patient. In the case of routine obstetric scans, the majority of patients are essentially 'normal', being 'low risk' and present with no indication of a complicated pregnancy. However, due to concerns about the health of the unborn child, the prospective parents' anxieties are frequently heightened. Conversely, some patients are poorly informed about the purpose of the scan, are not aware that a possible abnormality may be detected and are bewildered when a problem arises.

It is also important to consider diagnostic sensitivity and specificity issues during obstetric scanning, as this can be responsible for causing great psychological distress for patients. Ultrasound is very good at detecting non-normal anatomy but is often not very precise at providing a definitive diagnosis. Unlike the situation in non-obstetric ultrasound, where other imaging modalities can be used to provide an accurate diagnosis, obstetric scans often have no such fall back. This may result in invasive testing that can put the pregnancy at risk of miscarriage. This presents a dichotomy, in that the patient expects a scan in pregnancy to see the unborn child, while there is also the potential for unnecessary distress should a false positive scan result, resulting in further invasive testing. There is a need for continued staff education and evidence-based practice in order to minimise the negative impact on the patient.

The manner in which obstetric scan findings are explained to parents is important as often the first words of 'bad news' are the ones the patients remember most clearly. This is not an easy task for the sonographer and support should be offered to all professionals involved in breaking bad news. As part of sonographic training, theoretical methods of breaking bad news are taught. However, in clinical practice it can be challenging to put this theory into practice.

Perspectives on what constitutes 'bad news' may differ from patient to patient and also between health professionals. For instance, when multiple pregnancies are identified, this could be variously regarded as a joy or a burden. For some parents, this may be exciting news and many might consider multiple pregnancies to be a gift – something special. However, for some the prospect of twins might be daunting, since the responsibility of two or more babies, along with the financial implications might be devastating news. The sonographer needs to choose their words carefully in such situations and gauge the patient's reactions in order to inform how their discussion during the scan may continue.

While the majority of pregnancies are uneventful and result in a normal healthy baby, complications occur in some cases. When a fetal abnormality is detected, it needs to be explained to the patient alongside the implications for the continued pregnancy and the baby's health in a non-judgemental and empathetic manner. A sonographer does not always have the depth of knowledge to be able to answer all questions the patient may have – however, they are often the first health professional to explain the abnormality to the patient. There is research which supports the belief that the patient prefers and expects the sonographer to be the professional who breaks the bad news first. A timely referral procedure needs to be in place to provide the mother and her family with the information and ongoing support they need in the decision-making process that follows.

The sonographer needs to develop the skills to be able to explain and manage all situations causing least distress for patients. Differences between departmental protocols indicate that different people might be present during the ultrasound examination, in different hospitals or clinics. While a sonographer's communication of bad news is frequently directed towards the woman and her partner, other friends, family and children may be present and might be equally shocked and affected by the news. On the other hand, a woman might be alone in the room when the bad news is explained. She might benefit from her partner, friend or relative being present during the examination to support her. While there is no correct answer as to the number and type of people present during ultrasound examinations in pregnancy, careful consideration should be given to the implications if a problem arises.

While the patients' wellbeing is a sonographer's priority when breaking bad news, they should also be aware of the psychological impact on themselves and any other healthcare professionals or students present. Any students present when a problem is detected in pregnancy may be affected by this but may not feel that they can react in front of the patient. Debriefing of staff present in such situations is important for their continued wellbeing. Counselling is available in hospitals for staff that are affected by these situations and its use should be encouraged.

Making the decision to continue with a pregnancy or to have a termination is difficult. Some women choose to have a termination following the detection of a fetal abnormality. Termination of pregnancy may also be chosen for other reasons. In these cases, women often attend for an ultrasound dating scan. When undertaking a pre-termination scan, some women do not want to be able to see the ultrasound monitor, whereas some women will want to have the baby and heart beat pointed out to them. The sonographer needs to ensure that they undertake the scan as per the patient's wishes and any 'slave' monitor present for patient viewing will need to be turned on or off accordingly.

The waiting area for patients also needs to be considered. Is it acceptable for a waiting room to simultaneously hold women attending for routine antenatal scans, early pregnancy complication scans and pre-termination scans?

ORGAN SPECIFIC SCANNING

The British Medical Ultrasound Society issues guidelines on the organs which should be scanned during an ultrasound examination.[14] For an upper abdominal scan, their guidance advises that all organs should be examined regardless of clinical indications. Organ-specific scans should be avoided in most instances. Clinicians examining patients presenting with abdominal pain cannot always identify which organ is causing the pain, and therefore a targeted scan might miss the underlying pathology. However, there is some pressure for organ-specific scanning to be undertaken in an attempt to reduce scan examination times and increase throughput in order to reduce waiting times.

Organ-specific scanning can be argued not to be in the best interest of the patient, as many pathological symptoms can have a host of differential diagnoses. For instance, ovarian pathology can present with pain in the right hyperchondrium and shoulder, mimicking pain which could also be associated with gallstones.

KEY POINTS

When considering patient centred care in ultrasound, there are some fundamental qualities that are required to ensure that we meet expectations. Core standards to ensure safe practice, excellent communication skills to empower the patient and a flexible working environment are key to providing patient centred care. However, this does not come at no cost. Investment in evidence-based practice and continued training and development of sonographers are essential in the drive to make healthcare responsive and meet the demands of the twenty-first century.

Chapter | 20 |

Nuclear medicine

F.I. Peer

INTRODUCTION

Nuclear medicine employs small amounts of radioactive substances to diagnose or treat a variety of medical conditions. Radionuclide studies are relatively non-invasive for patients,[1] since radiation doses are normally small and there are very few reported adverse reactions to nuclear medicine agents. These agents, which we call *radiopharmaceuticals*, are administered either orally, by inhalation or by intravenous injection and accumulate in the body, giving off gamma rays. Once emitted from the body, this radiation may be externally detected by gamma cameras, positron emission tomography (PET) scanners, gamma probes or gamma counters. This results in no pain or discomfort for patients. The amount of radiation present in the various body areas may generate images that provide details of the function of the relevant organs. Thus, some medical conditions may show up earlier than with other tests and the most suitable treatment can begin as soon as possible.

In the more modern nuclear medicine facilities, images from gamma cameras and PET scanners may be fused with those obtained from computed tomography (CT) or magnetic resonance imaging (MRI). This allows for correlation of information from two different modalities to provide a more comprehensive diagnosis. Some centres also offer laboratory procedures, e.g. *in vitro* glomerular filtration rate (GFR) studies for kidney function, where at set intervals after the administration of the radiotracer, blood samples are obtained. The amount of radioactivity in samples is then analysed and calculations related to function are obtained.

Therapeutic procedures, where radioactivity is administered to treat certain medical conditions such as an overactive thyroid gland, are also employed. Since the aim in this instance is often to destroy target tissues locally 'from the inside out', higher radiation doses might be administered. But the benefit of the administered radioactivity will always exceed the risks of the procedure.

RADIATION DOSES IN NUCLEAR MEDICINE

As in any other medical imaging or treatment procedure, the patient's experience is enhanced when they are well informed about the study. There needs to be open communication (see Chapter 2, Communication with specific patient groups) between the patient and the healthcare practitioner,[2] providing clear guidelines and patient information. Ionising radiations, in the form of gamma rays and beta particles (see Chapter 9, Ionising radiation) are used in nuclear medicine procedures. These procedures are regarded as 'low dose' and expose the patient to a small dose of radiation similar to the range of doses received from many common X-ray investigations. The patient presents only a very minor hazard to other members of their family or to hospital staff.[3] This is because the activities of administered radionuclides are kept 'as low as reasonably achievable' (ALARA) and their radioactive 'half-lives' are short, leading to a rapid decay. In addition, the radiopharmaceuticals are quickly excreted from the body.

However, before and after radionuclide therapeutic treatment, special precautions have to be taken. All radionuclides have a 'half-life', that is the time that it takes for the radiation undergoing decay to decrease by half. Thus, patients may continue to emit detectable levels of radiation for different lengths of time, depending on the identity of the radionuclide that has been used. After any radiopharmaceutical administration, the patient should be encouraged to be both well-hydrated and to empty the bladder as often as possible.

The radiographer/technologist or nuclear medicine physician should inform patients that they may emit radiation after their procedure and mention how long this radiation may be detectable. This is important when a patient has to travel – such a patient should be given a letter indicating the name of the nuclear medicine study, the radioisotope used, the date of administration of the radioisotope, its half-life and the amount administered. Also included should be the patient's name and the contact details of the facility that administered the radioactive dose.

The radiation dose to the patient from a typical nuclear medicine procedure may be compared to about 1–4 years of natural background radiation, depending on the type of study (Table 20.1). However, the value of medical imaging is great and hence, the risks are negligible compared with the health benefits of having the nuclear medicine procedure.

Table 20.1 Average radiation doses from various activities

Activity	Average dose in millisievert (mSv)
Cosmic radiation at sea level (from outer space)	0.2/year
Air travel	0.01 for every 1600 km travelled, e.g. London to New York = 0.03
Living in a stone, brick, concrete building	0.07/year
Average annual exposure living in the USA	3/year
Watching television	0.01/year
Chest X-ray (single view)	0.1
Abdominal CT scan	10
Mammogram (four views)	0.7
Thyroid (isotope) scan	0.14
Bone (isotope) scan	2
PET scan with F-18-FDG	10

Pregnancy and breast-feeding

It is the duty of the radiographer and the healthcare practitioner authorising the procedure to check whether a patient is pregnant or breast-feeding before administering any radioactive substance. The patient must advise the staff before any nuclear medicine procedure if she is breastfeeding, or could be pregnant (a pregnancy test must be done). A pregnancy test may be done if there is any doubt. Breastfeeding needs to be stopped before starting certain radioactive therapy treatments as there is a possibility of damaging the fetal thyroid gland.[3,4] So as to minimise radiation to the breastfed child, if possible the test may be delayed until the mother has stopped breastfeeding. Failing which, the radiopharmaceutical chosen must consider the secretion of radioactivity in breast milk.[4]

The patient may be advised to avoid pregnancy for at least 6 months after certain therapeutic nuclear medicine procedures.[4] Male patients are advised to avoid fathering a child for several months following some radioactive therapy doses. Children under 10 years of age are not usually given iodine therapy.

The following general guidelines[5,25] may be given for recommended interruptions of breastfeeding:

- 3 weeks after I-125 radiopharmaceuticals except labelled hippurate, and after Na-22, Ga-67 and Tl-201
- 12 hours after iodine-labelled hippurates and Tc-99m compounds except labelled red blood cells, -phosphonates and -DTPA
- 4 hours after Tc-99m compounds labelled to red blood cells, -phosphonates and -DTPA
- 2 hours after F-18-FDG
- Total avoidance after I-131 administration for therapeutic purposes.

DURING THE PROCEDURE

During most nuclear medicine procedures, there are no pain or side-effects. Some discomfort, in the form of a 'cold sensation', may be experienced where a radiotracer is injected intravenously. Some tests require the taking of blood samples and others require the patient to breathe in the radiopharmaceutical, which is similar to breathing in room air. The radiotracer, which is usually tasteless, may also be given orally in food or drink.[6] Some slight discomfort might be experienced while the images are being taken as the patient has to lie still during the acquisition of the images. Most nuclear medicine procedures may be performed on an outpatient basis. Each procedure in nuclear medicine is different and requires different patient preparation (see Table 20.2) radiotracers, administration routes and actual scan or therapy protocols.[6]

Table 20.2 Summary of indications and patient preparation for nuclear medicine examinations

Nuclear medicine examination	Indications	Patient preparation
Bone scan: Tc-99m MDP	Location of tumours and/or metastatic bone lesions, trauma, sports injuries, avascular necrosis, arthritis, loosening/ infection of joint prosthesis	Increased hydration
PET whole body scan: F-18-FDG	Tumour staging, response to treatment, pyrexia of unknown origin	Controlled diet (high protein – no carbs) day before and day of scan; nil per mouth from midnight on night before the examination; no strenuous exercise on the day before and on the day of scan; diabetic patients – special prep steroids to be stopped
In-111 pentetreotide	Neoplasms that express somatostatin receptors Gastroendocrine tumours	Suspend octreotide therapy
I-123 MIBG	Phaeoglioma or paraganglioma and other neural crest tumours	Block thyroid, stop other interfering drugs (tricyclics and Ca channel blockers)
Tc-99m nanocolloid	Sentinel node location Lymphatic obstruction	None
Thyroid scan Tc-99m pertechnetate	Hyperthyroidism Palpable nodules	Stop antithyroid drugs and iodine-containing substances
Parathyroid scan: Tc-99m sestamibi	Parathyroid adenoma	None
Myocardial perfusion: SPECT Tc-99m labelled agents (sestamibi, tetrofosmin, teboroxime)	Diagnosis and prognosis of coronary artery disease, prognosis after infarction,	Stop cardiac drugs (β-blockers, rate limiting calcium-channel blockers) for 2 days prior,
Tl-201	postintervention, viable myocardium	no nitrates at least 6 hours before study, no caffeine before vasodilator is given
Radionuclide ventriculography: Tc-99m RBC	Evaluation of patients with coronary artery disease, effect of cardiotoxic drugs	None
Lung scan: Ventilation (Tc-99m DTPA particles or Xe-133 gas or Kr -81m gas) Perfusion (99mTc-MAA)	Pulmonary embolism, assessment of regional ventilation and perfusion	None (for pulmonary embolism – recent chest radiograph)
Renal scan: Tc-99m MAG3 Tc-99m DTPA Tc-99m DMSA	Differential function, outflow obstruction, vesicoureteric reflux, renovascular hypertension, cortical scarring	Well hydrated, for renovascular hypertension – check specific preparation with nuclear medicine department
Gastrointestinal bleed study: Tc-99m RBC	Evaluation of bleeding in upper and lower gastrointestinal tract	None
Meckel's scan: Tc-99m pertechnetate	Meckel's diverticulum	None

Continued

Table 20.2 Summary of indications and patient preparation for nuclear medicine examinations—cont'd

Nuclear medicine examination	Indications	Patient preparation
Gastric emptying study – Solid and Liquid: Tc-99m sulphur colloid	Motility, gastroparesis, evaluation of effects of drugs	Fast overnight
HIDA scan: Tc-99m HIDA	Acute cholecystitis, functional status of hepatocytes, biliary excretion	Fast for 6 hours
Brain scan: SPECT: Tc-99m HMPAO PET: F-18-FDG	Assess cerebral blood flow, dementia, epileptic focus localisation	None
Gallium scan: Ga-67 citrate	Lymphoma, chronic infection, inflammatory process	Bowel prep
Radiolabelled white cell scan: In-111 or Tc-99m HMPAO	Infection or inflammation of prosthesis, grafts, suspected abscess, inflammatory bowel disease	None
Glomerular filtration rate: Tc-99m DTPA	Renal function on diabetics and oncology patients for nephrotoxic chemotherapy	Well hydrated

Depending on the procedure, if necessary the patient may be required to change into a patient gown and to remove any metallic objects from their person. Scans may be obtained immediately after the radiopharmaceutical is given, and/or a few minutes later; a few hours later or up to a few days later. As each test is different, different protocols will be followed. It is the duty of the healthcare professional to inform the patient of the protocol and to ensure prior to the study being booked that the patient will be able to attend on the different days.

Musculoskeletal Imaging

A radionuclide bone scan is a diagnostic study used to evaluate the distribution of active bone formation. Various Tc-99m labelled radiopharmaceuticals such as diphosphates or diphosphonates are available for bone imaging. Usually the radiopharmaceutical is administered intravenously followed by the acquisition of images. There are various available procedures, including multiphase bone imaging with dynamic/blood flow images, immediate blood pool images and delayed images, or single photon emission computed tomography (SPECT). which produces tomographic images of a portion of the skeleton[7, 8] As well as being useful in detecting and staging cancer, a bone scan may be requested to assist in the diagnosis of occult fractures, sports injuries, trauma, avascular necrosis, loosening and/or infection of joint prosthesis. It is also useful in patients with arthritis for the assessment of joints, unexplained bone pain and for patients with back pain.

No special preparation is required for a bone scan. The patient should be requested to drink plenty fluids before, during and after the procedure. Most of the radioactive material which does not accumulate in the skeleton will be rapidly excreted by the kidneys. The patient must be advised to empty his/her bladder as often as possible after the injection and again just before the scan is started. The amount of radiation used is small and similar to that given by other diagnostic X-ray tests. The patients must urinate frequently on the day of and after the test to reduce radiation exposure. The patient may be in close proximity to other people and go to the toilet normally without causing risk to others.[7]

Oncology scans

The most commonly performed nuclear medicine studies in oncology are bone scans acquired on a gamma camera and PET scans to assist with staging of tumours, detect metastases and evaluate response to treatment. Oncology patients may be experiencing pain and discomfort, especially post-therapy and may be receiving various drug treatments. Bone scans for oncology patients usually comprise delayed whole body imaging with planar and SPECT images of certain areas if necessary. The most commonly employed radiopharmaceutical is Tc-99m methylene diphosphonate (MDP). Because glucose metabolism is increased in many malignancies,[9] PET imaging with F-18-fluorodeoxyglucose (FDG) is a sensitive method for detecting, staging and monitoring treatment for many malignancies. PET imaging is usually combined with CT to obtain fused images which provide both the metabolic information from F-18-FDG PET and the anatomic information from CT in a single examination. Whole body imaging with Iodine-131 (I-131) is used mainly to detect residual or recurrent thyroid disease in patients with certain types of thyroid cancer.[10] Tumours that express somatostatin receptors, such as, adrenal medullary tumours, gastroenteropancreatic neuroendocrine tumours and insulinomas are best imaged using Indium (In)-111 pentetreotide, which is a somatostatin analogue. The purpose of somatostatin receptor imaging is to detect and localise neuroendocrine tumours in patients with elevated neuroendocrine tumour markers, and in some non-neuroendocrine tumours. This imaging may also be useful in the preoperative evaluation, staging and restaging of these tumours.[11] Planar and SPECT imaging is advised at 4 hours and 24 hours post-intravenous injection of the In-111 pentetreotide dose, as this may be helpful in distinguishing physiologic bowel activity from pathologic lesions.[7,11]

Lymphoscintigraphy is employed in identifying the sentinel node/s and lymphatic drainage in melanoma and breast cancer patients. The administration of the radiopharmaceutical (Tc-99m-nanocolloid) is usually by four intradermal injections made either directly into the tumour, peritumorally, into the scar where the tumour was removed or in the case of breast cancer in the periareolar region.[7] These patients are imaged immediately prior to surgery (0.5–4 hours), so that a gamma probe may be utilised in theatre to identify the area/s of increased activity. In theatre, correlation is made with the images. Iodine -123 (I -123) labelled to Metaiodobenzylguanidine (MIBG) has a high sensitivity for neural crest tumours such as neuroblastoma and phaechromocytoma1 as MIBG concentrates in sympathoadrenal tissue.

In vitro studies, such as, red cell mass and plasma volume may be used to differentiate polycytemia rubra vera from pseudo-polycythemia.

Endocrinology

Thyroid scintigraphy is usually requested to relate the general structure of the thyroid gland such as nodular or diffuse enlargement to thyroid function. This could assist with differentiating Graves' disease from toxic nodular goitre. Imaging is also useful to determine the degree of function by correlation of the clinically palpable nodules with scan findings, in differentiating thyroiditis from hyperthyroidism and in locating ectopic thyroid tissue.[12] Thyroid images are obtained after the intravenous administration of Tc-99m-pertechnetate or after the oral ingestion of radioactive iodine (I-131). The routine use of I-131 for thyroid imaging is being discouraged due to the large radiation dose to the thyroid gland unless thyroid therapy using I-131 is a consideration.

In patients with thyroid cancer, thyroid scintigraphy is helpful to determine the presence and location of functioning thyroid cancer and the presence and/or extent of residual functioning thyroid tissue. Imaging for the detection of thyroid metastasis and/or residual functioning thyroid tissue usually follows 48 hours after oral administration of I-131. Other radiopharmaceuticals such as I-123, Tl-201 and Tc-99m sestamibi also provide useful information.

Parathyroid scintigraphy usually employs dual isotope or subtraction imaging, where protocols using 2 different radiopharmaceuticals, such as, Tc-99m sestamibi and Tc-99m pertechnetate, for image acquisition are used.[13] This imaging is indicated to localize hyperfunctioning parathyroid tissue, for example, adenomas or hyperplasia in primary hyperparathyroidism or in patients with persistent or recurrent disease.[7,13]

I-131 therapy may be indicated for the treatment of Graves' disease, toxic multinodular goitre, or toxic autonomously functioning thyroid nodules. It is also used for the treatment of residual thyroid cancer and metastatic disease and for the ablation postoperatively of thyroid remnants after thyroidectomy.[10]

Prior to booking patients for thyroid scintigraphy or therapy, certain patient preparation is necessary. The use of certain medication such as antithyroid drugs, thyroid hormones and iodine containing medication may need to be discontinued a few days prior to the scan.

Cardiology scans

Nuclear medicine myocardial perfusion imaging (MPI) using one of the many radiopharmaceuticals available is a relatively non-invasive study to assess myocardial perfusion. MPI identifies areas of reduced myocardial blood flow associated with ischaemia or scar. Perfusion imaging is indicated to assess the presence, location, extent and severity of myocardial perfusion abnormalities; to detect viable ischaemic myocardium and to assess the significance of anatomic lesions found on angiography.[14] The relative regional distribution of perfusion may be assessed at rest, cardiovascular stress or both.[14,24] Some of the radiopharmaceuticals used for cardiac perfusion imaging include Tl-201, the Tc-99m-labelled pharmaceuticals such as sestamibi, tetrofosmin and teboroxime for SPECT imaging and Rb-82 for PET imaging. Hibernating myocardium is seen optimally on PET imaging, especially in patients who fail to demonstrate myocardial viability with conventional SPECT techniques may benefit from F-18-FDGPET, particularly those patients with marked left ventricular dysfunction. Global and regional ventricular function and assessment of the relationship of perfusion to regional function may be obtained using SPECT imaging with ECG gating.[14] Patient preparation in terms of stopping certain medications is essential prior to cardiac imaging[7,24] (see Table 20.2). Also cardiac patients may experience breathlessness and pain on exertion and may require careful monitoring.

The assessment of left ventricular function is obtained from multigated acquisition (MUGA) scans, where red blood cells are labelled *in vivo* with Tc-99m-pertechnetate. A MUGA scan is indicated for the assessment of left ventricular function (ejection fraction) prior to the administration of chemotherapy, for monitoring the effects of cardiotoxic chemotherapy and for the evaluation of dyspnoeic patients who are difficult to assess on echocardiography.[7,24]

Pulmonary scans

Lung scintigraphy is a diagnostic imaging procedure that utilises ventilation or, perfusion imaging or both to evaluate cardiovascular and pulmonary disorders.[15] Ventilation-perfusion lung scans are most commonly indicated to detect pulmonary emboli. However, for accurate interpretation, comparison with a chest X-ray taken within 24 hours of the lung scan is necessary. The ventilation study either with a radioactive aerosol, such as Tc-99m DTPA aerosol or radioactive gas, such as Xenon-133 or Krypton-81m, or pseudo-gases like Technegas is usually performed before perfusion imaging as it is more difficult to deliver a larger dose of the Tc-99m aerosol than it is to deliver a larger dose of Tc-99m macroaggregated albumin (MAA). Should both ventilation and perfusion agents be labelled with Tc-99m, it is extremely important that the count rate of the perfusion scan is at least three times the count rate of the ventilation study.[15]

Renal Studies

Dynamic renal imaging using tracers eliminated by glomerular filtration such as Tc-99m diethylene triamine pentaacetic acid (DTPA) or tubular secretion, e.g. Tc-99m mercaptoacetyltriglycine (MAG 3), may be employed to evaluate renal function, renal obstruction, reflux and for renal transplant assessments. This imaging may be supplemented by the use of a diuretic such as furosemide. Diuretic renography is considered a safe and valuable method for the assessment of renal function and to differentiate between obstructive and non-obstructive causes of renal or ureteral dilation.[16] Patients need to be well hydrated prior to these studies.

Tc-99m dimercaptosuccinic acid (DMSA) is employed for renal cortical scintigraphy for the detection of cortical defects of acute pyelonephritis and scarring related to chronic pyelonephritis.[17] Other common indications include: differential renal function estimation; assessment of the horseshoe, solitary or ectopic kidney; assessment of renal function in the presence of an abdominal mass and the detection of focal lesions (pseudotumours).

In vitro measurements of glomerular filtration rate that do not involve imaging may also be employed where the radiopharmaceutical, e.g. Tc-99m-DTPA, is injected intravenously and blood samples drawn at specific times analysed.

Gastrointestinal scans

The evaluation of hepatocellular function and the biliary system may be accomplished by performing hepatobiliary imaging using a combination of dynamic images followed by planar, SPECT and if necessary SPECT-CT images of the liver, biliary tree and bowel.[18] The production and flow of bile from the liver, and its passage through the biliary system into the small intestine may be traced. The indications for hepatobiliary imaging include; biliary atresia, acute cholecystitis, bile leaks, patency of the biliary system and functional biliary pain syndrome.[7,18]

Liver–Spleen imaging with Tc-99m labelled to a colloid may be used for determining the size and shape of the liver and spleen as well as for detecting functional abnormalities of the reticuloendothelial cells of these organs. Haemangiomas of the liver may be studied by liver blood pool imaging with Tc-99m labelled red cells. As damaged red blood cells are selectively taken up by splenic tissue, splenic imaging is possible using Tc-99m labelled to heat damaged red cells.[19]

Gastric emptying studies using a meal (egg sandwich) labelled with Tc-99m sulphur colloid is a comprehensive means to evaluate motility and gastric motor function in adults.[20] A liquid phase study may also be done in conjunction with this study. Dynamic imaging of the gastrointestinal system to detect the site of bleeding is performed with Tc-99m labelled red cells. For the localisation of Meckel's diverticulae to identify ectopic gastric mucosa, Tc-99m pertechnetate is the radionuclide of choice as it avidly accumulates in gastric mucosa.[21]

Neurology Scans

Radionuclide brain studies using SPECT and/or PET imaging are commonly used to assess cerebral blood flow, dementia and to locate epileptic foci. Tc-99m exametazime (HMPAO) or Tc-99m ethyl cystine dimer (ECD) are commonly employed in brain SPECT imaging .[7,22]

PET brain images with F-18 FDG may provide unique information related to function that is most times complimentary to the anatomic imaging information obtained from CT and MRI; as functional impairment may exist without anatomical change or often precedes structural changes.[23]

Infection-Inflammation

Patients presenting with fever of unknown origin may be studied with labelled white cells scans or more recently with PET scans. Gallium scans are routinely performed on patients with suspected inflammatory prosthetic joints.

PET-CT IMAGING

PET-CT provides the special benefits of the combination of both PET and CT studies in one procedure. The information from each scan is different but complementary.[25] The PET scan shows the region of high metabolic activity, while the CT scan helps to anatomically locate the area. The result of this combination is that highly defined 3D images are obtained on a single scan. The PET scans provide functional or metabolic information of organ tissues. Obtaining this functional information gives the physician an excellent tool in diagnosing both the presence and extent of disease and in determining the appropriate methods of treatment or therapy. Also, because the PET is combined with CT images, it is easier for the healthcare professional to pinpoint the exact location of interest and determine its functional status, which may ultimately reduce the risk of invasive surgery. Most PET scans use F-18-FDG as the radiotracer and because of its short half-life of 110 minutes, the radiation exposure is reduced. The effective radiation dose from the F-18 is modest, while the effective dose from the CT can vary. The CT dose would depend on whether it is used simply for localisation of the PET images or if high resolution diagnostic images are acquired. In many patients, the PET-CT may be repeated at intervals to check the response to treatment.

The patient preparation before a PET-CT scan is important so as to get optimal images. The patient needs to follow the instructions carefully.

After a PET-CT scan the patient is considered safe to be in the public environment but should limit contact with children and pregnant females.[10]

To enable rapid clearance of the radiotracer from the body, the patient should drink as much liquid as possible for the rest of that day and the day after the scan and empty his/her bladder as often as possible.[7,25]

LABORATORY STUDIES

Different studies employ different techniques. One of the most common procedures done is the glomerular filtration rate (GFR). This test is usually done on diabetic patients, oncology patients requiring certain chemotherapy and on patients with certain renal pathology.[7] The patient is advised to drink fluids and to empty his/her bladder as often as possible to minimise the radiation dose. The patient is considered safe to be in the public environment during and after the test. Other tests include red cell mass and plasma volume, red cell survival time and ferrokinetic studies.

THERAPEUTIC NUCLEAR MEDICINE

A nuclear medicine therapeutic study involves the use of different radiopharmaceuticals to treat certain medical conditions. It is considered an effective and safe treatment for these conditions.[26] Therapy is commonly employed to treat thyroid problems such as an overactive thyroid gland or patients with cancer of the thyroid. Radiotracers may also be used for the relief of pain from cancer that has metastasised to bone, to treat some types

of arthritis and some cancers. These tracers kill most cancer cells and may help control joint inflammation in patients with arthritis, as cancer cells and some other cells affected by disease are more sensitive to radiation than normal cells. Patient preparation instructions for the various nuclear medicine therapy studies are different and instructions relevant to the test need to be followed. Patients for example with cancer of the thyroid might be required to remain in hospital for at least 2–4 days after the radiopharmaceutical is administered. This is so that the radiation levels are low enough and that the radioactive materials leaving the patient's body may be safely discarded.

Patients requiring therapy for arthritis or joint pain usually receive an injection of the radiotracer into the fluid surrounding the affected joint. The joint is stabilised with a splint and the patient discharged. Therapy to relieve pain from cancer that has spread to bone is usually by an intravenous injection. These patients are seen on an outpatient basis.[26] Depending on the therapy administered, the nuclear medicine healthcare worker must discuss with the patient the safety measures required for that therapy after discharge. The safety measures may need to be implemented from 24 hours to 10 days depending on the therapy. Since most of the radiotracer leaves the body in the urine, patients should empty their bladders frequently. Attention should be given to the use of the toilet; spills should be cleaned up and the paper flushed. Toilets should be flushed twice. Males should use the toilet instead of urinals. The time spent in close contact with others should be limited. If possible, the patient should keep an arm's length away from people and sleep in a separate bed. Contact with pregnant females and children should be avoided. With certain therapies, some minor side-effects may occur. The doctor must discuss these with the patient.

The nuclear medicine healthcare providers are trained to communicate with the patient and provide the appropriate patient care and comfort before, during and after the study. They should behave in a professional manner and recognise patients' rights.[27] Before commencing a procedure, the nuclear medicine practitioner must review the appropriateness of the study ordered, check that the patient complied with the patient preparation instructions prior to the study, check that patient consent (if necessary) is obtained and explain the procedure to the patient.

KEY POINTS

- Nuclear medicine procedures are relatively safe and non-invasive
- The principal hazards to patients and staff derive from ionising radiation, not from any side-effects of the radiopharmaceuticals themselves

- The patient acts as a source of radiation during and after the administration of radioactive isotopes
- With some high dose procedures there may need to be special precautions especially with regard to disposal of urine as well as breast-feeding
- Patients may arrive in nuclear medicine with a wide range of conditions, including cancer, heart problems and respiratory disease
- Procedures may be time-consuming and require repeat visits to the department
- Patient management has been revolutionised by non-invasive imaging that leads to early, more precise and much less morbid diagnosis

- From a cost point of view, nuclear medicine is less expensive and may give more precise information than exploratory surgery
- As medical care is the largest source of human exposure to ionising radiation outside of nature, it is important to maintain a balance between the potential benefits and possible risks from radiation exposure, especially in the paediatric population
- Diagnostic nuclear medicine procedures have been used for over 50 years with no known long-term adverse effects, since the radiation exposure from the administered radiotracers is very low

Chapter 21

Magnetic resonance imaging

Johnathan Hewis

CHAPTER OUTLINE

This chapter will consider:

- MRI screening
- Static magnetic field and the missile effect
- Gradients, noise and ear protection
- Radiofrequency and heating
- Claustrophobia/anxiety in clinical MRI
- Unconscious patients, sedation and general anaesthesia
- Pregnancy and MRI
- Medical emergencies in clinical MRI
- Cryogens
- MRI training and education

INTRODUCTION

Magnetic resonance imaging (MRI) is an exciting and rapidly developing imaging modality that has seen an enormous growth in the number of referrals and clinical installations over the last decade.[1] The ability to acquire multiplanar images while combining functional and anatomical imaging in one examination, all without the use of ionising radiation, makes MRI a highly appealing imaging option. MRI is a key diagnostic tool for many care pathways and is the primary diagnostic method of choice for several neurological and musculoskeletal disorders. MRI creates a unique and highly hazardous environment that must be afforded respect. During a scan, a patient is simultaneously subjected to three types of electromagnetic field (EMF) (as mentioned in Chapter 10, Non-ionising radiations and ultrasound). At present, the general consensus is that there is no evidence for a *genotoxic* or *carcinogenic* risk from MRI exposure.[2] However, MRI presents a clear risk to patients with certain biomedical implants or devices, or when unsafe objects are taken into the MRI environment. Numerous deaths and serious injuries have occurred within this environment and therefore a primary role of the MRI practitioner is to apply constant diligence and maintain safety. The MRI environment can also place psychological stresses on patients due to its confined nature. This chapter will explore patient centred care considerations specific to the MRI environment, focusing on common physical, biological and psychological risks, while providing practical solutions for risk reduction and recommendations for best practice.

MRI SCREENING

The static magnetic field of a super-conducting magnet is *always* turned on; it cannot just be turned off at the end of the working day. Therefore, access to the MRI environment has to be strictly controlled at *all* times and *all* staff, patients, visitors and objects entering this environment (Fig. 21.1) must first be checked or *screened* by trained MRI practitioners. A rigorous and successful screening process should aim to identify *all* individuals with biomedical implants/devices or loose objects that may not be MRI-safe (Box 21.1). Screening prior to scanning is the most critical means of safeguarding patients in MRI.

From the patient's perspective, the MRI can be a daunting and a scary looking environment. The patient may be distressed prior to their scan appointment due to anticipation of the scan results (see Box 21.2); a previous negative imaging experience or fear of the unknown. Unfortunately, there are also many misconceptions about MRI safety held by the general public and some hospital workers may inadvertently heighten this fear. It is therefore important to discuss the procedure carefully with the patient, provide a clear justification for the MRI screening process and not presume that the patient is already fully informed.

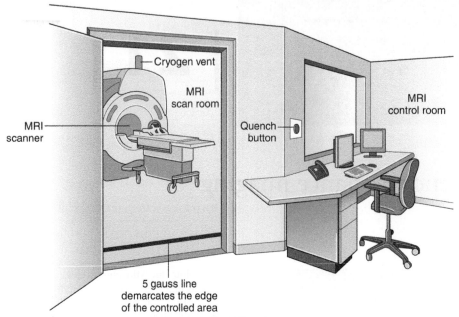

Figure 21.1 The MRI environment.

Box 21.1 **Terms used for safety in an MRI room**

There are several important terms used to describe the safety status of items that might be brought into an MRI scan room:

MRI-safe – an object that is MRI-safe does not pose any safety risk and is not a potential projectile. The object may however, cause artefacts if it is within or close to the area of examination and/or the function of the object may be disrupted when within the MR environment, e.g. a dedicated MRI-safe ECG monitoring unit

MRI-compatible – an object that is MRI-compatible does not pose any known safety or projectile risk *and* it will not cause any artefact during imaging nor is the function of the object disrupted, e.g. an MRI-compatible trolley.

MRI-unsafe – an object that is known to pose a hazard in all MRI environments.

Note: Many practitioners wrongly use **MRI-safe** and **MRI-compatible** interchangeably, which can create confusion and can be dangerous.[3]

MRI-conditional – is a term being used increasingly, where an object does not pose any known safety or projectile risk but under defined *field* conditions, the behaviour and safety of the object is clearly defined for a specific MRI environment or set of conditions. Outside of these conditions it may pose a hazard.

Box 21.2 **Case study**

I can vividly recall MRI safety screening one particular patient, a middle-aged professional gentleman who we will call Simon. Simon had been referred for an urgent scan of his internal auditory meatus (IAM) following the sudden onset of unilateral hearing loss. Simon had answered a range of initial safety questions with the referring clinician who completed the MRI request card. He had answered a series of safety questions with the MRI booking clerk who made his appointment on the telephone and he had also completed and signed an MRI safety questionnaire on arrival to the MRI department. All of these indicated no cause for concern. I completed the final safety check with Simon by explaining the importance of the safety questions and reaffirming each of his responses to the detailed safety questionnaire only to reveal that Simon actually had a cardiac pacemaker!

This particular case raises many concerns, including why the referring clinician did not know the full medical history of their patient, and reinforces the need to remember that patients may not be thinking completely rationally when presenting for their scans. It is important to give all patients adequate time to complete the screening process and that the patient is fully informed and aware of the implications of their answers. An MR practitioner needs attention to detail when considering MRI safety!

No MRI screening process can be infallible and it is highly dependent upon the patient's ability to accurately recall any previous surgery or relevant injury/trauma. Emotional distress, memory loss, reduced mental capacity and language barriers may significantly hamper the accuracy of the screening process. Where there is doubt, the patient should *not* be scanned. When screening an individual for whom English is not their first language and there is a clear communication issue, a professional interpretation service should be employed to allow safe completion of the screening process.

STATIC MAGNETIC FIELD AND THE PROJECTILE EFFECT

All substances are affected to some degree when placed inside a powerful magnetic field; the scientific term for this is magnetic susceptibility. Human tissue is only mildly affected by a powerful external magnetic field and we take advantage of this phenomenon to create MR images. Certain materials are greatly affected by a magnetic field, e.g. *ferromagnetic* objects are highly attracted to the static magnetic field. If you were to take a standard iron oxygen cylinder (iron being *ferromagnetic*) into the *controlled area* of an MRI scan room (Fig. 21.1), the strong attractive force of the static magnetic field would wrench the cylinder out of your hands and it would fly across the room with considerable force and strike the scanner. Such *translational* forces

are commonly referred to as the projectile (or 'missile') effect and pose a significant risk to anyone in the path of the object; worldwide this has led to several fatal injuries and many near misses.[4] Many everyday objects are not safe to take into the MRI environment and *all* screened individuals must remove loose everyday ferrous objects before entering the scan room. Figure 21.2 provides examples of loose everyday objects that are *not* MRI-safe and need removing prior to entering the MRI environment. *All authorised staff working in the MRI environment must ensure they are vigilant in removing any potential projectiles from their own person.*

Missiles, trapped individuals and quenching the magnet

The strict *screening* process described earlier is designed to stop non-MRI-safe ferromagnetic objects entering the *controlled area* of the MRI environment.[5] The *controlled area* is defined as any area where the magnetic field exceeds 5 gauss (0.5 milliTesla). The controlled area should ideally be contained within the MR scan room and a *5 gauss line* demarcated on the floor as a visual reminder of the edge of the main magnetic field (Fig. 21.1).

A loose ferromagnetic object can potentially become a missile and fly into the scanner. Anecdotally, minor incidents are quite frequent within a busy clinical MRI department, e.g. it is relatively easy for a solitary ferromagnetic coin to be missed in a patient's pocket if they are allowed to wear their own clothing during a scan. Ideally, all patients

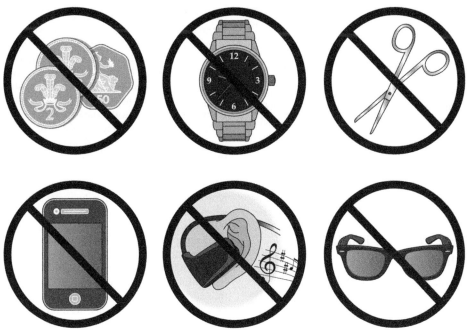

Figure 21.2 Examples of everyday objects that are not safe in MRI.

should change into MRI-safe clothing provided by the MRI department and leave all their clothing and possessions in a locker. This eliminates the risk of patients accidentally carrying potential projectiles into the MRI environment and would also remove potential image artefacts caused by inappropriate clothing.

Small ferromagnetic objects which have become stuck to the magnet can be easily removed by hand, with care, from the scanner. *The patient should first be removed from the bore of the magnet before attempting to retrieve a small ferromagnetic object.*

If a person is trapped in or pinned to the scanner by a large ferromagnetic object such as a non-MRI-safe wheelchair, this cannot be removed manually due to the huge attractive forces of the static magnetic field. In this situation, the MRI practitioner will need to reduce the static magnetic field by instigating an *emergency run down* or *quenching* of the static magnetic field. This is performed by purposefully pressing the *quench* button located in either the MRI scan room or the MRI control room (Fig. 21.1). A superconducting magnet contains cryogen coolants such as liquid nitrogen or helium, in order to achieve such large field strengths. Cryogens are rapidly released during an emergency *run down* or *quench*. The cryogen should boil off and be vented outside via cryogen vent piping (Fig. 21.1) resulting in a significant reduction in the static magnetic field to allow the recovery of the trapped individual. *It should be noted that quenching the static magnetic field may result in permanent damage and should ONLY be performed in an emergency situation.*

Minimising the risk of projectiles can be achieved by:

- Adequate training and high diligence of MRI personnel
- Maintaining restricted access to the *controlled area* and ensuring the MRI environment is supervised at all times
- Ensuring that the door to the controlled area is locked when there is no MRI practitioner present
- Clear labelling of MRI-safe accessory equipment, e.g. MRI-safe wheelchair
- Ensuring that non-ambulatory patients are transferred to a dedicated MRI non-ferromagnetic wheelchair or trolley/gurney.

Metal detector warning systems can be installed in clinical MRI and used in addition to a rigorous *screening* programme. Metal detector systems must not be relied upon as the sole method of *screening*; this could be fatal. If used appropriately, such systems can help increase detection of potential missiles and non-MRI-safe devices and implants.[5]

Biomedical devices, implants and foreign bodies

Many individuals have biomedical implants or devices that cannot just simply be removed and may not be safe in the MRI environment; these first need to be identified and checked by MRI staff. The vast majority of medical implants, such as most orthopaedic implants and intravascular stents, are MRI-safe. Active implants with electrical or magnetic components are typically unsafe and a magnetic field of 5 gauss or greater can disrupt the function of active biomedical implants.[6] *Individuals who have a cardiac pacemaker are NOT safe to enter the MR environment; doing so can result in death*. Ferrous implants can also experience *translational* forces as already described or *torque* (twisting) forces associated with passing through the static magnetic field. Torque forces can potentially result in significant harm. Table 21.1 provides current guidance on safety considerations for several common medical implants/devices.

This list is far from exhaustive; you should consult your MRI department for current advice and local guidance regarding the safety of a specific biomedical implant or device. The screening of biomedical implants and devices is not a rigid science, since new devices appear constantly and each new device or model requires additional safety testing. Recently, there have been dramatic increases in the number of high field strength magnets (e.g. 3 Tesla or greater) installed for clinical examinations. High field strength scanners provide beneficial increases in the signal to noise ratio (SNR) for imaging compared with lower strength magnets. The higher SNR can be traded off to either allow quicker scan times or enable increases in spatial resolution. But also, the higher field strength increases the magnitude of any safety risks. *It is important to note that a biomedical implant/device or an item of equipment tested to be MRI-safe at 1.5 Tesla MAY NOT be safe in a higher field strength, e.g. 3.0 Tesla.*

Patients can also present with a wide range of foreign bodies, e.g. shrapnel injuries. Each patient needs to be considered on an individual basis and may need referring for an X-ray examination prior to MRI. Metallic intraocular foreign bodies (IOFB) can be a concern in the MRI environment, particularly if they have penetrated the orbit to a significant depth and lie in close proximity to the optic nerve. There are less than half a dozen published reports of complications from metallic IOFBs in clinical MRI but they include pain, discomfort, cataract formation and unilateral blindness.[8] Routine X-ray screening to exclude metallic foreign bodies is controversial and some research suggests that it may not be cost-effective.[9] The potential risk is hard to determine but MRI centres in the UK routinely perform IOFB X-ray examinations as a precautionary screening tool typically for patients with a known history of eye injury when working with metal where the patient is *unsure* if the IOFB was fully removed by a medical professional.

Working clinically in a region with a large steel industry, I have scanned many patients with a previously unknown metallic IOFB that have been identified as incidental findings, whilst scanning their head/brain. Surprisingly, an individual can easily be unaware of a having a high-speed penetrating eye injury. When scanning the head/brain of these patients, the metallic foreign body will cause an area of magnetic susceptibility artefact within the orbit.

Table 21.1 Common biomedical implants and their MR safety considerations[5-7]

Medical device/ implant	MRI-safe/compatible	Considerations
Cardiac pacemaker	*Not* MRI-safe	A static field greater than 5 gauss can disrupt a cardiac pacemaker; this can lead to a cardiovascular event and death. MRI-safe pacemakers are being developed but are not currently available in the UK
Orthopaedic implant, e.g. hemiarthroplasty	Considered safe once *in situ* for 6 weeks; odd exceptions exist – such as for certain cervical spine internal fixations	Such implants will also cause magnetic susceptibility artefacts. Ferromagnetic implants should be *in situ* for at least 6 weeks to allow them to become embedded by fibrous tissues. Large implants may experience translational forces and vibrate with patients, sometimes reporting the feeling of heating (more marked at higher field strengths)
Intravascular stents	Almost all considered safe once *in situ* for 6 weeks	Such implants will also cause magnetic susceptibility artefacts. Ferromagnetic implants should be *in situ* for at least 6 weeks to allow them to become embedded by fibrous tissues to reduce the risk of migration
Aneurysm clip	Dependent upon year and model	Older aneurysm clips can be ferromagnetic; these may experience torque when moving the patient into the scanner. Or the aneurysm clip may be safe on the first visit but become permanently magnetised and present as a risk at a subsequent scan. Twisting a ferrous aneurysm clip can result in intracranial haemorrhage and death
Intrauterine device (IUD)	MRI-safe	No safety considerations
Skin staples (used for surgical wound closure)	Typically *not* MRI-safe	Potential heating risk, therefore must be removed prior to scan

As a precaution such individuals should be removed very slowly from the bore of the magnet once the scanning is complete. Withdrawing the patient slowly may help limit movement of the foreign body caused by *torque* forces. When scanning patients with a known metallic foreign body, it is important to provide clear instruction to the patient to alert the MRI practitioner if they experience any discomfort or heating sensations in that anatomical area.

GRADIENTS, NOISE AND EAR PROTECTION

During scanning, MRI uses additional magnetic fields or *gradients*, which are turned on and off rapidly. Gradients produce the loud characteristic sound of MRI during image acquisition. The majority of sequences produce noise within acceptable safety thresholds but faster pulse sequences (e.g. echo planar pulse sequences) can exceed 100 decibels that may potentially result in more permanent hearing impairment during prolonged exposure.[6] All people present in the scan room during image acquisition

must therefore wear ear protection, e.g. earplugs or ear defenders, that reduce or attenuate the MR noise to acceptable levels (Fig. 21.3). Active noise cancellation ear protection systems are normally installed in high field strength MRI systems (e.g. 3 Tesla or above) because they subject patients to increased levels of acoustic noise.[10]

The acoustic noise of MRI can be particularly distressing for specific patient groups: children, confused patients or individuals suffering with psychiatric disorders may all suffer anxiety due to the high ambient noise levels.[11] One of the biggest problems with high acoustic noise levels in MRI is the negative impact on communication. Due to the physical nature of the MRI equipment, the patient is scanned remotely from the MRI practitioner and that can result in a feeling of isolation for the patient.[12] Effective communication is essential to provide emotional support and enable the practitioner to provide the patient with clear scan instructions. More importantly, two-way communication is required to gain feedback from the patient regarding their comfort and to enable them to raise any safety concerns. MRI ear defenders enable two-way communication and the ability to play the patient music that may help provide psychological comfort. Some patients will only tolerate

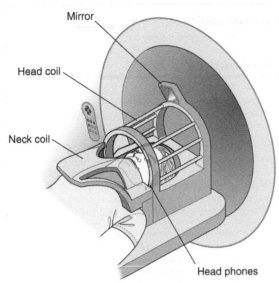

Figure 21.3 Coil positioning for a head and neck MRI examination.

earplugs and this will significantly limit any two-way communication compared with scanning with two-way ear defenders. *Note that it is important to still provide ear protection to unconscious, anaesthetised or sedated patients.*

Gradients can also create various potential short-term side-effects during scanning, which could be disconcerting for a patient, including peripheral nerve and muscle stimulation, which manifests as involuntary twitching; or a sensation of flashing lights at the back of the eye caused by stimulation of the retina when scanning in the head region. These are particularly pronounced at higher field strengths and occur with fast or strong gradient pulse sequences. MHRA guidelines[5] for gradient exposure levels should be adhered to, to minimise these phenomena.

RADIOFREQUENCY WAVES AND HEATING

MRI uses radiofrequency (RF) electromagnetic waves to transfer energy into the patient to stimulate hydrogen protons to create an image; this energy transfer is called *resonance*. Depositing energy into the patient can cause localised heating and/or increase the patient's core body temperature. An increase in core body temperature is particularly dangerous in children, the elderly, pregnant women, hypertensive patients and unconscious or uncommunicative patients. Excessively increasing the core body temperature can potentially trigger a cardiovascular event.[6] Manufacturer software will alert the MRI practitioner when a high *specific absorption rate* (SAR) has been selected

for a specific imaging sequence. An accurate patient weight needs to be inputed with the scan details to ensure an accurate SAR estimation. MR practitioners should monitor SAR levels during a scan and be mindful of software warnings. Good airflow through the bore of the magnet is essential to help patients regulate their body temperature.

Highly conductive objects that are inside the patient or in direct contact with the patient's skin can potentially lead to excessive heating and ultimately RF burns. Examples of reported causes of RF burns include damaged RF coils, large tattoos, standard monitoring devices and transdermal medication patches left *in situ*.[13] Furthermore, certain shapes can concentrate RF currents and therefore the MRI practitioner needs to carefully consider the position of the patient, RF coils and any cables associated with equipment to avoid creating conductive loops.

Excessive heating and potential RF burns can be avoided by:

- Adequate patient preparation, e.g. removal of metallic objects such as jewellery and transdermal medication patches
- Rigorous patient screening to exclude certain biomedical implants/devices that present risk of heating
- Use of insulating padding to prevent skin on skin contact points
- Use of insulating padding to prevent direct contact between the patient and RF coils, equipment cabling and the bore of the scanner itself
- Use of dedicated MRI-safe accessories, e.g. MRI-safe monitoring equipment
- Correct positioning of cables – ideally parallel and close to the centre of the bore
- Not using faulty equipment.

Providing clear instructions and maintaining effective communication with the patient throughout the scan is important to help minimise the incidence of RF burns.

CLAUSTROPHOBIA/ANXIETY IN CLINICAL MRI

Claustrophobia can be considered as a potential contraindication for clinical MRI. Patients can experience claustrophobic or anxiety symptoms immediately prior to or during an MR examination. A patient experiencing claustrophobia/anxiety may not be able to commence the scan; may prematurely terminate the examination or the images acquired may be suboptimal due to movement artefact and lack of cooperation. The reported incidence rate of claustrophobia/anxiety of MRI varies significantly but it is a commonly reported phenomenon, ranging from mild anxiety to a panic attack.[14] Claustrophobia is characterised by a persistent and marked fear of enclosed spaces, resulting in severe psychological distress. Labelling *all* patients who experience anxiety during MRI as claustrophobic is inappropriate and it should be noted that many patients will present with pre-existing anxieties unrelated to the MRI environment. Effectively caring and managing patients experiencing anxiety symptoms with varying levels of *psychological distress* is an essential skill required by all MRI practitioners.

The presenting symptoms for claustrophobia/anxiety can be multifaceted but may include: feeling faint/dizzy; nauseous; feeling hot/sweating; trembling; choking; perceived difficulty in breathing/suffocation or even a fear of dying.[12] The common symptom is a perceived lack of control due to a sense of confinement. These symptoms can be triggered by various contributing factors that include:[12,14,15]

- The restricted bore dimensions and restricted movement
- Close proximity of MRI RF coils (notably head and neck coils)
- Prolonged examination times
- Acoustic noise
- Sensory deprivation
- Temperature of the MRI environment
- Anxieties of pre-existing medical conditions
- Underlying psychiatric illness
- Fear of the MRI results.

Knowledge and an understanding of the aetiology of anxiety are required to be able to provide effective care. For example, the anatomical area under MRI examination has to be placed in the centre of the opening or *bore* of the magnet, the *isocentre* being the most homogenous and therefore diagnostically useful portion of the magnet. The aperture of the bore is fairly limited and can feel restrictive and enclosing. Patients undergoing examinations of the head and neck region are particularly prone to feeling enclosed or trapped. The *coils* used for head and neck imaging, are required to be in close proximity to the patient to achieve good quality images (Fig. 21.3). This close proximity provides the high signal to noise ratio (SNR) required. For many anxious patients, the close proximity of the coil and bore can heighten the sense of confinement (Fig. 21.3). Mirrors can and should be fitted to the head coil to enable the patient to see out into the scan room and will help reduce sensory deprivation. A modern MRI installation incorporates a short bore magnet, an internal fan to create air flow through the bore and is well lit to help reduce the feeling of enclosure. Patients are also given an emergency trigger to hold, that sounds an alarm in the scan room to signify an urgent problem.

Managing patients suffering with claustrophobia/anxiety will depend upon the individual's level of psychological distress. Anxious patients require good communication throughout their scan to provide reassurance. From personal experience, anxious patients need to progress with the examination at their pace. Trying to rush an anxious patient will normally heighten their distress and result in premature termination of the examination. It is also important to give the patient as much control of the situation as possible, reassuring them they are able to terminate the scan at any point and to actively involve the patient in the procedure.[14] Modern

scanners allow greater flexibility in RF coil and patient position/orientation; wherever possible, the MRI practitioner should choose a position/orientation that provides the patient with the least physical and psychological discomfort.

Anxious patients may need emotional support after the MRI examination and this can often be ignored. A patient may feel a sense of failure and can be upset or angry if they fail to complete the examination. This may also be combined with a sense of frustration that an opportunity to reach a diagnosis for their symptom or condition has been lost. It is important to spend time with these individuals, particularly if the examination is incomplete or failed and provide them with an opportunity to ask questions once they have regained their composure. Beyond these immediate concerns, individuals who experience anxiety during MRI can develop long-term clinical anxiety disorders such as clinical claustrophobia.[15]

It is imperative not to force a patient to attempt an MRI examination if they appear highly anxious or distressed, this may cause more harm than good.

UNCONSCIOUS PATIENTS, SEDATION AND GENERAL ANAESTHESIA

Patients in these categories should only be scanned in dedicated MRI centres able to provide appropriate and experienced medical support. Patients who fail to complete an MRI examination due to psychological distress may be considered for intervention that includes sedation and general anaesthesia. Sedation and general anaesthesia significantly increase the risks associated with a diagnostic scan and this requires careful justification. Other diagnostic tests should first be considered where possible.

Anaesthetists and supporting staff administering sedation and general anaesthesia for MRI examinations require dedicated education and training in MRI safety. Patient *screening* should occur prior to administration of any sedation/anaesthetic agent. Careful and continuous monitoring is required for all unconscious patients using dedicated MRI monitoring equipment and MRI-safe accessories, e.g. MRI-safe ECG electrodes. There are many specific safety considerations that are beyond the scope of this chapter. Recent research into alternative claustrophobia/anxiety interventions such as neurolinguistic programming (NLP)[16] suggests that non-invasive therapies may be a potential alternative to sedation/anaesthesia in adult patients.

PREGNANCY AND MRI

Potential heating effects and acoustic noise are both concerns when scanning a pregnant patient, but both can be limited to some extent by the MRI practitioner when setting scan parameters. It is possible to scan pregnant women but elective and non-emergency procedures are normally deferred until after the pregnancy. Prudence is normally exercised and scanning is generally avoided in the first trimester (period of organogenesis) due to the indeterminate long-term risks of clinical MRI.[2] Some published case studies suggest that acoustic noise can result in permanent hearing impairment at birth in children exposed *in utero* to MRI; however, recent research[17] suggests that at 1.5 Tesla, there is no increased risk of substantial neonatal hearing impairment during the second and third trimester of pregnancy.

Pregnant MRI personnel should normally be given the option of not entering the MRI controlled area during the pregnancy, particularly during the first trimester and should not remain within the *controlled* area during scanning.[5]

MEDICAL EMERGENCIES IN CLINICAL MRI

Unstable patients should not be scanned within the MRI environment due the remoteness of the scanner from the scan console, long scan times and complexity of providing effective monitoring. Acutely ill inpatients are routinely scanned; many patients are also administered intravenous MR contrast agents (e.g. gadolinium) and various patient categories receive sedation or anaesthesia to achieve diagnostic MRI scans. Therefore, the likelihood of a medical emergency is still present in this environment, although hopefully infrequent (see Box 21.3).

MRI practitioners must instigate basic life support while removing the patient from the scan environment as quickly as possible. Maintaining a secure *controlled* area is challenging during a medical emergency but is essential, to protect the patient and staff.

Box 21.3 **Scenario**

Location: MRI department
Patient: An elderly male inpatient goes into cardiac arrest during the administration of an intravenous gadolinium contrast injection.
Imaging to be performed: The MRI examination is abandoned and an urgent crash call is placed.
Practical considerations: Despite being an emergency all aspects of MRI safety *must* still be strictly observed for the safety of staff and the patient. The patient must be recovered from the MRI scan room as swiftly as possible by the MRI team. The patient is moved out of the MR scan room to a safe environment to allow access to the patient by the crash team.
The crash team should *not* enter the MRI scan room or attempt to take any equipment into the room, e.g. a defibrillator or the crash trolley.

CRYOGENS

Cryogens are extremely cold liquids which maintain the MR magnet in a superconducting condition. They could be dangerous if they were to escape into an enclosed space. If the emergency venting fails and the cryogen were to enter a sealed scan room it poses a risk of asphyxiation to individuals present due to the displacement of oxygen.[6] Leakage of cryogens into a sealed room will also cause over pressurisation and may make it difficult to enter the MRI scan room to rescue individuals present. Some MRI scan room doors incorporate a dedicated emergency hatch for this purpose. An oxygen alarm should be fitted in all MRI scan rooms to alert when oxygen levels are depleted.[7] If cryogens leak into the MRI scan room, the area should be evacuated and the room well ventilated.

MRI TRAINING AND EDUCATION

In the UK, the MHRA (Medicines and Healthcare Regulatory Agency) provide safety guidelines for clinical MRI[7] and clearly outline the responsibilities of MRI practitioners. All *authorised* persons are required to have a good knowledge of MRI safety and to receive regular training. Currently, there are no national educational or training standards required for MRI practitioners, often training is performed 'in house' only. It would seem prudent that all MRI practitioners undergo formal postgraduate education in the field of MRI as well as structured clinical training to provide practitioners with both adequate theoretical knowledge and understanding, combined with clinical competence.

KEY POINTS

- Although MRI is often regarded as a non-invasive imaging method as it does not use ionising radiation, there is a wide range of potential hazards in MRI, some of which can lead to severe injury or even death if operating procedures are not followed correctly
- All patients and staff entering the MRI environment must be safety screened
- MRI staff need to be fully aware of all safety risks and keep up-to-date with new developments, since MR procedures are constantly advancing
- Hazards are presented by flying external objects, cessation of pacemaker function, internal movement of ferromagnetic particles or surgical clips, induced currents in nerves, tissue heating and burns, claustrophobia, noise and supercooled cryogens

Mammography

Patsy Whelehan

This chapter will focus on:

- Skills for promoting wellbeing in mammography
- Physical risks to the patient/client
- Psychological risks to the patient/client
- Informed consent and the benefits and harms of breast screening

INTRODUCTION

Mammography is a branch of diagnostic imaging which exemplifies the complexity and the demanding nature of the practitioner's role in patient/client centred care. There is a convention that women attending for screening mammography are not referred to as patients because they are not presenting with a medical problem. They are therefore known as 'well-women' unless and until shown to be otherwise and will be referred to here as 'clients'. Optimisation of the client experience requires high levels of knowledge and understanding, as well as excellent technical, clinical and communication skills. The mammography examination is one of the most intimate to take place under the auspices of the imaging department and breast cancer is one of the most emotive conditions encountered by medical imaging practitioners.

The two domains of mammography, screening for breast cancer in the 'well-woman' population and investigating breast symptoms, differ in many aspects when one considers the holistic care of the patient/client. A woman's decision to respond to a recommendation or invitation to participate in a breast screening programme is influenced by many factors, including the cognitive, psychosocial and emotional. Her decision to return for subsequent screening is influenced in part by the practitioner's role in providing a satisfactory mammography experience. In addition, the delicately-balanced and often controversial nature of the relationship between the benefits and harms of screening for breast cancer with mammography confer challenging informed consent responsibilities on individual practitioners as well as on screening programmes. In the 'symptomatic' clinic, patients can be considered to have driven the process to a greater extent than women in a screening programme, by actively seeking help for breast-related problems. This subtle difference in the relationship between the patient and the service, and the effects on emotions, perceptions and expectations, is perceived by many practitioners to be a formative aspect of the mammography encounter.

Clearly, it is of prime importance in caring for our patients that practitioners achieve excellent clinical imaging techniques in order to maximise accurate detection and diagnosis of abnormalities in the breast. In the UK, it generally takes at least a year's specialist postgraduate academic and clinical training for practitioners and at least a year's vocational clinical and theoretical training for assistant practitioners to achieve success in an assessment of competence in mammography.[1]

KEY SKILLS REQUIRED FOR PROMOTING WELLBEING DURING MAMMOGRAPHY

Mammographic positioning has famously been referred to as an art as well as a science[2] and many newcomers to the speciality are surprised by how challenging the technique is to master. There is artistry as well as science involved in the practitioner's clinical–technical skills and the communication skills required to gain the confidence and contribution of the patient/client in achieving optimum positioning.

Too often, we have talked and written of the patient/client's 'cooperation' and 'compliance' in achieving high quality mammograms. Women may feel a lack of power during screening mammography, which may arise from being in a state of undress as well as from being 'pushed' or manipulated into position.[3] Talking the patient/client through the positioning procedure can reduce the amount of physical guidance required, potentially reducing feelings of disempowerment in the patient/client and at the same time, decreasing musculoskeletal strain for the practitioner. These considerations are probably even greater in the case of physically disabled clients/patients, as a result of the extra challenges involved in achieving optimal demonstration of the breast tissue (see Chapter 14, Moving and handling).

Compression of the breast in mammography not only contributes to image quality by reducing the risk of unsharpness from motion and geometric effects but is important in reducing radiation dose to the breast tissue. Of course, with compression comes the notorious possibility of pain or discomfort. The practitioner's role in maximising effective tissue compression to limit radiation dose and optimise image quality, while at the same time minimising discomfort, pain and distress, requires both excellent positioning skills and skilful communication (see Chapter 1, Principles of communication).

PHYSICAL RISKS TO THE MAMMOGRAPHY PATIENT/CLIENT

Radiation exposure

In this age of automated selection of exposure factors by sophisticated equipment, practitioners should not forget that they still have a responsibility to ensure that parameters are optimised through the correct set-up and use of the equipment. In addition, there are certainly some occasions when expertise can enable the operator to make a better decision than the machine's software on, e.g. the optimum beam energy (see also Chapter 9, Ionising radiations).

In mammography the radiation doses are so low that deterministic effects are not expected to be at issue. Risk of radiation-induced breast cancer – a stochastic effect – is the key issue to be addressed and is particularly crucial in breast cancer screening, which involves a number of mammograms over time in women who generally have no clinical signs of breast cancer. The risk of inducing a breast cancer and the risk of a radiation-induced breast cancer leading to death can only be estimated by the use of theory, extrapolation and modelling because it is impossible to know what exactly led to any particular breast cancer and the risk of dying from breast cancer is variable. In turn, extrapolation and modelling rely on a number of

assumptions. The estimated likelihood of inducing a breast cancer from screening with mammography depends upon a number of variables, including the dose used, the screening age range and the total number of mammograms – or screening frequency. Additional complications arise from the risk–benefit ratios being expressed in a variety of ways in the literature.

In the UK, the National Health Service Breast Screening Programme (NHSBSP), for regular 3-yearly two-view screening between the ages 50 and 70, the ratio of cancers detected to cancers induced by screening, has been estimated to be greater than 10:1.[4] This estimate was based on film-screen mammography, so is likely to be slightly better following the introduction of digital mammography because of lower radiation doses to the breast. The overall benefit–risk ratio of screening will be affected by a complex array of factors including breast cancer mortality rates but is expected to be somewhat lower than the detection:induction ratio.[5] Of course the majority of women attend for breast cancer screening without receiving any life-expectancy benefit because they do not have breast cancer and therefore cannot benefit from early detection. At the same time, the current lifetime risk of breast cancer for women in the UK is approximately one in nine. Therefore, for the practitioner who may be asked by women attending for screening to explain the radiation risk in the context of the potential benefit, it is relevant to consider the number of cancers induced by screening in a given number of women screened alongside the baseline incidence of breast cancer.

It has been estimated that if 100 000 women were screened every 2 years between the ages of 50 and 74, with a radiation dose of 1.3 mGy per view, there would already be over 1500 cancers in the women screened for every cancer induced by the screening. Thus, because the risk of breast cancer in the female population is high, the additional risk from regular mammographic screening is extremely low in comparison. Nevertheless, the estimated risk of being screened has to be weighed against the *potential* benefit of having a cancer detected early and surviving as a result. Reduction in mortality from breast cancer as a result of screening is another complex and contested question.

> **!** Notwithstanding the complexity of this area, practitioners should develop a sufficiently good understanding to convey a reasonably accurate impression of current estimates of risk. The primary aim is not to reassure women but to give them the best available information to enable them to make a decision whether to accept the benefit–risk ratio of screening.

In-line with general radiographic principles and because, as described above, the risk of inducing a breast cancer is related to the radiation dose, it is important to keep doses in mammography as low as reasonably achievable. However, in digital systems, some aspects of image quality will suffer if doses are set too low and this could jeopardise cancer detection and thereby adversely affect benefit–risk ratios in screening. Practitioners need to be guided by their medical physics colleagues in the optimisation of digital systems prior to use but must take responsibility for routine quality control to ensure that the dose versus image quality balance is maintained at an optimum level. Further than this, there are two main aspects of radiographic practice which limit radiation doses in mammography – exposure factor selection and compression of the breast tissue.

Although modern automatic exposure control (AEC) systems are very effective, there are occasions when the practitioner may wish to override the AEC in order to achieve better dose control and/or better image quality. For example, a young woman with large firm breasts may benefit from a higher beam energy than the mammography machine would automatically select. The practitioner should be alert to such situations and exercise judgement in switching to semi-automatic and overriding either the kilovoltage (kV) or the filter setting. A combination of experience, understanding of the science of exposure factor selection and a thorough understanding of the mammography machine will enable practitioners to make the right decision in such scenarios. In addition to minimising the radiation dose, raising the beam energy will shorten the exposure time and thereby reduce the risk of motion blur. Another example of where practitioners should consider using higher beam energies than may be automatically selected is in magnification mammography. Radiation doses are relatively high when magnification is used because the breast is nearer the X-ray source. By increasing the kV, not only will the dose to the breast tissue be reduced but the likelihood of motion blur and consequent risk of diagnostic difficulty or repeat exposure will be minimised. It has been shown that, because of the effectiveness of the air-gap technique in reducing the effect of scattered radiation on the image, good image contrast levels in magnification mammography can be maintained with values up to 34 kV.[7,8]

> ! Compression of the breast tissue to minimise tissue thickness reduces the radiation dose dramatically and therefore will also reduce the risk of inducing a breast cancer. It has been shown that radiation dose to the breast increases by 21% and by 66% when tissue thickness changes from 4.4 to 4.8 cm and to 5.4 cm, respectively. The challenge for the practitioner is to achieve effective thickness reduction with minimal pain for the patient/client.

Pregnancy and lactation

There is no radiation protection requirement to ask women whether they are pregnant before performing mammography because the primary beam will not irradiate the pelvis. However, changes to the breast tissue during pregnancy and lactation mean that mammography is considerably more difficult to interpret. In the case of pregnant or lactating women with breast symptoms, the status is clinically relevant and should be elicited during the clinical consultation and noted on the request form. However, sometimes a woman will identify herself to the practitioner as pregnant or lactating, without this having previously been made clear and at this point, the practitioner should refer to the radiologist for guidance on how to proceed. Ultrasound scanning is usually employed as a first-line imaging technique, with mammography only used if there is a very high level of suspicion of malignancy or after malignancy has been diagnosed. In the NHSBSP, pregnancy and lactation have hitherto only rarely been at issue because the age at which women become eligible for screening has been 50 years. However, with the recent randomised introduction of a starting age of 47, and indeed in many independent sector breast screening settings where screening is provided at earlier ages, the likelihood of women presenting for screening when pregnant or lactating is slightly greater. Current NHSBSP guidance is that asymptomatic women should not be screened while pregnant or until at least 6 weeks after lactation has ceased because it is expected that mammography will be considerably less sensitive than usual and that the potential benefit of screening is therefore reduced.

Pain in mammography

There have been many studies investigating various aspects of the phenomenon of pain in mammography but they report a very wide range of rates of pain. Most of the variation can probably be attributed to methodological problems and heterogeneous study design.[9]

> ! Although it is often assumed mammography pain arises purely from compression of the breast tissue, it is likely that pressure from the edges and corners of the imaging surface on the ribs and axilla also plays a part.

Many factors have been suggested as potential determinants of the severity or rate of mammography pain. These include factors specific to the women themselves – both physical, such as breast density[10] and psychological such as anxiety levels.[11] However, radiographic practice also seems to be important, both in terms of clinical technique and more general standards of care.

One example of the influence of clinical technique is the importance of full mobilisation of the breast medially for the mediolateral oblique projection.[2] This is expected to reduce discomfort by equalising tissue thickness and reducing the dragging of the compression paddle across the chest wall. In addition, there is a need to avoid further compression of the breast once the tissue thickness has been maximally reduced.[14]

> **!** The practitioner's communication skills appear to be an important factor in the quality of the patient experience of mammography, including perceived pain.

For example, it has been shown that if women understand that they may say stop during the procedure, if the compression is becoming too painful, they are less likely to report that the mammogram was painful.[12] It has also been shown that pain is more likely if the patient feels the practitioner did not pay her enough attention.[16] Following general principles of good practice in communication, e.g. making eye contact when speaking and listening attentively, will tend to increase levels of trust and enable patients to feel more at ease. However, it is also important to explain the procedure fully, including the reasons for compression, to minimise feelings of lack of control. For example, the practitioner can say, 'Please let me know if you feel the compression is becoming too tight and I will stop'.

In the screening setting, there is some evidence that painful mammograms are implicated in women's decisions whether to return for subsequent screening.[13,14] The importance of the practitioner's responsibility to minimise pain thus goes beyond the quality of care at the time.

The only interventions that have been shown in prospective trials to have an effect in reducing pain levels are patient controlled compression and use of cushioning pads.[15] In both these interventions, blinded controlled trials are clearly not possible, so there may have been a placebo effect but the precise mechanism of the effect is perhaps relatively unimportant.

Physical injury from mammography

Anecdotal evidence suggests that bruising can occur following mammography, particularly over the ribs where the lateral chest wall is in contact with the edge of the imaging surface during positioning for the mediolateral oblique projection. One published case report was interpreted by the authors as an instance of mammography causing bruising with subsequent fat necrosis within the breast itself.[16] The patient in this case reported a lifelong history of bruising easily and was taking regular aspirin. Even if the interpretation of the

facts on this occasion was correct, it is likely to be a very rare occurrence but serves to emphasise the need for gentle and careful handling and positioning technique. This is further reinforced by occasional claims from patients that injuries to their necks or shoulders have occurred during mammography. Attention should be paid to the potential for image quality degradation with use of these two interventions.

Some women, particularly those with large, more pendulous breasts, can suffer from skin candidiasis (thrush) under the breast. This can cause the skin to be thin and friable and breakdown can occur when the breast is lifted for mammographic positioning. When this condition is noticed or reported, practitioners should warn patients of the possibility of skin breakdown during the examination and offer the option of re-booking the appointment once the skin condition has been successfully treated. Situations such as this should always be documented in the record of the examination.

POTENTIAL ADVERSE INCIDENTS IN MAMMOGRAPHY

Pacemaker damage

Although some pacemaker pulse generator units are implanted abdominally, it is not unusual for them to be placed at thoracic level, under the skin and subcutaneous fat but superficial to the pectoral muscle. Such implants can interfere with mammographic positioning and with demonstration of the whole breast.[17] Opinions differ on whether mammographic compression of a pacemaker risks causing damage and therefore local policies vary on whether it is obligatory to avoid this. There are very few published reports of pacemakers being damaged by mammography so it is probably a rare occurrence. However, a recent case was reported where a lead was believed to have been dislodged during mammography.[18] Compression in the presence of a superficially implanted pacemaker unit is at least likely to be uncomfortable and may also cause anxiety for the patient. Departmental policy, NHSBSP policy or practitioner judgement may therefore dictate that it is better to compromise the amount of breast tissue visualised rather than compressing the pacemaker. As always in such situations, an open discussion is required with the patient/ client to ensure the limitations are understood before proceeding. Where the pulse generator is implanted within or behind the pectoral muscle or in a fascial pocket posterior to the breast tissue, mammography is less problematical.

Breast implant damage

Recent publications have highlighted adverse incidents relating to breast implants. A large number of incidents involved breast implant rupture during mammography. Other adverse events included mammographic compression crushing implants, pain during mammography attributed to implants, inability to perform mammography because of capsular contracture or fear of implant rupture, and delayed detection of cancer attributed to implants. The Royal College of Radiologists' guidance on screening and symptomatic breast imaging[20] suggests that the risk of prosthesis rupture as a result of compression during mammography is extremely small. They do, however, advise that the presence of any visible breast asymmetry should be recorded before mammography is performed[2] in case the examination is blamed for producing an existing abnormality. Usual practice is for only minimal compression to be applied to implant-bearing breasts, if the implant is within the compressed field.

Most breast implants are composed of radiopaque silicon compounds preventing any useful image being obtained of tissue overlying the implant but radiographic technique can be adjusted to maximise the amount of tissue visualised *around* the implant. One option is to take a third image in the lateral projection to profile additional tissue not seen in the craniocaudal or mediolateral oblique projections. In some cases, an implant displacement technique can be performed. This involves pushing the implant back towards the chest wall behind the compression paddle and drawing the breast tissue forwards, allowing more effective compression of the breast tissue anterior to the implant than would otherwise be possible. This is usually not feasible where there is only a very small proportion of natural tissue present or where a hard fibrous capsule has formed around the implant. Conversely, augmentation silicon implants inserted posterior rather than anterior to the pectoral muscle allow for effective compression of the breast tissue separate from the implant.

> **!** It is important that women with breast implants are aware of the limitations of mammography and can make an informed choice whether to proceed. This is particularly important to discuss during the appointment when the practitioner is taking note of the patient's medical history.

Any patient who has an older type of implant called 'Trilucent™' should not have a mammogram because the implants are at high risk of breaking down; most women who had this type of implant have now had them removed. In the presence of a focal symptom, ultrasound scanning can be used for first-line imaging but in the NHS-BSP there is no alternative to mammography for detection of asymptomatic abnormalities in the breast.

PSYCHOLOGICAL RISKS TO THE MAMMOGRAPHY PATIENT/CLIENT

In patients presenting to a breast clinic having noticed a symptom which they think may indicate the presence of cancer, the fear of cancer and its consequences can give rise to high levels of anxiety and distress. These can manifest in a number of ways, including anger or irritability, so practitioners need to be sensitive to the patients' difficulties. Patients vary greatly in the amount of anxiety experienced in the face of suspected breast cancer, under the influence of factors such as the level of social support they have. Consideration should also be given to the particular feelings men may experience when attending a breast clinic, as the environments tend to be very female-orientated and this can give rise to embarrassment. For men and women, mammography is a very intimate examination, not only because the practitioner has to handle the breast but also because of the bodily proximity and contact involved in positioning for mammography. Mindful of this, practitioners should aim to minimise the intrusiveness of the examination by careful technique, clear explanations and maintaining a professional manner throughout. On occasions, women who have severe claustrophobia or, more rarely, fear of being touched may present for mammography. These women require sensitive and supportive care from the practitioner who should adapt to their needs rather than relentlessly pursuing the habitual practices used in routine situations. This will only be achieved by listening to the patient/client and offering the opportunity to suggest how undue distress may be best avoided.

> **!** The practitioner should not be afraid to try something different. For example, fully explaining and demonstrating the positioning with oneself as the model can enable the highly anxious patient/client to make a remarkably good job of at least starting to position herself. This is likely to minimise feelings of panic by promoting a sense of control over the situation.

Anxiety has been linked to higher perceived pain from mammography but this has mainly been observed in the screening setting[21] with many practitioners believing that women who have presented themselves for investigation of breast symptoms tend to display greater tolerance of mammographic compression than asymptomatic women responding to an invitation to be screened.

Anxiety in the breast screening context is at issue with regard to the extent to which breast screening causes anxiety about breast cancer. Studies examining this effect report that mammographic screening does not appear to create anxiety in women who are given a clear result after a mammogram and are subsequently placed on routine recall.[22] However, women who have further investigations following their routine mammogram experience significant anxiety in the short term, and possibly in the long term. Services and practitioners must therefore do everything possible to care for the psychological wellbeing of women recalled for investigations following screening mammography. Once again, this largely depends on quality of communication.

INFORMED CONSENT AND THE BENEFITS AND HARMS OF BREAST SCREENING

The duties of the practitioner in respect of consent to imaging examinations are laid out by the Society of Radiographers and discussed elsewhere in this volume. For the mammography practitioner, the issue is arguably more problematical in breast screening than in clinics where patients have presented with symptoms. This is because breast cancer screening is based on a delicate balance of rather complex benefits and harms. Decisions to implement screening for a given population depend upon the balance of benefits and harms for that population, whereas the balance for an individual woman will be different from the population level and will vary across individuals. Breast screening is designed to reduce mortality from breast cancer in the population. Although most experts would agree that it achieves mortality reductions, the number of breast cancer deaths prevented by mammographic screening is controversial.[24] The disadvantages of breast screening include radiation exposure, pain and anxiety and imperfect sensitivity and specificity. In addition, breast cancer screening inevitably leads to the detection in some women of cancers which would never have become clinically apparent in their lifetimes.[25] Because of uncertainties over the rates of progression of such lesions, treatment is usually offered, despite ultimately being unnecessary. The size of this problem has also been the subject of much debate. Against this background, the practitioner's duty to ensure informed consent to mammography is challenging, despite being shared with policymakers. Conveying the complex benefits and harms of screening, both of which are *potential* effects at the individual level, mostly has to be achieved before attendance, so that a woman can decide whether to accept a screening invitation. However, practitioners should still check that patients/clients are satisfied with the information received and should answer any questions that may remain. The 'implied' consent of attending the screening unit should at no point be taken for granted. The issues are, of course, even more challenging when the potential patient/client has a learning disability (see Chapter 3, Communication with patients with disabilities and additional needs).

OTHER PROCEDURES IN THE BREAST IMAGING DEPARTMENT

Although it is beyond the scope of this chapter to consider interventional breast procedures in detail, the principles covered with respect to caring for patients in standard mammographic examinations also apply to interventional procedures. These include X-ray-guided tissue biopsy and lesion localisation procedures. Practitioners should not feel that their responsibilities are in any way diminished by the additional presence of a radiologist or advanced/consultant practitioner. A key consideration in interventional techniques is infection control (see Chapter 16, Methods of infection prevention).

KEY POINTS

- Mammography is a challenging procedure for patients, clients and practitioners
- There are some distinctions between caring for well-women attending for breast cancer screening and patients attending for investigation of breast symptoms
- In all cases, promoting psychological and physical wellbeing and protecting those in our care from harm are inseparable from, and equally as important as, achieving excellence in image quality

Chapter | 23 |

Computed Tomography

Aladdin Speelman

CHAPTER OUTLINE

This chapter will consider:

- Principles of care before, during and after CT
- Special procedures and circumstances
- Interventional CT
- Physical and radiation risks
- Radiation dose reduction

INTRODUCTION

This chapter will highlight the importance of patient care and will provide some practical aspects of patient care in the computed tomography (CT) department.

Effective patient care encompasses all aspects of healthcare. Radiography is a people-oriented profession and requires proficiency in a wide variety of communication techniques, which is a key component of good patient care. The most skilled and proficient practitioner will become inept if effective communication, which accentuates patient care, is not provided. Modern day patient care elevates the patient to the core of our radiographic responsibilities.

Patient care in CT departments is aimed at enhancing the patient's wellbeing through the duty of care provided. It is imperative that the techniques and protocols applied in CT departments validate this principle. The information explosion of the twentieth century has resulted in better informed patients, well aware of the level and type of service expected. Practitioners should ensure that the patient is informed of all aspects pertaining to the CT examination and their subsequent management. This chapter will provide tips on patient care before, during and after CT examinations. The second part of this chapter deals with the physical and biological risks for patients undergoing CT examinations.

APPROACHES TO GOOD PATIENT CARE

When performing CT examinations, practitioners need to consider the following fundamental points of patient care: Namely that all patients be:

- Treated with respect and dignity
- Treated fairly, irrespective of their social status, race, gender, mental or physical status, sexual orientation, religion or beliefs.

Practitioners should further take cognisance of the patient's emotional state; a patient in severe pain is less likely to cooperate or be in the mood for light-hearted conversation. The way patients are treated should thus befit their mood.

PATIENT CARE BEFORE IMAGING

Before patients are brought into the scanner room, practitioners need to ensure that they:

- Introduce themselves to the patient by their name and title
- Address patients according to their titles. It will be discourteous to address an unmarried female as 'Mrs' and vice versa
- Always correlate the identity of the patient to prevent a CT examination performed on the wrong patient. A good and safe method is always to check the age and sex of your patient. It is important that patients are called Mr Peter Smith, as it will prevent Mrs Smith from responding in the waiting area. Patients with names or

surnames that sound similar, will often respond when called in the waiting area. Confirm their identity by asking them their date of birth (which you would have checked already). Knowing the sex and age of your patient before they are called will alert you when the wrong patient responds to your call. Performing a CT examination on the wrong patient will have serious medico-legal risks for the practitioner, and should be prevented at all costs

- Check that the request form and folder (if you are not employed in a paperless hospital) is accompanying the right patient. If your CT department employs a Radiology Information System, ensure that all the necessary administrative duties such as entering of the patient, billing for the procedure and transfer of patient data to the CT department has occurred. It is also important to check whether previous radiological procedures and results are available. Previous radiographic examinations and results are needed to compare progress or regression of disease

- Determine whether the clinical history justifies the clinical examination. By knowing the clinical indications and associated radiographic appearance of the pathology on CT, practitioners will ensure that the correct CT examination is requested

- Understand the medical terminology on the request form, as this will guide your radiographic approach. If a patient has a clinical history of claustrophobia, practitioners will know to attend to their fear for narrow spaces by pointing out to them that the gantry is in fact an open entity

- Ensure that all relevant patient details such as the patient's name, hospital identity number, examination number were correctly entered on the Radiology Information System (RIS) or Picture Archiving and Communication System (PACS) or control panel of scanner. Incorrect entering of patient's details may cause confusion and may pose a medico-legal risk if wrong results are matched with the wrong patient. Incompatible patient data will lead to non-integrity of patient data, which will hamper merging CT examinations with other imaging studies, when using RIS or PACS.

Explanation of the CT procedure

A patient centred healthcare philosophy demands that patients be informed of all matters related to their management. When explaining the procedure, the practitioner should refrain from using scientific jargon. Some aspects that need to be conveyed to the patient are:

- In which position they will be placed on the scanner table
- Whether they will be palpated during the CT examination

- For how long the examination will take place
- Whether any breathing or other instructions will be requested
- Warn patients about the table and gantry movements that will take place. Patients unfamiliar with CT scanning often get frightened once the table or gantry movement occurs
- Whether there will be a need for delayed sequences
- Patients should be encouraged to indicate to the practitioner when they feel uncomfortable by showing a hand or lifting their feet.

Good patient care should determine that no procedure will be explained to patients in the waiting room, especially where other patients can hear you. Similarly, personal details of patients should never be asked in front of others, including staff, as this will be violating their right to privacy. Personal questions should be asked in the privacy of the scanner room, behind closed doors. Where there is a need for contrast media administration, the patient should be informed about the risks and side-effects of contrast media. Informed consent should be obtained prior to administration thereof. (To read more about contrast media reactions and contrast nephrotoxicity, see Chapter 11, Drugs and contrast agents.)

The need for informed consent

Every patient is entitled to provide informed consent before any procedure can be performed. This doctrine is underscored by the patient's right to know and participate in his/her own healthcare. Informed consent is therefore needed for all invasive procedures performed in the CT department such as those requiring contrast media administration.

In order for a patient to give an informed consent, the patient has to be informed of:

- The nature of the treatment
- Any risk, complication and expected benefits or effects of such treatment
- Any alternatives to the procedure and their risks and benefits.

Other procedures in CT imaging that require informed consent are for:

- Fine needle aspiration biopsies (FNAB) of the lung nodules, liver lesions or abscess drainage
- Facet block injections.

Practitioners have a duty to ensure that informed consent is signed for such invasive procedures, as they will not be exempt from any lawsuit that may arise from failure to obtain informed consent. (See Chapter 29, Ethical and legal considerations in professional practice, for more background on the medico-legal responsibilities of the practitioner.)

Patient preparation before the CT examination

Patient preparation is an important but often overlooked part of the CT examination.

- It is important that patients are appropriately dressed for all CT examinations. No metal objects should be worn over or near the anatomical area to be examined. Metal objects will cause artefacts, which will result in a repeat of that sequence and additional radiation dose to the patient
- Patients should be dressed in a disposable non-transparent gown for all CT examinations, except for a CT of the brain, sinuses and/or facial bones
- Bowel cleansing should be adequate to ensure a CT examination of diagnostic value. The presence of stool may mimic an endoluminal mass lesion or mask the presence of either a polyp or colonic carcinoma. Fluid residues can cover the colonic mucosa, covering areas of internal bowel surface
- Any residual barium from previous barium studies should be identified to prevent streak artefacts, which may lead to a repeat or suboptimal CT examination. It is therefore important to verify whether the patient underwent any barium study prior to the CT examination. If this is the case, a conventional antero-posterior radiograph of the abdomen should be performed to establish whether the bowel is free from any residual barium. If barium is evident in the GIT, the CT examination will need to be postponed.

Patient preparation for CT of the brain, sinuses or facial bones

- Metal objects such as rings, nose or tongue studs, hairpins, dentures containing metal and glasses and hearing aids, should be removed before starting the CT examination, as they cause unwanted streak artefacts.

Patient preparation for CT of the chest

- Ensure that patients remove metal objects such as nipple rings or underwear containing metal.

Patient preparation for CT of the abdomen/pelvis

- Patients who will undergo CT imaging of the abdomen need to remove metal objects such as navel rings, as if discovered only during the surview (topogram), it will require a repeat surview, which will cause an unwanted additional dose to the patient

- Do not assume that the patient is aware that money should be removed from pockets when wearing underwear or tracksuits
- Ensure that the patients followed the bowel preparation prescribed by your department
- It is essential that the 10-day rule be applied to all females within childbearing age. The 10-day rule is used to prevent unintended exposure of the child *in utero* to radiation. Embryos between 2 and 15 weeks' gestation are considerably more sensitive to adverse radiation effects, such as microcephaly (and accompanied mental retardation), central nervous defects and growth retardation.

Room preparation

Preparing the scanner room in the CT department is essential and should be completed before the patient enters the room. It is not proficient professional radiographic practice to invite a patient into a scanner room that is untidy or disorganised. Practitioners should therefore refrain from preparing the scanner bed, or tidying the room when the patient has already entered. If the room is disorganised upon entering, it may result in patients becoming distrustful towards you. It is imperative to aim to deliver a first class service to your patients.

In preparing the scanner room, the practitioner should consider:

- Clean linen has been placed on the bed prior to the patient entering the scanner room
- Remove any foot pedestals/objects which may compromise the patient safety or transfer onto the scanner bed
- Ensure that a drip stand or drip hook is available, if needed
- If contrast media is to be administered, ensure that emergency drugs and accessories are available. Emergency drugs should be unexpired. Ensure that other accessories such as laryngoscope and sphygmomanometer is in a working condition and available on the emergency cart
- When preparing for contrast media administration, accessories such as cotton wool, tourniquet, syringes, butterfly, Jelco needle or other appropriate needles should be available
- Ensure that ventilators are in a working condition, and that oxygen supply is available
- If the pump injector is to be used, it should be free from contrast media or blood
- Gonad shields are available and clean
- Sponges needed for patient support, and immobilisation straps are available and clean
- Ensure that you are aware of the emergency evacuation procedure for the scanner on which you will perform the examination. Most scanners have a manual override at the foot end of the scanner bed. This is used to

pull the bed out of the gantry in an emergency, such as when a patient experiences a cardiac arrest or convulsion, or when technical errors occur such as malfunctioning of the gantry, or power failures

- Also ensure that you are well aware of where the emergency power disconnection switch is located, so that power can be disconnected should mechanical malfunction of the scanner occur.

PATIENT CARE DURING THE PROCEDURE

- Before transferring the patient onto the scanner bed, the practitioner needs to ensure that the patient's privacy is protected by closing all doors leading to the scanner room
- During the CT examination, the patient should be observed, as they can move, lift their head or move their arms over the area of interest, causing unwanted artefacts and exposure to their limbs
- Ensure that easy venous access will be available by removing excess clothing. Remove any long sleeves which will hamper venous access
- For invasive procedures such as rectal catheter placement or (therapy procedures) close curtains covering the lead glass between the control area and the scanner room
- Scanner beds are hard and every effort should be made to ensure that the patient is comfortable on the bed. For support and comfort, a supporting pillow or knee rest can be placed under the knees
- Placing of a sponge or pillow under the shoulders of terminally ill patients, who often have little subcutaneous fat, is also recommended. Patients who are comfortable on the bed are more likely to lie still
- Ensure that all limbs are secured/immobilised and are not hanging off the side of the scanner bed. This is particularly crucial for para- or quadriplegic patients
- The comfort of the patient on the scanner bed can be further enhanced if the procedure is performed in the shortest time possible, without compromising quality of care
- Patients positioned on the scanner bed should always be covered with a bunny blanket or sheet. This will portray a level of professionalism expected from all practitioners
- Ensure that the patient understood breathing or other instructions when needed
- During positioning of the patient, the patient's eyes should not be exposed to the laser light as this may be harmful to the eyes.

CT of chest or abdomen

- When positioning a patient for a chest CT, ensure that their arms are placed on a supporting sponge or pillow above their head, as their arms will become fatigued if not properly supported. The patient's elbow should be straightened as bending the elbow may hamper the flow of contrast media, especially if the needle is inserted in the antecubital vein
- Never leave the patient on the scanner bed without informing them of the reason why they need to be kept on the scanner bed, e.g. when performing delayed sequences.

Care for escorts

- Ensure that patient's escorts are wearing lead rubber aprons to protect sensitive organs against scatter radiation
- It is advisable that escorts stand as far as possible from the gantry to minimise their exposure to scatter radiation. The use of thyroid shields is also recommended
- Escorts accompanying restless patients should be informed not to place their arms inside the gantry aperture, as this will expose their arms to ionising radiation and may cause artefacts over the anatomical part to be scanned
- It is equally important to apply the 10-day rule to female escorts to prevent unintended exposure to an unborn child *in utero*. No pregnant escort should be allowed in the scanner room.

AFTERCARE OF THE PATIENT

- All patients should be assisted off the scanner bed by lending support. Supporting them with your hand will show compassion, which is a sign of good patient care
- Elderly patients often suffer from postural hypotension and may feel dizzy when getting off the scanner bed. The hypotension and dizziness is caused by a slight drop in their blood pressure while being supine on the scanner bed. It is recommended that the elderly be allowed to sit up for a minute or two, to allow their blood pressure to recover
- All personal belongings, removed before the examination, should be returned
- If contrast media was administered, there may be a need to check for delayed contrast media reactions. Inform the patient if this is the case. Remove butterfly/needles safely. Apply firm pressure on the puncture site to prevent bleeding. Any blood spilled at the puncture site should be cleaned using cotton wool. Ensure that the drips for inpatients are opened using the roller clamp
- Discard used needles and syringes safely by placing them in the sharps container

- Patients should never leave the CT room if they are not completely dressed. It is unprofessional practice to allow patients to leave the CT room half dressed
- Enquire whether your patient has follow-up visits or referral to other departments
- Inform the patient when the results of their CT examination will be available and how it will be relayed to their referring physician
- Always ensure that the scanner room is clean and tidy for the next examination, especially when working in busy CT departments, as this will render the room available for the next patient and practitioner
- All equipment and accessories used should be stored safely and neatly
- Outpatients should be provided with a contact number of the CT department should they wish to contact them, especially in cases of delayed contrast media reaction.

PATIENT PREPARATION FOR CONTRAST MEDIA ADMINISTRATION

Contrast media in CT imaging is usually administered to enhance, inter alia, pathological processes such as neoplasms, inflammatory conditions, e.g. abscesses, cysts, encephalitis, meningitis, tuberculous meningitis or congenital diseases such as aneurysms and arterio-venous malformation. Most pathological processes trigger an increase of blood flow at their location. Since contrast media travels in the bloodstream, enhancement of these pathologies is often evident due to the higher than usual blood flow (and thus contrast media) in that region.

Contrast media should only be administered if there is clinical justification. Even though contrast media in use is relatively safe today, there is still a potential risk of a patient experiencing an allergic reaction to contrast media (see also Chapter 11, Drugs and contrast agents).

The following aspects should be considered when preparing patients for contrast media administration:

- Practitioners need to ensure that the patient needing contrast media administration is informed of the side-effects thereof
- Written consent should be provided prior to administration
- The volume/dose to be administered should be appropriate for the CT examination
- The iodine concentration should be appropriate for the CT examination. In CT angiography or CT venography studies, contrast media with a higher iodine concentration (e.g. 300 mgI/mL) should preferably be used. This is to ensure adequate opacification of vasculature
- Contrast media allergies must be established before contrast media administration

- Establish whether the patient's renal function is adequate. Contrast media administration is usually contraindicated for patients with renal impairment, dehydration or cardiac failure. (See also Chapter 11, Drugs and contrast agents.)
- Patients with a hypersensitivity to contrast media should preferably be examined without the use of contrast media to reduce their risk of an allergic reaction.
- Hypersensitivity to previous contrast media administration is a good predictor for a patient at risk of an allergic reaction. Where contrast media is required for such patients, they can be treated with appropriate antihistamines or anti-anaphylaxis to reduce their risk of an allergic reaction
- Contrast media to be used should not be expired. It is the duty of all practitioners to check the expiry date before administration.

Contrast media administration for paediatrics

- Ensure that the dose to be administered for paediatrics is safe. As a guide, the formulae of 1 millilitre of contrast media for every 2 kilograms of body weight can be applied.

Pump preparation prior to contrast media administration

Every effort should be made to use the pump injector safely. The incorrect use of the pump injector can potentially be lethal to patients. The three major risks in the unsafe use of the pump injector in CT are the following:

- Accidental injection of air can cause an embolus, which may lead to an infarct of tissue distal to the embolus
- Passing of bacteria or other pathogens into the patient's body (which can cause septicaemia). This can occur when an aseptic technique was not followed during drawing up and injection of contrast media
- Rupturing of veins if flow rate of the pump is too high. Rupturing of veins can cause a local haematoma or extravasation of contrast media

The following guidelines can be used for the safe use of the pump injector:

- Ensure that correct settings (flow rate and volume) are selected on the pump injector for each examination. A flow rate of 3 mL/second is usually employed. Younger patients and those receiving chemotherapy, requires a slower flow setting on the pump injector
- Remove as many air bubbles as possible by turning knob underneath pump injector
- Care should be taken that the extension tube is connected using an aseptic technique. No contamination

of the tip of the extension tubing should occur, such as falling on the floor or touching the scanner bed

- Pump is turned upside down (nozzle pointing downward) to ensure that any residual air bubbles are transferred to the top (back) of pump injector. This will prevent injection of tiny amounts of residual air bubbles
- Ensure that the heat wrap (cover) is placed around the syringe of the pump to heat up contrast media, to prevent injection of contrast media that is too cold, which may disturb the thermodynamics of the blood
- Practitioners should ensure that the pump injector activation is synchronised with the acquisition of the CT sequences, to prevent mistiming of intravenous injection.

Contrast media extravasation

- Extravasation is caused when contrast media leaks into the soft tissue surrounding the puncture site
- Extravasation is mostly caused by needles not correctly placed in the lumen of the vein. Extravasation of contrast media will lead to a suboptimal enhancement of vascular or pathological processes, as an inadequate volume of contrast media will be travelling through the patient's body
- Extravasation of contrast media may result in a repeat dose of contrast media and even a repeat CT examination which means an unwanted radiation dose
- Extravasation may also cause a haematoma at the puncture site which can be painful
- Patients receiving chemotherapy generally have fragile veins, which often blow up during contrast media administration. Care should be taken that the pump injection is halted once any blowing up of the vein is noted
- It is imperative that the correct flow rate is selected for the pump injector to prevent rupturing of the veins.

CARE FOR INTRAVENOUS DRIPS

- Practitioners should always ensure that the intravenous drips of patients are in working order
- Ensure that infusions do not occur too fast or too slow by closing or opening the roller clamp where appropriate. A too slow infusion may result in patients not getting the required medication or fluids in time, while a too fast infusion may cause medication overload which may compromise homeostasis
- If the roller clamp is left open, blood will flow into the tubing which may block the tube, requiring replacement of such tubing

- If infusion does not occur, the vein may become thrombosed, which will necessitate another phlebotomy and unnecessary pain
- For trauma patients in shock, infusion needs to be maintained in order to restore the required electrolyte balance especially after severe blood loss
- The tubing should never be kinked, or placed underneath the patient, as it will restrict flow of medication (or fluid), compromising patient treatment
- Drip bags should never be placed on the scanner bed, or hanging too low, as this will result in retrograde flow of blood into the extension tubing.

PATIENT CARE FOR CRITICALLY ILL OR TRAUMATISED PATIENTS

Critically ill patients from the resuscitation departments, intensive care units (ICU), or terminal wards, need to receive preferential treatment and require a high level of care. These critically ill patients should always be accompanied by a nurse practitioner. A seriously ill patient may react differently due to pain, stress or anxiety. If patients are coherent, communication should occur as with normal patients. It is important to work quickly and efficiently while continuing to communicate with the patient even if they do not respond. Informing the patient of what is about to happen may be reassuring even in the absence of a verbal response.[1]

The following aspects should be considered when examining critically ill patients in the CT department:

- Always give preference to critically ill or traumatised patients
- Keep a close watch over their vital signs as this may drop in a short space of time, which will require emergency resuscitation
- The scanner room should be unoccupied when they arrive, so that the examination can be performed immediately upon arrival
- Ensure that the ventilators and suction apparatus are in working condition
- Assist escorts with the transfer of the patient by ensuring that vital stats monitors are safely positioned on the scanner bed, as these may fall off during table movement
- Ensure that the breathing tube of the ventilator, extension tubing of drips and other lines, will not be stretched beyond capacity during table movement
- The patient should be taken off the bed immediately after the scan and transported back to the ward. Post-processing functions such as copying or transfer of images, should occur only after the patient has left the department.

PATIENT CARE FOR THOSE UNDER THE INFLUENCE OF SUBSTANCES

CT practitioners who work after hours or do call, will often need to examine patients under the influence of alcohol or drugs. The practitioner will via communication establish their level of coherence. Some patients will be able to cooperate fully, whilst others might be irrational, hyperactive or even aggressive. The secret is not to provoke any bad behaviour.

Practitioners should:

- Work as speedily as possible in order to get them back to their department
- Do not counter aggression with aggression as it may lead to violence or reprisal from aggressive patients
- If the patient is restless, and if their composure allows, apply immobilisation of the limbs (if required)
- Often it is useful to postpone the CT examination until the patient's level of cooperation has improved, provided that the patient's clinical condition will not be jeopardised by the postponement.

PHYSICAL RISKS IN CT

The risks for patients undergoing CT examinations can be classified into two categories – direct physical risks (to the patient's self), and biological risks posed by the ionising radiation. Practitioners should aim to minimise these risks at all costs. Each of these risks poses their own challenges and will be discussed separately.

Handling of restless patients

There is always a danger of the patient falling off the scanner bed. Patients most at risk from falling off the bed are restless children, the elderly, psychiatric, patients under the influence of substances (alcohol and drugs), critically ill patients who have suffered cerebrovascular accidents or serious trauma. It is imperative that restless patients be immobilised using immobilisation straps. Immobilisation straps should not be applied too tightly as it may compromise blood flow to immobilised limbs. Restless and confused patients should never be left alone in the scanner room (or the waiting room) as they may try to climb off their beds.

During the CT examination, practitioners should always watch these patients during scanning, especially if a gantry tilt or bed movement is to occur, as they can move if not watched closely. It is important to work quickly, without compromising patient care. If a CT exam takes too long, these patients may become more restless which may cause movement artefacts which may require repeat scanning.

Restless psychiatric patients should never be left unsupervised as they can injure themselves or wander and may get lost. This will be tantamount to negligence and may result in litigation. Sedation should only be considered once all efforts to immobilise or scan restless patients have been exhausted.

Transfer of patients

Patients who are being transferred to and from the scanner bed are at risk of physical injury and this should be prevented at all costs. It is therefore important that practitioners apply safe transferring techniques. Paraplegic or quadriplegic patients, or those who have undergone neurosurgery, should be transferred carefully as any physical injury to their skull or body will be exacerbated. A safe way of preventing any injury to their heads is to support their heads when transferring them to or from the scanner bed. This will prevent their heads from knocking the scanner bed or head rest during the transfer, which may cause further intracranial or extracranial damages. The same would apply for their limbs. (For more tips on how to transfer patients, please refer to Chapter 14, Moving and handling.)

Transfer of the patient with confirmed or suspected spinal injuries

Remember that patients with any confirmed or suspected spinal injuries should be treated with the outmost care. Patients with unconfirmed spinal injuries should be treated the same as patients with confirmed injuries, as the possible risk of causing damages to the spinal cord is equally high for unconfirmed spinal injuries.

Every effort should be made to maintain spinal stability during patient transfer.

- As a rule, patients with spinal injuries should never be turned unless it is absolutely necessary. Even if there is clinical justification, the transfer of these patients, should be done by experienced staff. (Refer to Chapter 14, Moving and handling, for guidelines on how to transfer patients safely.)

Physical risks during interventional CT procedures

Biopsies of small lesions (e.g. lymph nodes, pulmonary nodules, focal liver lesions) require precise needle placement to attain a secure position for therapeutic or diagnostic purposes.[5] Interventional procedures in CT such as conventional fine needle aspiration biopsy (FNAB), facet joint injections, and CT fluoroscopy assisted biopsies, pose potential risks to the patient. Even though the practitioner is not directly responsible for the execution of these interventional procedures, they do have some responsibilities with regards to the success of the examination and the patient's wellbeing.

FNAB of the thorax

FNABs are performed to obtain cells from lesions within the thorax. FNABs are thus done so that these cells can be analysed by cytology in order to establish the type of lesion present. These procedures can be long, especially if the lesion is small, or are located at odd anatomical sites. Practitioners should ensure that the patient is comfortable on the bed, to ensure cooperation. Practitioners should ensure that once the needle is advanced, the correct table position is selected. This can be done by matching the light marker to the site at which the needle enters the skin, to prevent scanning at the incorrect level. If the needle cannot be introduced parallel to the scan plane, compensation should be made for the angle at which the needle is placed.

There is always a potential risk of causing a pneumothorax or haemothorax during passing of the needle into the thorax. Practitioners should encourage patients to hold their breath when the needle is passed through the chest wall to minimise possible injury to the pleural membranes or soft tissue. Once the needle is *in situ*, patients should be encouraged to maintain shallow breathing, as deeper irregular breathing may cause the needle to shift out of position, or even break with subsequent risk of haemorrhage or damage to underlying soft tissue. A broken needle will need to be removed by surgery.

Practitioners should further ensure that an aseptic technique is applied during all interventional procedures. No contamination of any of the accessories should occur during the procedure. Care should be taken that the needle does not touch the gantry, as this too may cause shifting of the needle and will in addition increase the risk of cross infection to the patient. Remember that even although local anaesthetics are used to anaesthetise the skin, underlying structures such as the lungs and deep thoracic wall muscles cannot be anaesthetised due to their relative deep anatomical location. Repositioning of the needle is inevitably painful.

Practitioners should ensure that all patients who underwent a FNAB of the chest, should have a chest radiograph within an hour after the procedure, to rule out any pneumothorax or haemothorax.

Facet joint injections

Facet joint pain is attributed to segmental instability, inflammatory synovitis, or degenerative arthritis.[6] The use of CT in management of facet joint pain has become routine in clinical practice. CT guided techniques has brought about an increase in the precision of these procedures and help to confirm needle placement. The patient is placed in the prone position, and several images are obtained at the level of interest to determine entry site and angle of approach. The entry site is marked on the skin, and a 22-gauge needle is advanced into the joint.

Possible complications of facet joint injections include inter alia: infection, haemorrhage, pneumothorax, anaphylactic (idiosyncratic), reaction to iodinated contrast material or anaesthetic and nerve damage. The practitioner role in minimising the risk would be similar to that described for FNABs, above.

BIOLOGICAL RISKS IN CT – RADIATION DOSES

Regardless of scanner model or make, all CT scanners consist of a gantry, X-ray tube and detectors. When X-rays pass through the body part, the incident beam is attenuated in a manner dependent on the local tissue composition. Tissue with higher densities such as bones or calcifications absorbed more of the beam than soft tissue organs such as the liver or spleen. The beam exiting the patient will fall on a set of detectors. These detectors will generate a signal that is used to reconstruct the image. The X-ray beam energy (determined by tube potential) and photon fluence (determined by the product of tube current times the tube rotation), are important factors that affect radiation exposure to the patient.[7]

Studies have shown that CT examinations account for only a small percentage of all imaging examinations but contribute to a very large percentage of the total medical radiation dose to the population.[8] This can be ascribed to the fast growth in the clinical use of this imaging modality, brought about by the improved volume coverage, improved z-axis resolution and the speed of the latest multislice scanners.[10] It is imperative for practitioners to ensure that the 'As Low As Reasonably Achievable' (ALARA) principle is upheld when performing CT examinations.

Bio-effects associated with radiation exposure can be divided into two main groups: the deterministic risk which relates to the death of cells and the stochastic risk which relates to cancer induction or genetic damage (see Chapter 9, Ionising radiations, for more information). Recently, deterministic effects of CT radiation have been reported, where patients have suffered temporary hair loss after undergoing multidetector CT (MDCT) brain perfusion studies.[11] The estimated lifetime risk of cancer death for those undergoing CT of the abdomen has been estimated to be about 12.5/10 000 population for each CT abdominal scan in adults.[12] Risks for children are higher.

Dose reduction in CT

Even although practitioners are not always directly responsible for vetting requests for CT examinations, they can play a role in ensuring that where CT examinations are not clinically justified, that they are not performed.

Establishment of clinical guidelines to advise referring doctors, radiologists and practitioners about the appropriateness and acceptability of CT examinations helps eliminate inappropriate requests for CT.

CT examinations should not be repeated without clinical justification. Imaging modalities such as ultrasound and magnetic resonance imaging (MRI), should be used for appropriate clinical indications when equal or greater diagnostic information can be obtained. Once a CT examination has been clinically justified, each examination should be optimised for each patient. The principle of optimisation should be applied on an individual basis, so as to achieve an image quality sufficient for a particular patient, in order to obtain diagnoses with the minimum dose to the patient.[13]

Optimal use of CT scanning is governed by:

- The diagnostic quality of the examination
- The radiation dose to the patient
- The choice of CT technique.[14]

The benign condition of complicated acute pancreatitis is thought to be responsible for the largest cumulative radiation dose from CT, and imaging thereof, may be substituted by MRI.

CT images are often acquired before, during and after intravenous administration of contrast material. When medically appropriate, multiphase studies should be kept to a minimum and where possible, pre-contrast sequences should be eliminated. This may be relevant in the evaluation of liver and bowel wall conditions, where pre-contrast sequences can frequently be omitted without affecting the interpretation of the imaging study.[7]

Practitioners also need to ensure that repeat examinations due to double booking of patients, or lost CT results, does not occur. Practitioners should also ensure that topograms (scout views) are only covering the area of interest and do not extend beyond the anatomical area to be examined. In addition, CT sequences should also only include the anatomical area of interest and should not be acquired purely out of curiosity.

Use of appropriate CT parameters

Various CT parameters can be manipulated by practitioners to minimise the dose to patients. These are:

- Low dose CT
- Automatic exposure control
- Tube rotation
- Section thickness
- Pitch and dose.

Low dose CT

Low dose CT protocols are now routine in many CT departments. Studies have shown that the dose delivered to patients can be lowered by lowering the tube potential

(kV) or tube current (mA) during image acquisition, without reducing image quality. A 50% reduction in tube current is considered to reduce radiation dose by half. Other studies have shown that a four-fold decrease in the radiation dose occurs when the kilovoltage is dropped from 140 to 80 kVp, for both body and head CT protocols.[15] Reduction in the tube current is the most practical means of reducing CT radiation dose. Practitioners should, where possible, reduce the tube current (milliamperes, mA) in order to reduce the dose to patients. For example, when scanning for abdominal aortic aneurysms, the tube current can be lowered as low dose protocols will not influence the ability to diagnose aneurysms.

Automatic exposure control (AEC)

AEC is analogous to acquisition timing in general radiography. All scanners employ AEC. The user determines the image quality requirements (with regards to the noise or the contrast-to-noise ratio), and the CT system automatically determines the right tube milliampere-seconds (mAs).[16] Various tube current modulation strategies have been developed by CT manufacturers to reduce dose to patients during image acquisition. The two modulation strategies were developed in response to large variations in patient body diameter and subsequent variation in radiation absorption along certain anatomical regions. Tube current modulation is therefore aimed at ensuring even image quality (noise reduction) along the full sequence, with a lowered dose.[16]

Longitudinal (z-axis) modulation

Longitudinal modulation involves variation of dose (mA) between anatomical regions in the z plane, e.g. between shoulders versus abdomen versus pelvis. The aim of varying the tube current along this plane is to ensure uniform noise levels (with lower dose) across the various anatomic regions. The operator chooses a desired level of image quality for input to the algorithm that will calculate the required mAs.[16]

Angular (x–y) modulation

The purpose of angular current modulation strategies is similar to the z-axis modulation, i.e. to ensure uniform dose over areas of varying thickness. The diameter of the lateral plane at the shoulder region is much larger then the antero-posterior (AP) diameter of the same region. Angular current modulation ensures that the exposure during image acquisition is automatically lowered for areas with shorter diameters (in this case the AP plane of the shoulder region). This angular modulation occurs in real time as the tube rotates about the patient. The use of angular (x–y) or longitudinal (z-axis) current modulation is a valuable tool that can reduce doses to patient.

Tube rotation

The longer the tube rotates around the patient, the higher the dose will be and vice versa. Where a shorter tube rotation is selected, anatomical structures will be exposed to radiation for a shorter time. There has been a dramatic decrease in tube rotation times with recent technologic innovations, most notably with the development of sixty-four slice scanners. If the tube rotation time is decreased (faster gantry rotation), the radiation exposure decreases, and tube current may thus have to be increased to maintain constant image quality.[17] Practitioners should therefore always select a shorter tube rotation, provided that this will not automatically increase the mA. Practitioners should therefore be knowledgeable about their scanner configurations in order to reduce dose without compromising the diagnostic quality of CT examinations.

Section thickness

Section thickness in CT refers to the thickness of the slice obtained. Thin collimation can lead to a higher dose, especially if tube current is increased to maintain image noise at a level similar to that of thicker sections.[7] Thinner slices further require more rotations around the patient for the same volume coverage compared with larger slices, which increases the dose imparted. Thus, it is important to employ thicker beam collimation where possible, in order to reduce dose.

Pitch

With MDCT scanners, beam collimation, table speed, and pitch are interlinked parameters that affect the diagnostic quality of an imaging study. In MDCT, detector pitch can be defined as the distance in table movement (in mm) divided by the detector width in mm.[18] Increasing the pitch is another useful method for reducing radiation dose. Faster table speed for a given collimation, resulting in higher pitch, is associated with a reduced radiation dose (especially if other scanning parameters, including tube current, are held constant) because of a shorter exposure time, whereas narrow collimation with slow table speed, resulting in a longer exposure time, is associated with a higher radiation dose. In other words, an increase in the pitch decreases the duration of radiation exposure to the anatomic part being scanned. Studies have shown that increasing the pitch from 1.0 to 1.5 can decrease the radiation dose by 33%, without any apparent loss of diagnostic information.[17]

Shielding of superficial organs

Superficial radiosensitive organs, such as the eye lens, thyroid gland and breast can be shielded using bismuth material or the more commonly available lead apron. The aim of using shielding is to prevent scatter radiation to sensitive organs.[11]

CT radiation risks in children

Radiation risks to children in CT are far greater than for adults. This can be attributed to three factors:

- The increased organ radiosensitivity of children relative to adults
- The longer lifetime risk for radiation-induced cancer
- Lack of adjustment of paediatric CT parameters based on size or region of scanning.[9]

Most manufacturers now incorporate dedicated paediatric protocols into their scanners, and these act as a useful guide for children's dose reduction.[11] Practitioners should employ paediatric protocols when examining children as the exposure (dose) required is far less than for adult protocols.[19] Adult protocols should under no circumstances be used when scanning children. Use of dedicated paediatric protocols and large beam collimation is strongly recommended. The use of thin slice beam collimation when scanning children should be kept to an absolute minimum.

Body weight and habitus

Body weight and habitus are used in some clinical departments to choose appropriate CT parameters in order to reduce dose.[3] Some experts believe that using patient diameter will provide the best approximation of tissue length traversed during the examination because body weight alone does not account for body habitus or height, which can vary with identical body weight, resulting in incorrect selection of parameters and thus dose imparted.[20]

CT in pregnancy

CT is often used for emergency indications such as suspected pulmonary embolus, abdominal perforation, renal colic or trauma among pregnant patients.[21] CT examinations on pregnant females should only be performed where strong clinical justifications exist. Where possible, other imaging modalities such as ultrasound and MRI should be employed as the risks to the unborn child are much lower with these modalities, compared to CT imaging.

The fetal dose delivered by MDCT for pulmonary embolism in pregnant females is mainly attributed to scatter radiation and is lower than direct scanning of the uterus in the first trimester. The major risks to the fetus, with direct scanning of the uterus using MDCT, is that of neurologic deficit and carcinogenesis.[21]

Optimal CT parameters should be selected such as scanning only the anatomical part in question. The use of larger beam collimation, higher pitch and or low dose protocols should be selected. Applying the ALARA principle in pregnant patients are therefore crucial as dose to the unborn fetus can be potentially harmful and should be applied with care. Lead protection of sensitive organs such as of the uterus, breast and thyroid is strongly recommended.

KEY POINTS

- Patient care in the CT department is aimed at enhancing the wellbeing of patients
- All patients should be treated with respect and dignity, irrespective of their social status, race, gender, mental or physical status, sexual orientation, religion or beliefs
- Before a CT examination, practitioners need to correlate the identity of patients
- Practitioners should ensure that the clinical history justifies the CT examination
- Patients should always be informed about the procedure, namely: how long the examination will take or whether any breathing or other instructions will be requested
- Informed consent is needed for invasive procedures prior to starting the examination
- Patients undergoing CT of the abdomen need to have bowel free from barium or faecal matter

- Patients should be made comfortable on the scanner table
- The 10-day rule should be applied to escorts accompanying patients in the scanner room
- Critically ill patients must be given preference in any CT department and should be examined upon arrival
- Restless patients need to be immobilised on the scanner bed using immobilisation straps
- Radiation dose in CT can be minimised by the following:
  1. Performing only CT examinations that are clinically justified
  2. Using low dose protocols
  3. Using tube current modulation strategies
  4. Faster pitch
  5. Larger beam collimation
  6. Shielding of sensitive organs
  7. Using dedicated paediatrics protocols when examining children.

Section | 7 |

Cancer therapy procedures

Chapter | 24 |

External beam therapy

Louisa Clark, Paula McLean, Sindy Singh

THE PATIENT REFERRAL PATHWAY

External beam radiotherapy (EBRT) is the medical use of ionising radiation to treat disease, particularly cancer. The purpose of EBRT is to deliver a therapeutic dose of radiation to a particular region while minimising the damage to surrounding, healthy structures. Modern EBRT primarily uses photons and electrons, produced by linear accelerators.

Most patients consult their GP when they notice symptoms or experience health problems. For some tumour types, symptoms occur early in the course of the illness (e.g. hoarse voice from larynx cancer) – resulting in presentation to the GP with early-stage disease. However, for some tumours, the symptoms tend to be more ill-defined (e.g. abdominal discomfort with pancreatic cancer) and the diagnosis is only made when the disease has reached late-stage. The GP has a number of options for patient referral. If a cancer diagnosis is suspected from the outset, the patient can be referred by an expedited route to the appropriate medical team at a local hospital. At present, such patients with suspected cancer can be referred according to the '2-week rule' and this ensures that they are seen within this period of time at the hospital. If the GP does not suspect cancer, the patient is referred through the normal channels and this can lead to a wait of weeks or months in the patient being seen. Irrespective of the mode of referral, once a patient has been assessed by a medical or surgical team, they will normally be sent for specific investigations – usually comprising blood tests and radiological procedures. These investigations will then be reviewed at a multidisciplinary team (MDT) meeting at which point a definitive diagnosis may be made or further tests may be arranged to define the nature and stage of the disease. The patient does not attend this MDT meeting but, instead, is seen at a clinic appointment at a later date. Once a final diagnosis of the site, type and stage of cancer has been made, the MDT recommends a plan of treatment, with referral to the appropriate member of the team who becomes the patient's lead clinician. In the case of patients for whom radiotherapy is the treatment of choice, this involves referral to a clinical oncologist. Figure 24.1 summarises the patient's journey from the point of referral by the GP to the formulation of a treatment plan by the MDT. Beyond this, the patient has a consultation with a clinical oncologist who subsequently writes a referral for radiotherapy. The steps involved in that process are illustrated in Figure 24.2.

The flowchart in Figure 24.2 demonstrates the patient journey from the MDT to follow-up. There will be a separate detailed explanation of each part. The highlighted sections do not involve the patient directly.

The multidisciplinary team involved in treatment

This multidisciplinary team (MDT) consists of a group of professionals with specific expertise in managing the disease affecting the patient. Each MDT comprises a core membership and a group of extended members. The precise make-up of the team will vary depending on the tumour type. The core membership will frequently include a pathologist, cytologist, radiologist, nuclear

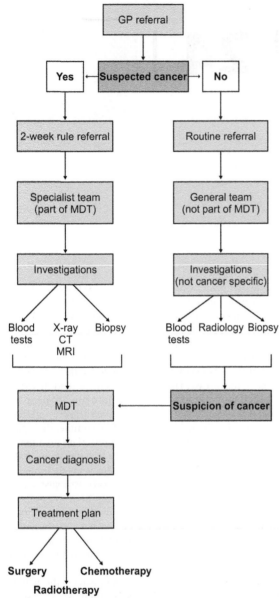

Figure 24.1 The patient journey from referral to treatment planning.

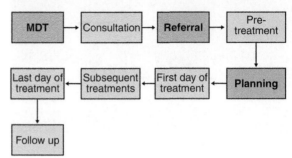

Figure 24.2 The patient journey from treatment to follow-up.

the plan of treatment is decided is defined as the 'decision to treat' date and is important, as it is used for calculating waiting times with regards to government targets. Currently, the MDT in the UK is required to meet a target of 31 days between the decision to treat and the actual start date of radiotherapy, although this may be extended at the patient's request or if there are medical reasons (e.g. neoadjuvant hormone therapy, recovery from surgery) for a delay. Each patient will be allocated a 'key worker' (usually a clinical nurse specialist) who takes responsibility for helping the patient and the family to come to terms with the diagnosis and who coordinates the subsequent hospital appointments.

Consultation with the lead clinician

Following a decision to treat with radiation, patients will be referred to a clinical oncologist who explains the rationale for treatment and the practicalities of radiotherapy planning and delivery. Particular emphasis is given to the likely acute (early) and chronic (late) side-effects of treatment. In most cases, this will involve a candid discussion of the risk–benefit balance of withholding or delivering the treatment. Thereafter, the patient is asked to provide written informed consent for treatment. Women of childbearing age will be asked if they might be pregnant and, if not, will be asked to take precautions against this occurring during treatment and for up to 6–12 months afterwards. If the irradiated area includes the pelvis, both women and men will be warned that the treatment may affect future fertility. They do have the option of storing their eggs or sperm. Patients have the opportunity to seek a second opinion if they feel it is required. In most cases, there is also a time interval between the clinical oncologist giving the patient their treatment information and the actual start of radiation treatment. The patient's next routine appointment is in the pre-treatment area.

Written information that describes the treatment and the side-effects should be routinely offered to patients and their families. Different hospitals will also have access to other information sources for their patients (e.g. Macmillan and Cancer, Information Prescriptions and Welcome Evenings). Macmillan and Cancer offer an extensive resource of written information regarding a wide range of specific

medicine specialist, surgeon, clinical oncologist, medical oncologist, clinical nurse specialist and an MDT coordinator. In addition, extended membership may include a psychologist, physiotherapist, dietician, speech and language therapist and dentist. This complex team is involved in discussing, arranging, performing, reporting and reviewing all the necessary documentation and investigations in order to allow the team to arrive at a rapid and accurate diagnosis. These steps are essential for prognostication and selection of the optimal treatment. The point at which tumour types. 'Information Prescriptions' is a Department of Health-funded online resource that provides reliable information that can be used to augment patient care (www.nhs.uk/ips). In view of the fact that attendance at a radiotherapy department for the first time can be daunting, some Trusts run a welcome evening for patients, usually outside normal working hours. This is an informal session run by radiotherapy practitioners and volunteers. It is held for patients, relatives, carers and includes a tour of the radiotherapy department, demonstration of how a typical radiation treatment dose would be delivered and, perhaps most importantly, an opportunity to ask questions.

Referral for radiotherapy

Before the patient can begin the radiotherapy planning process, the clinical oncologist must complete a referral form for radiotherapy. This important document includes the patient's demographic details, the site of disease, its laterality (left, right, midline), the stage of the tumour and its histology. In addition, the patient's general medical details (including prior radiotherapy, presence of cardiac pacemaker or implantable defibrillator, joint prosthesis and any acute or chronic infections), their performance status and mobility should be recorded. Critically, the clinician must provide accurate details of the treatment intent (radical versus palliative), any immobilisation techniques that may be required and the proposed treatment prescription (total doses to each planning target volume and the number of treatment fractions).

The patient's pre-treatment and treatment appointments are booked according to the department's guidelines and in-keeping with the national waiting time targets. Wherever possible, the patient will be offered treatment times that fit in with his/her daily routine. For example, many patients will continue to work normally during radiotherapy and may prefer early morning or late afternoon time slots.

PRE-EXTERNAL BEAM RADIOTHERAPY PROCESS

Simulation

This step in the patient's journey for EBRT usually refers to a patient's visit to the computed tomography (CT) simulator or conventional simulator. This is the first time that a patient will attend the radiotherapy department and meet with radiotherapy practitioners. It is important to use this opportunity to create a good first impression of the department and professionalism of the staff. Prior to the simulation procedure taking place, the process will be explained to the patient, the patient's consent form is reviewed and re-confirmation of consent to proceed is required. In this setting, patients have the opportunity to ask questions.

It is important to achieve a reproducible patient position to ensure an accurate treatment delivery. The simulation couch and treatment couch are, therefore, identical; both flat and firm. Immobilisation equipment is also used. There are standard pieces of equipment, but as patients vary in age, size, shape, mobility and flexibility for any given tumour site, the immobilisation is tailored to the individual. In cases where the intent of the radiotherapy is for palliation, additional pieces of immobilisation are used to increase comfort. A beam direction shell (BDS) is a specialised piece of immobilisation equipment that is individually made for a patient requiring EBRT to the head and neck area. It is necessary for practitioners to consider the additional time and processes required to produce the BDS that the patient has had to endure. During the pre-treatment process, data for planning of the treatment are acquired. In some cases, intravenous contrast may be used to visualise anatomy more clearly on the CT image data. This involves the insertion of a cannula to administer a contrast agent. Dots are tattooed on the patient's skin as a permanent reference for treatment field alignment. Patients vary in their acceptance of this requirement, so a practitioner needs to be aware of possible alternatives or aid for referencing, e.g. marks drawn on to the skin protected by a tegaderm dressing or the use of a numbing spray. The immobilisation equipment used and patient position are recorded in the treatment card. The patient is then given the initial appointment for treatment. Most departments will also provide a tube of aqueous cream, which the patient is advised to start using on their skin included in the treatment area, once they commence treatment.

Planning

The data that is acquired from the pre-treatment phase is utilised to create an EBRT treatment plan on a radiotherapy computer planning system. The plan provides a visual reconstruction of the parameters that will be used to deliver treatment. The computer planning of a patient's treatment for EBRT occurs without the patient being present.

There are internationally accepted guidelines for the construction of treatment plans. It is the responsibility and duty of the planning staff to ensure that an optimum plan is produced. This involves outlining of the tumour volume and surrounding organs at risk. The treatment fields are positioned to achieve the prescribed dose to the tumour volume while minimising the dose to surrounding organs and normal tissue. Ultimately, this reduces the side-effects that the patient could experience. Each organ has a tolerance dose which relates to the portion of the organ exposed to radiation for a stated daily administered dose. The use of multi-leaf collimator (MLC) shielding allows a partial blocking of the radiation beam within the treatment field to minimise the dose to selected areas. MLCs are utilised to deliver intensity-modulated radiotherapy (IMRT). This is a complex technique, which relies upon an increased number of treatment fields, each from a different angle. While this increases the amount of tissue receiving a dose, the dose is of a lower amount. As the computer planning process develops and becomes more complex, it also becomes more time consuming. This has a knock-on effect on the workload in the planning area. Once a plan is produced and approved for treatment, data is input into the verification system and checked independently. Daily quality assurance (QA) checks ensure the machine is operating within tolerance and individual patient QA would verify that any required MLC configurations match those that are saved within the system.

EXTERNAL BEAM RADIOTHERAPY PROCESS

The first day

The first day of treatment presents many challenges. The patient must be reassured and their treatment must be checked and verified. Completing both these actions well will ensure a much smoother experience for the patient, resulting in their having increased confidence in their treatment. The early completion of these actions will also ensure that time is not wasted later on, since patient concerns will have been addressed and communication channels opened in case of any further problems or queries. In addition, any mistakes or omissions within the patient's treatment plan can be rectified before they arrive and verification of the treatment will minimise the risk of any adverse incidents later in the patient's course of radiotherapy. Communication is vital, not only with the patient, but also among the other members of the radiotherapy team and with the larger MDT. Communication with the patient on their first day of treatment usually includes a first day chat. Patients often experience a range of emotions on the first day of their treatment and good communication will help to make the patient feel more comfortable, with the added advantage of creating a bond with the practitioner, which will make communication easier throughout the remainder of their treatment.

It is important that the patient receives information regarding what to expect of their treatment and their treatment schedule, as well as reaffirmation of the potential side-effects and how to manage them. This also provides an opportunity for the patient to ask any questions they may have and for the practitioner to reconfirm consent and pregnancy status if appropriate. Relevant contact information should also be taken for the patient; this allows the practitioners to contact the patient should the need arise, e.g. in the event of a machine breakdown, to alter an appointment time. Allowing for patient choice should also be a priority. Allowing the patient to choose appointment times and, where possible, the gender of the

treatment practitioners and privacy to change into treatment gowns, will all allow the patient to feel more in control of their treatment and encourage patient centred care within the radiotherapy department.

A first day chat can be adequately provided in 10–15 minutes; however, it is important to tailor this to the individual patient. Some patients will want detailed information and will have lots of questions. If this is the case, it is important to allow them to talk freely and address any concerns they may have. Otherwise, they may feel that the practitioner is uninterested in them personally, resulting in the patient lacking confidence and possibly feeling that the practitioners do not really care about them and their treatment. This could lead them to hide any side-effects they experience, which would be detrimental to their health and their treatment. The opposite is also true and some patients will only want the bare minimum of information. If so, it is important to comply with their needs. Basic information and care advice can be dispensed; with the remaining information being given at the most appropriate times. This will ensure the patient does not feel overwhelmed and will allow them to digest the information given. It is important that the patient still feels comfortable with the practitioners so they can come to them if they are having any problems or if they decide that they do want some advice. However, it is also important that the other members of the team are made aware that for the time being, the patient does not want excessive amounts of information given to them. This will prevent the patient from getting frustrated with the other practitioners should they try to provide advice or information at another time.

Good communication between the team members on the treatment unit has many other advantages. There are many checks to be done prior to the patient starting their treatment. It is important that nothing is overlooked as well as avoiding the repetition of tasks by separate members of staff, which is time consuming and non-constructive. These tasks will ensure the treatment is given in an efficient, timely and accurate manner. The type of checks undertaken will vary depending on the department and the type of treatment to be given but can include: checking treatment schedules and appointments, ensuring all equipment necessary for the patient's treatment is on the unit prior to the patient's arrival and ensuring all appropriate forms and plans have been signed and checked by the relevant staff.

The MDT also has a part to play in the patient's first day of treatment; once again, this may depend on the treatment site and on individual departments' protocols. It is important to check whether any other teams need to see the patient either before or after their treatment, perhaps in relation to chemotherapy, dietetics or assessments by the consultant. The first day of treatment is often confusing for patients and the practitioner may be their initial point of contact in the department. The patient will rely on the practitioner to inform or remind them of any other appointments they may have. If the practitioner is not aware of these appointments, they are often missed, resulting in delays in treatment or the administration of drugs or dressings.

All of the above can be done prior to the patient receiving their treatment. There are still some checks, however, which can only occur once the patient has been set-up and the treatment is about to be delivered. These consist mostly of treatment site verification and dose verification. The treatment site can be verified by a series of images; these ideally occur before the treatment is delivered and can be checked online. Although this increases the amount of time the patient will spend in the treatment room, it will ensure the accuracy of the treatment delivery. Isocentre or beam's-eye view (BEV) images can be matched to planning digitally reconstructed radiographs (DRRs) to ascertain whether the set-up is accurate and, therefore, whether the treatment is about to be delivered to the correct area. It is also possible to verify using cone beam computed tomography (CBCT) which allows for soft-tissue matching against the original planning CT scans. Diodes or thermoluminescent dosimeters (TLDs) can be used to verify the amount of dose being received, either at the entry point of the field or to an organ at risk. This can reduce the risk of radiation incidents occurring as any discrepancies in the expected dose and the actual dose will be picked up early on in the treatment and can, therefore, be corrected.

As there is so much to do, both prior to and during the patient's first day of EBRT, good management and preparation is essential. Failure to complete some of these checks can increase the risk of incidents occurring as well as leaving the patient with little confidence in their team and feeling vulnerable and unable to discuss their concerns.

Subsequent treatments

Although the majority of the checks and information-giving procedures are carried out on the first day of the patient's EBRT, there are still subsequent verifications that must occur to ensure the continued accuracy of the treatment. It is also important that the practitioners are aware of any further appointments that the patient may have during their course of treatment so that the patient can be informed of these in a timely manner.

Further safeguards include the regular use of on-treatment verification images. These are essential to ensure that the set-up of the treatment remains accurate throughout the entire course of treatment. These images can also be used in the event of weight loss or gain or if there is any change in the patient's contour, as evidenced by checking focus skin distances (FSDs), to ensure that the external changes are not compromising the position of internal structures. The risk of an incident or near miss occurring will be greatly

reduced by a regular imaging regimen. These images can be looked at online prior to the patient's treatment or offline once the patient has received their daily treatment. Reviewing the images offline will minimise the time the patient has to spend on the treatment couch but will mean any discrepancies discovered cannot be corrected for until the next fraction of radiotherapy.

As discussed earlier, the patient will also have a variety of appointments to attend during their EBRT. These may include appointments with other health professionals, chemotherapy appointments and, most commonly, on-treatment review clinics. These can often take a considerable amount of time and will have implications for the patient, as they may need to organise extra time off work, child-care or give advance warning to whoever brings them in that they may be in the department longer on that particular day. Forewarning the patient of these extra appointments and the time they may take will enable them to prepare for them and feel more in control of their treatment. However, if they are not given adequate time to prepare it may result in the patient feeling frustrated and angry and possibly being unable to attend the appointment.

The final day of treatment

It is often in the weeks after the patient's final treatment that their side-effects will reach their peak. This is also the time when most patients find themselves with the least amount of support. Relevant information provided at this point may help to minimise the negative psychological impact on the patient during this time. This information could include making the patient aware that their side-effects may continue to get worse and how to manage this if it occurs. Also, providing them with a list of contact numbers so they know who to contact should they have any problems or concerns between the end of their treatment and their first follow-up appointment, which may not be for another 6 weeks. During this time, if the department has a practitioner in an advanced practitioner role in clinic, the clinic practitioner may contact the patient, via telephone, after a couple of weeks to check how they are coping and to answer any questions or concerns the patient may have. Although this practice is time consuming, it has several advantages, since the patient does not need to come into the department. Also, the patient feels well cared for and does not feel the sense of abandonment that can sometimes occur once their treatment has finished. It can also result in reduced time taken during their follow-up appointment, as they will already have had some of their questions answered. Finally, it provides the opportunity to address any possible issues earlier on. For example if the patient is experiencing excessive side-effects they may need to return to the department earlier than originally planned to have them assessed and treated.

FOLLOW-UP

The patient is followed up by their clinical oncologist and the referring surgical team at regular intervals after they have completed radiotherapy. Depending on the severity of the acute radiation effects, patients may need to return at weekly intervals during the resolution phase. This is particularly common for patients with very brisk cutaneous or mucosal reactions (e.g. head and neck cancer patients). However, for most patients, the first appointment will usually take place 4–6 weeks after treatment. At this initial follow-up visit, the medical team will confirm that the radiation reactions have settled appropriately (usually back to grade 0 toxicity) and will examine the patient for evidence of residual or recurrent cancer. In certain circumstances, especially with deep-seated tumours that are not readily accessible for clinical examination, the doctor may arrange a base-line CT or magnetic resonance imaging (MRI) scan to document the fact that a complete remission has been achieved. This scan also serves to define the altered anatomy following treatment (the patient may have surgical and post-radiation scarring) and can be used for future comparison in the event that the patient undergoes repeat scans. Depending on the site that was treated and the natural history of the disease, subsequent follow-up visits are arranged. Typically, for a patient with head and neck cancer, they will be seen monthly for the first 6 months; 6-weekly for the next 6 months; 2-monthly in the second year; 3-monthly in the third year and 6-monthly thereafter. In contrast, patients with breast cancer will be seen by their surgeon 3 months after their surgery and by the clinical oncologist 6 months after the end of treatment. They are then followed up 6-monthly by the surgeon and 6-monthly by the clinical oncologist for 5 years. By convention, patients will be regarded as having been cured of their disease if they reach 5 years of follow-up with no evidence of disease recurrence at the local tumour site or the loco-regional lymph nodes and no sign of distant metastases.

KEY POINTS

- The patient's experience starts from the moment they enter the department
- Practitioners have to be aware of the impact the staff and the environment have on the patient
- Staff need to maintain a professional image at all times; both on and off duty when they are in the department
- All areas of the department must be clean and in good order
- Patient choice based on up-to-date information, clearly communicated, is paramount in achieving patient-centred care

Chapter | 25 |

Brachytherapy

Pauline Humphrey

INTRODUCTION

Brachytherapy is a type of radiotherapy where a sealed radioactive source is placed close to or into a tumour or tumour bed. The word *brachy* comes from the Greek and means 'near to' or 'close'. It is often used in combination with external beam radiotherapy (EBRT), as a boost to the tumour site or tumour bed, but it can also be used as a primary treatment. It is used in approximately 3% of radiotherapy patients in the UK[1] and it is reported that across Europe, the majority of brachytherapy is used in treatment of gynaecological tumours (59% of all cases), followed by prostate (17%), breast (9%), lung/bronchus (3%) and oesophagus tumours (2%).[2]

Brachytherapy is used to treat a variety of cancer sites and can be divided into four main types of treatment:

- Intracavitary brachytherapy – into a body cavity, e.g. intravaginal or intrauterine brachytherapy for cancer of the cervix, endometrium or vagina
- Interstitial brachytherapy – into tissues, e.g. prostate or breast brachytherapy
- Intraluminal brachytherapy – into a lumen, e.g. oesophageal or endobronchial brachytherapy
- Surface moulds – e.g. skin or eye plaques

Depending on the type of radioactive source and the method of administration, brachytherapy can also be subdivided into:

- Low dose rate brachytherapy (LDR) – dose rates between 0.5 Gray (Gy) per hour to about 1 Gy per hour
- Medium dose rate (MDR) – dose rates between 1 Gy per hour and 12 Gy per hour
- High dose rate brachytherapy (HDR) – dose rate greater than 12 Gy per hour
- Pulsed dose rate brachytherapy (PDR) – where pulses of high dose rate are given at regular intervals, typically a pulse of a few minutes is given each hour.

When brachytherapy was first developed, radioactive radium sources were manually placed into the tumour. To minimise radiation dose to staff, afterloading techniques were developed, typically with caesium sources. This requires the placement of tubes or needles which are later loaded with the radioactive source(s). The development of remote afterloading devices from the 1960s means the treatment delivery can be given to the patient in a shielded room, controlled by staff outside the room.

The main advantage of using brachytherapy is due to the high intensity of radiation close to the source, and the rapid decrease in dose with increasing distance from the source, following the inverse square law. It means that high doses can be given to the tumour while little dose may be given to surrounding sensitive structures, organs at risk. Another advantage is that by placing the radioactive source in or close to the tumour volume, there is likely to be less chance of inaccuracies due to immobilisation of organ movement when compared with external beam radiotherapy.

PREPARATION FOR BRACHYTHERAPY

By its very nature, almost all brachytherapy techniques (excluding surface moulds) are likely to be quite invasive, and therefore, patient care is particularly crucial. Such invasive procedures will require appropriate patient preparation with information and support from skilled healthcare practitioners. It requires excellent team-working across many professional disciplines to ensure that the patient is able to comply and maintain safety and well-being throughout. Putting a radioactive source inside a patient can sound really scary and creates a certain amount of anxiety and fear for patients and their carers. Therefore, patient preparation is the key to successful completion of brachytherapy.

To prepare our patients for an invasive procedure we need to provide appropriate information and support. This will need to be given in a timely manner and tailored to the needs of the individual patient. The needs of patients vary widely; so many aspects need to be considered. (See Chapters 1–4 in the Communication section.)

Ideally, we need to bring this into the discussion of treatment options at the time of explanation of diagnosis. But can the patient take this much information in? Weighing up surgery, external radiotherapy and chemotherapy, brachytherapy may just be too much to take in, or seem so far away that it is not discussed or not remembered by the patient. If brachytherapy is to follow a course of external beam radiotherapy, then this may be an ideal opportunity to revisit the information a number of times.

Often diagrams are useful, especially in describing how and where brachytherapy applicators are going to be used. If patients can understand the basic principles of brachytherapy, getting a high radiation dose inside or close to the tumour, they are more likely to accept the benefits that this invasive technique brings. A well informed, consenting patient is far more likely to be compliant with the brachytherapy procedure, perhaps putting up with some discomfort or embarrassment if they are really aware of the rationale and benefits of the treatment. And hopefully, the better informed they are, then their levels of fear and anxiety can be minimised too.

Due to the invasive nature of brachytherapy it may be especially important to be aware of cultural or religious issues for patients. The gender of the staff caring for the patient may be a particular concern and would need to be discussed in advance. Patients with cognitive impairment need careful explanations of the procedure and appropriate assessment of capacity to consent; use of patient advocates may be required. This needs careful documentation, especially when the treatment involves the use of anaesthesia or sedation. (See also Chapters 5–7 in the Psychosocial aspects of patient care section.)

Sometimes psychological factors will influence whether a patient can tolerate brachytherapy. For example, with brachytherapy for gynaecological cancers, previous trauma such as bad experiences with cervical smears or vaginal examinations, difficulties in childbirth or a history of sexual abuse may make treatment difficult to cope with. Patients may need extra help and support to find a way to get through the treatment. The support of a clinical psychologist may help a patient find appropriate coping strategies.

Preparation may also need to include physical or pharmacological preparation, e.g. bowel preparation before prostate brachytherapy.

PRE-ASSESSMENT FOR BRACHYTHERAPY

This may be a simple questionnaire about medical history, current medication and allergies for a patient having outpatient or day-case brachytherapy, such as vaginal vault brachytherapy. It is really useful to know if a patient is diabetic, or epileptic, but also essential to know if, For example they have a history of depression, physical disability or hearing problems.

Current medication may indicate medical history which the patient has forgotten to give information about; again antidepressants or anxiolytics may just give a hint to underlying issues that we need to be aware of. It is also helpful to ask patients about their social circumstances. This can give clues to how a patient may cope and what support they have around them. Will they have a responsible adult at home after their admission for brachytherapy? Is there someone to provide transport?

For brachytherapy requiring anaesthetics, a more detailed pre-assessment may be required. We obviously have to consider the anaesthetic risks and what information the anaesthetist would require. This may include an Electrocardiogram (ECG) ECG for older patients, blood tests including a clotting screen, possibly a chest X-ray. Currently we are seeing an increase in the number of obese patients requiring treatment and it is good practice. to have an anaesthetic review. This may include an anaesthetist reviewing case notes or meeting the patient and discussing adaptations to the brachytherapy or anaesthetic techniques to ensure a safe procedure.

ANALGESIA/ANAESTHESIA

Another key component of good patient care in brachytherapy is getting the right analgesia or anaesthesia for the type of procedure, and tailored to the specific needs of the individual patient. There is very little information in medical journals about analgesia or anaesthesia in brachytherapy, so many techniques have developed through experience in individual centres.

For some brachytherapy procedures, such as vaginal vault brachytherapy, a simple applicator placed into the vagina may require no analgesia or anaesthesia. It is essential to encourage the patient to relax as much as possible, use plenty of lubricating gel, sometimes local anaesthetic gel can help, then careful placement of the applicator is usually well tolerated.

For more complex procedures such as intrauterine brachytherapy or prostate implants, then a much greater level of analgesia would be required. Whether a general anaesthetic or spinal anaesthetic or sedation is necessary, will depend on many different factors. Some departments have their afterloader treatment unit inside their operating theatre, or theatre suite, so a patient may be anaesthetised for the insertion, treatment and applicator removal. In broad terms, this may have an advantage that the patient can be asleep throughout the procedure, which they are likely to prefer. However, this can be a very lengthy procedure if imaging and complex planning is involved. If patients are anaesthetised for a number of hours this is extremely time consuming for the whole theatre team, and limits imaging to that which can be carried out within theatre; typically ultrasound or orthogonal images taken with a C-arm X-ray unit. This will also limit the number of cases that can be completed per theatre list. With developments in imaging and planning, the use of CT and MRI planning would require a patient to be moved from room to room, and therefore for practical reasons, anaesthesia would be limited to the insertion of applicators only. So analgesia during the imaging, planning and applicator removal needs to be sufficient if a general anaesthetic has worn off. This may have some advantage in allowing a shorter anaesthetic and if an afterloader unit is in a room away from the theatre, this may allow further theatre procedures to continue at the same time as imaging, planning and treatment of other cases.

Spinal anaesthesia

The use of spinal anaesthesia may be an advantage when the imaging, planning and applicator removal is expected to take a number of hours. This may be useful for prostate brachytherapy implants for high dose rate brachytherapy delivery and also intrauterine brachytherapy, where CT and MRI imaging are becoming more commonplace.

An anaesthetic agent such as bupivacaine can be instilled into the cerebrospinal fluid, providing a dense block for up to 3 hours (Fig. 25.1). The addition of diamorphine into the CSF can increase the duration of the regional anaesthesia further.

For intrauterine brachytherapy, some centres use a general anaesthesia for the first insertion, during which they place a cervical sleeve. This will stay in place after applicator removal and make the next applicator insertion easier so sedation may be used for any subsequent insertions. Other

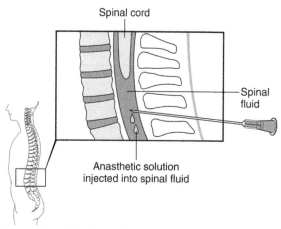

Figure 25.1 Spinal anaesthesia.

centres may choose to use general or spinal anaesthesia for every applicator insertion.

Typical pre-meds and general anaesthesia for intrauterine brachytherapy

Sometimes getting the right level of analgesia in intrauterine brachytherapy can be difficult. A typical preparation may be a premed of a loading dose of paracetamol (1.5–2 g) and a non-steroidal anti-inflammatory such as Meloxicam. The applicators may then be inserted while the patient is under a short, light, general anaesthetic, such as a propofol syringe driver. While asleep, they are given fentanyl and the vast majority wake-up with no pain, often describing the feeling of the urinary catheter in place, feeling like they need to pass urine. In some cases, as the fentanyl wears off, they begin to experience an aching or gradual onset of pain, like a period pain or sometimes cervical spasms. They can be given a top up of an analgesic depending on the severity of the pain they are describing. We usually ask them to rate the pain on a scale between 1 and 10. Although this is quite subjective, it can help as a rough guide and also to monitor if they feel the pain is subsiding or increasing. As a top up, they may be given opiates such as morphine i.v., oramorph, tramadol or further i.v. fentanyl. It is also worth bearing in mind how long till applicator removal when choosing which analgesic. If using a standard plan with fixed geometry applicators, it may only take 30 minutes from leaving recovery to complete treatment delivery and applicator removal. For a customised plan, with CT and MR imaging, it can take a number of hours to produce a plan. Sometimes re-imaging as a final check before treatment may be required. If a patient is waiting on a ward during this time, then ward staff often need guidance on offering appropriate postoperative analgesia.

PRACTITIONER-LED SERVICES IN BRACHYTHERAPY

Another way to improve patient care may be to train practitioners to take over some of the tasks that doctors have traditionally carried out. In the UK, many practitioners have been trained to carry out vaginal vault bachytherapy. As long as this is done in a safe way, with experienced practitioners with specialist underpinning knowledge, a clear protocol that states which cases can be practitioner-led and where the boundaries are, when to seek medical advice or support, then there can be benefits to patients and patient care. It may be possible to schedule patients at times when doctors are doing the more complex planning tasks, or in clinics. So there may be fewer delays in starting treatment, possibly more flexibility in appointment times. And many patients say they like seeing the same person each time for their treatment and perhaps it is less daunting for them to see a practitioner rather than a doctor, makes brachytherapy a bit less frightening. As a role development for practitioners it can be very rewarding work.

Typically, practitioners spend more time per patient than in EBRT, and some of this is getting to know the patient, so they feel understood and supported, to make this invasive treatment psychologically manageable. And vaginal vault brachytherapy accounts for 75% of our gynae-brachy cases, so it releases doctors' time for the more complex brachy cases such as recurrent disease or MRI planning for advanced cervical cancer.

KEY POINTS

- There are many aspects to providing good quality care in brachytherapy
- These can only work if you have good teamwork, a sharing of the responsibilities and workload, and a common goal
- With a good understanding of each other's roles and boundaries and understanding the individual needs of our patients we can achieve good outcomes for our brachytherapy patients

Chapter | 26 |

Chemotherapy

Laureen Hemming

INTRODUCTION

Staff working in medical imaging and radiotherapy will come across patients receiving chemotherapy on a regular basis. Chemotherapy as a treatment for cancer developed as an unexpected consequence of experience with exposure to mustard gas[1] during the Second World War. At this time, sailors were accidently exposed to mustard gas which was discovered to lower their white blood cell count. Doctors wondered whether the mustard gas could be beneficial in treating rapidly dividing white cells in lymphomas and an experiment was instigated which worked sufficiently well to warrant further trials and research. Chemotherapy has developed a reputation for side-effects which has sometimes overshadowed its efficacy in the treatment of cancers.[2,5] Paradoxically, chemotherapy can pose problems for patients and health professionals, since it provides a cure but at a cost, which is often called into question.[3] Staff have to administer chemotherapy and remain positive for the patient's sake, while knowing that most people will experience side-effects which may compromise their quality of life. However, the use of chemotherapy is now much more sophisticated than previously and many of the side-effects are effectively controlled. This has had the beneficial result that some cancers are now viewed as long-term conditions rather than fatal ones. It is a major treatment for cancer and many people with cancer are prepared to manage the consequences, as it may give them a good chance of surviving.

The aims of chemotherapy are to:

- Effect a cure of certain cancers that respond well to treatment
- Treat certain cancers palliatively, thus containing disease and symptoms
- Work concurrently with other treatments such as radiotherapy so as to eradicate as much cancer as possible
- To shrink tumours prior to other treatment such as surgery, thus containing the disease to a manageable size.[5-6]

To fully appreciate the manner in which chemotherapy agents work, an understanding of the mechanics of cell replication is essential.

THE MECHANISMS OF CHEMOTHERAPY

The cell cycle

The cells in the body are constantly being regenerated, via a cycle controlled by a variety of factors governed by enzymes and hormones. Some cells are replaced and renewed more rapidly than others and the process of regeneration can take between 15 and 120 hours, the average being about 48 hours.[5] Regeneration and replication of cells occurs in five cyclical phases:

- G_1 – the cell prepares for regeneration, proteins accumulate to make RNA
- S (synthesis) – here the cell doubles its DNA content
- G_2 – the cell prepares for division, which is the next phase of mitosis. In between each of these phases, checks are made: a significant protein involved in these checks is p53, which is inactivated in many cancers. If faults are detected in the chromosomes during these

checks, then apoptosis (programmed cell death) occurs and the regeneration process is stopped. In the absence of detected faults, the cell proceeds to the mitotic phase

- M (mitosis) – the cell splits in two, these are referred to as 'daughter cells'
- G_0 – the new cell enters a resting phase which lasts until the cell receives signals to recommence regeneration.[2,5]

Tumour cells develop when this process of regeneration and replication becomes altered and out of control. DNA mutations in affected cells cause regeneration rates to vary – rapidly in leukaemias and lymphomas, slowly in sarcomas and carcinomas. The normal control mechanisms of removing damaged cells through apoptosis are lost so these cells continue to regenerate while losing the shape and function of the originals, becoming undifferentiated and cancerous.

There are over 50 different chemotherapy agents, which are usually referred to as cytotoxic (because they kill cells). These are divided into those which are 'phase specific'[7] (acting at a particular point in the cell cycle) or 'nonspecific' (acting at several points of the cell cycle). They work best on cells that are in the process of dividing, during the mitotic phase.[8] The person being treated will therefore require several cycles (or courses) of chemotherapy if an effective kill rate of tumours is to be achieved,[2,6] since cells are regenerating at different speeds.

Chemotherapy targets all the cells in the body, normal and abnormal. Normal cells recover and renew from chemotherapy much quicker than tumour cells, taking approximately 3 weeks.[6] Therefore, chemotherapy is given in 'cycles', which are timed in intervals that allow for the optimum recovery of normal cells while hitting tumour cells before they have recovered, thus effecting a greater abnormal cell kill. Most people have at least six cycles and are monitored after every two or three, to ascertain whether the agents are having the desired effect.[2] However, people may undergo many more cycles with different agents being used, especially if the cancer is responding to treatment.

Tumour response to chemotherapy

Chemotherapy is not the preferred option for the treatment of all cancers, as some cancers do not respond as well.[5] The cancers that respond best to chemotherapy are:

- Acute lymphoid leukaemia in children
- Acute myeloid leukaemia
- Hodgkin's disease
- Germ cell testicular cancers
- Choriocarcinoma
- Ovarian cancer
- Wilms' tumour
- Embryonal rhabdomyosarcoma
- Ewing's sarcoma.

In other cancers, chemotherapy is used as an adjuvant therapy, that is in addition to surgery and radiotherapy, or palliatively, to reduce unpleasant symptoms and control disease without curing the person.

Table 26.1 shows a classification of chemotherapy agents, according to their mode of action.

Table 26.1 Chemotherapy agent classification

Grouping	Action	Examples
Alkylating and platinum agents[1,5,6,8]	Prevent DNA splitting in the G_2 phase but are also active throughout the cell cycle, thus inhibiting the formation of two daughter cells in mitosis	Carboplatin Chlorambucil Cisplatin Cyclophosphamide
Antimetabolites[1,5,6,8]	Affect the synthesis phase of the cell cycle in two ways, by modifying nucleic acid affecting the formation of new DNA strands (1) or by preventing a reduction of folic acid (2), which is required for DNA synthesis to continue	Capecitabine (1) Gemcitabine (1) 5-fluorouracil (1) Methotrexate (2)
Mitotic inhibitors[6]	Affect the spindle formation between the strands of DNA during mitosis	Vinca alkaloids Taxanes Camptothecin analogues
Antimitotic or cytotoxic antibiotics[5]	Affect the formation of RNA and DNA (called intercalation)	Anthracyclines Non-anthracyclines
Topoisomerase inhibitors[1,6]	Enzymes that interrupt the uncoiling of DNA strands	Epidophyllotoxins Etoposide Irinotecan

ADMINISTRATION OF CHEMOTHERAPY

Traditionally, chemotherapy is given as an intravenous infusion[6,8] that requires cannulation (insertion of a needle) of the person, which when repeated frequently, can become painful. If the person requires several cycles of chemotherapy, more permanent devices can be fitted, such as Hickman catheter or porta caths. The dosage is calculated according to the person's body surface, which is derived from their weight and height and is expressed as mg/m^2.

Drug companies have been developing oral preparations of the various cytotoxic drugs, which have proved equally as effective as intravenous drugs; however absorption of the drugs may be affected by food and digestion. If the drugs make the person nauseous to the extent that they vomit, it raises questions about whether the full dosage has been absorbed. While patients report preferring oral chemotherapy, they are reluctant to continue if they feel it compromises the efficacy of the treatment.[23] Healthcare professionals worry about the person's determination to comply with the regime, particular if they experience undesirable side-effects and stop taking the drugs, so even although oral therapy may prove more cost-effective in view of reduced hospital contact, both parties prefer intravenous administration because it increases contact and support.

Chemotherapy in the UK is usually administered in specialist outpatient or chemotherapy departments, with many cancer centres making these environments more comfortable with reclining chairs and 'smell free' to reduce people's experiences of nausea.[8] Many people express a preference for day-care as they feel they are less in the 'sick' mode; it normalises life and some have compared it to 'going to the hairdressers'. Instead of being placed under a hair dryer, they are hooked up to a giving set with a chemotherapy infusion, reading magazines.[4] However, some people are frightened, and feel lonely when managing the side-effects of the drugs at home.

Clinics may be called 'one stop' or 'two stop'; one stop clinics can involve spending a whole day in the department as the person receiving chemotherapy usually requires a full blood count assessment and a creatinine clearance test (which measures the function of the kidneys) before treatment commences.[8] Most chemotherapy

---

Box 26.1 Required blood values for commencement of chemotherapy[8]

- Haemoglobin: >10 g/dL
- Total white blood count: >3.0 × 10^9/L
- Total neutrophil count: >1 × 10^9/L
- Platelets: >80 × 10^9/L

---

agents are excreted through the kidneys, but some are metabolised in the liver. If the kidneys are not working efficiently, a build up of toxic waste occurs in the body. Waiting for results before treatment commences is frustrating. Box 26.1 outlines the blood values necessary for chemotherapy to proceed.

'Two stop' clinics require the person to attend twice, 1 day for a blood test and the following day (or 2 days later) for chemotherapy, which reduces waiting times as the blood results and chemotherapy regime are ready for delivery as soon as the person arrives in the department for treatment, but does entail two visits to the hospital. The negative aspect of reducing waiting times and increasing the number of people treated in a day is that people have reported feeling dehumanised.

Resistance

An individual can develop resistance to a chemotherapy agent, and the first dose of any agent is carefully monitored to ensure the person does not suffer an allergic reaction.[8] These are not common but given the toxicity of the agents, risks are not taken. Cancers themselves can become resistant to treatment; they produce chemical enzymes called cytokines which can make the cells less receptive to the chemotherapy agents.[1,7,22] The larger the cancer and tumour burden, the less effective chemotherapy becomes.

Combination chemotherapy

Treatment with a single chemotherapy agent may have limited results, especially as resistance can develop. To improve the curative potential of chemotherapy, many regimes are based on using a combination of drugs, as this means a greater 'cell kill'. By using a mixture of phase-specific agents and cycle-specific agents, more cells are targeted at a given time increasing the potential effectiveness of the treatment. Within the combination, other drugs that are not specifically chemotherapy agents but which improve their action, can be given. Combination therapies are usually known by their acronyms, which usually derive from the first letter of each drug used, e.g. CHOP – which includes 'cyclophosphamide, doxorubicin (formerly called hydroxydaunomycin), vincristine (formerly called Oncovin) and prednisolone. Another combination is FEC – fluorouracil, epirubicin and cyclophosphamide.[9]

Pre-treatment advice and information

Chemotherapy regimens are all individualised to meet a person's specific needs and are modified according to the response to the treatment. It is important that each person understands the full implications of their treatment. Each person is invited to attend the clinic before chemotherapy treatment starts so they can become acquainted with procedures, meet the staff that will be part of the care team and have an opportunity to express concerns. One frequently asked question usually relates to hair loss. It is at this point that they are asked to sign a consent form agreeing to the treatment. Information is given regarding precautions that need to be taken; such as using a soft toothbrush to avoid mouth ulcers and recording their temperature. An increase in temperature is often the first signal that they may have acquired an infection, their resistance to fighting infection having been lowered as a consequence of the chemotherapy.

SIDE-EFFECTS OF CHEMOTHERAPY

Chemotherapy agents cause numerous side-effects which result in treatments becoming curtailed and therefore less effective; however, if side-effects are managed well or prevented through the use of medication, the person can continue, giving the agents a better chance at eradicating the cancer cells. The main side-effects are now discussed in greater depth.

Neutropenia (reduced neutrophil count)

Neutropenia is a serious side-effect of chemotherapy, requiring immediate action, because if untreated, it can prove fatal. Chemotherapy depresses the function of the bone marrow and its production of blood cells, in particular neutrophils. When neutrophil levels are lowered, the person is at risk of developing infections. The infections in the most part come from the patients themselves. If the oral mucosa is breached, the person can develop ulcers and sores, which are a source of infection.[6] It is recommended that soft toothbrushes are used to clean teeth, as this reduces the chances of damaging the gums.

Neutropenia, a reversible condition, is said to occur when the neutrophil count is lower than $1 \times 10^9/L$; febrile neutropenia occurs when the person's temperature is greater than 37.5°C. Neutropenic events can occur in approximately 40% of people receiving chemotherapy and are a significant reason why chemotherapy may be reduced in intensity and halted for a while until the person recovers.[10] The person receiving chemotherapy needs a thermometer and needs to keep a record of their daily temperature. If their temperature is raised, they must contact their healthcare team immediately or report to hospital for a possible emergency admission.[6,10] Everyone receiving chemotherapy is given a card detailing local arrangements and the emergency telephone numbers of who they should contact.

People at greater risk of developing neutropenia may be given a course of granulocyte stimulating factor (GCSF) over a period of 10 days, which helps the neutrophil production to recover quickly. A 'neutropenic diet' in which uncooked foods such as salads, blue cheeses, unpasteurised milk products, and undercooked meats is advocated, as this also reduces the risk of opportunistic infections.[6] People are also advised to avoid mingling in crowded areas when shopping or having visitors who have an infection, while their immune system is lowered by chemotherapy.

Alopecia (hair loss)

Alopecia is the most visible sign that a person may have cancer and is unwell; however, this side-effect occurs only with some chemotherapy agents, such as cyclophosphamide, etoposide, methotrexate, taxanes and vinca alkaloids.[11] As treatments often involve a combination of agents, it is more than likely that there will be some hair loss. While the hair does grow back after treatment, at the time, alopecia is a significant problem for both men and women, as all body hair is lost. It affects the person's confidence, sense of self, body image, perception of their sexuality and can inhibit social interactions. When the hair grows back, it may be changed in texture, colour and curliness, which can affect the person's sense of self.[12]

There are several ways in which people may manage this side-effect. Men are more likely to shave their heads rather than cope with thinning hair as the hair loss may not be uniform, and the subsequent regrowth will be uniform. Men and women can be fitted for wigs or choose to wear hats or scarves to minimise the effect of baldness. Some acrylic wigs are available from the NHS; the Cancer Research website has a list of wig suppliers.[12] Other ways to manage this are to have hair cut short before treatment starts, reduce the frequency of hair washing, avoid hair dyes and having perms.

Alternatively, people can opt for scalp cooling. Initially, scalp cooling was achieved by wearing gel filled caps that had been frozen, which were periodically changed as they warmed up.[6,11] Now, scalp cooling is achieved mechanically, where the machine keeps the cap at a constant temperature. Optimum results are achieved when the cap fits snugly to the head, so the right size needs to be selected for each person. The cap has to be worn for at least 15 minutes before treatment starts and continues for at least 30 minutes after treatment has stopped.[6] The person wearing the cap may need extra blankets to keep warm while the scalp is being cooled. The caps are heavy and the cold may be a deterrent from persevering with the cooling process. Scalp cooling is not a guarantee against hair loss; some people still experience hair loss or thinning, especially if the cap does not fit snugly, which can be very distressing having coped with all the discomfort of the cold cap. Healthcare professionals are often reluctant to advocate scalp cooling knowing that it is not always successful.[11] Cooling of the scalp reduces the uptake of the chemotherapy agents in the hair follicles. However, fears that the cancer will metastasise in the scalp because of scalp cooling are ill-founded, as there is no research-based evidence to support this claim.[6,11]

Nausea

Chemotherapy-induced nausea (CIN) is described by many as the worst side-effect; it affects approximately 60–70% of people having treatment.[13] Some agents are known to be more ematogenic (causing nausea and vomiting) than others; cisplatin being at the top of the range and the vinca alkaloids at the bottom.[6,13] Sometimes the nausea is accompanied by vomiting and although nausea is frequently described as nausea and vomiting, they are two separate conditions requiring different approaches in care.[14]

Nausea is a subjective, individual experience that has been previously described as queasiness, unease in the stomach, a feeling that they need to vomit, retching, heaving.[14] Following chemotherapy, the nausea may be acute, in that it occurs within the first 24 hours, or delayed, occurring 48 hours later. If acute nausea is untreated, the person may develop anticipatory nausea, where the very thought of attending for chemotherapy may induce nausea and this is very difficult to manage. Nausea, a complex symptom to manage, is associated with a range of other interrelated symptoms such as fatigue and constipation, anxiety, taste changes in the mouth and heightened perception of smells. As the symptom occurs after treatment, the person invariably has to cope with this at home on their own; it is exhausting, disrupts sleep and prolongs the recovery period between treatments.[14]

As the symptom is an individual experience, thorough assessment is crucial before treatment commences. Critical questions are:

- How often do you feel nauseous?
- How long does it last?
- How severe is it?
- What other sensations and symptoms accompany it?
- What makes it better?
- What makes it worse?[13]

Keeping a record in a journal or diary is useful, as a pattern usually develops. If very severe, it may curtail treatment making good management of this distressing symptom essential.[24]

Most people prescribed chemotherapy will be given a premedication of an antiemetic, usually Ondansetron 8 mg and a steroid, Dexamethasone 8 mg up to an hour before the chemotherapy is administered, as the main goal is to prevent the symptom developing.[15] Newer drugs such as neurokinin type 1 receptors are being used as they remain in the body for a shorter time.[13] Antiemetics cause drowsiness and constipation, which add to the symptom burden.

There are non-pharmacological approaches that can be used in conjunction with the drugs. There is evidence suggesting that using music for distraction alleviates feelings of nausea. Progressive muscle relaxation; meditation and controlled breathing have also proved effective. Guided imagery, where the person is encouraged to focus on a pleasant scene or an enjoyable calming experience of their own experience is effective because the person has a sense of control over their situation.[13] The research-based evidence for non-pharmacological interventions is limited but they do have the advantage of being relatively inexpensive, easy to learn and to apply.[13,14] These techniques can be used in other situations where tension and anxiety mount, such as waiting for test results.

Constipation

The vinca alkaloids (vincristine and vinblastine) have a direct affect on the bowel which affects bowel transit time and lengthens the time food products remain in the colon, resulting in more water being reabsorbed into the body, so stools become harder and constipation is the end result.

Most of the time, constipation occurs secondary to other side-effects, such as nausea, where the person's dietary intake may be diminished and they have not had sufficient fluids. Vomiting also results in a poor food intake and it is more difficult to sustain a high fibre nourishing diet when feeling nauseous. The medication that is used prophylactically to minimise the experience of nausea is constipating, as are all analgesics that are taken to control pain.

Constipation is a significant problem, requiring proper assessment to establish the cause. If it is related to the chemotherapy regime using vinca alkaloids, it is known that the problem disappears 10 days after treatment has stopped.[6] However, if the constipation is secondary to other treatment (iatrogenic), the person needs laxative therapy in combination with the analgesics and antiemetic. The bulk forming laxatives are not advised because they require the person to drink plenty of water, which is difficult when feeling nauseous, and the preferred treatment options are to increase fluid intake (espresso coffee is a natural purgative) and exercise; if that fails, laxatives which both stimulate the bowel and soften faeces are required.[6,16]

Diarrhoea

Chemotherapy agents are most effective on cells that rapidly divide, which includes those lining the gut, resulting in diarrhoea. Some of the drugs most likely to cause diarrhoea are:

- Capecitabine
- Cisplatin
- Cyclophosphamide
- Daunorubicin
- 5-Fluorouracil
- Irinotecan

The diarrhoea may start very soon after the first treatment, i.e. within hours, and can prove acutely embarrassing for the person. Its severity can result in dehydration so it is very important to treat it effectively with drugs such as loperamide or codeine. If the diarrhoea does not subside, it may be necessary to reduce the drug dosage or stop treatment until the person recovers. Their compromised immune status may mean that they are more susceptible to developing infections due to *Clostridium difficile* and neutropenia.

Fatigue

It is believed that 60–95% of people having cancer treatment experience fatigue severe enough to interfere with their expressed quality of life.[17] This symptom does not only occur in people receiving chemotherapy but can occur after surgery and radiotherapy as well, and can persist even after treatment has been completed.[18] Unfortunately, people with this symptom often do not report it as they consider it to be an inevitable consequence of the disease. It is a 'subjective feeling of tiredness, weakness or lack of energy' that is not relieved by resting.[17] Approximately 50% of newly diagnosed cancer patients report suffering from insomnia, which results in feeling fatigued but insomnia does not explain why many people receiving chemotherapy report feeling fatigued.[17] Cancer-related fatigue (CRF) is complex, unlike normal (non-cancer-related) experiences of fatigue, which is relieved by rest, and can be the result of numerous factors such as:

- Psychological distress, anxiety and worry
- Anaemia
- Increased levels of cytokines (enzymes produced by the tumour)
- Insomnia.

The person with CRF may express it as a mental fatigue, where they find it difficult to think and concentrate or physical fatigue, where they feel weak, tired and listless. Assessment can take various forms and there are numerous different scales that could be used which may determine the severity of the fatigue.[18] Assessment is crucial, in that certain factors like anaemia, once identified can be treated and thus eliminated.

Resting is not always the most helpful solution to fatigue; simple exercise like a short walk can enhance feelings of wellbeing and thus reduce the sensation of feeling fatigued, although the research evidence on the effect of exercise in fatigue reports mixed findings and sample sizes are too small to make a conclusive case.[18]

Cognitive behavioural therapy (CBT), where the person is encouraged to reframe their thinking about their cancer experience, has had some reported success. CBT occurs over a period of months and is individually tailored to meet a person's specific needs.[19]

Peripheral neuropathy

Chemotherapy-induced peripheral neuropathy affects 30–40% of people, occurring with high doses of chemotherapy agents such as the platinum drugs, the taxanes and vinca alkaloids or combination therapies including those agents which can damage the nerves and are felt in the feet and hands as tingling (paraesthesia) or altered sensations (dysaesthesia), numbness and shooting pain in the fingers and toes.[20] The condition can be painful and this neuropathic pain can be difficult to manage. Experiences of tingling in the fingers and toes should be reported at once to the healthcare team, as reducing the dose or stopping treatment for a short while can reverse the problem, however, it is not always reversible and it can be a major factor in people opting out of further treatment. Taking supplements such as vitamin E and B may help, but should only be taken following consultation with the medical team. People who have been heavy alcohol drinkers may be more susceptible to the condition.[20] The neuropathic pain can be treated with analgesics, which are combined with antidepressants or anticonvulsant drugs such as gabapentin, which are more efficient in controlling nerve pain than analgesics alone.

'Chemobrain' and 'chemofog'

Some people observe that during the treatment period, they experience memory problems, where they may forget words when they are talking, or forget appointments. They usually find reliable solutions like making lists, keeping a diary, etc. Others report difficulty in concentrating on reading and absorbing information. There may be a variety of reasons for 'chemobrain' and 'chemofog'; people may be anxious, have sleep problems or feel fatigued, all of which can affect concentration levels. In general, people report this as a passing problem. More significant side-effects may detract from the focus on concentration, or they may feel that they adapt to a world of treatment and recovery. Researchers into this topic found that it is a problem that is rarely shared with healthcare professionals but is openly discussed with others in a similar position in clinics in chemotherapy department waiting rooms.

KEY POINTS

- Treatment of cancers with chemotherapy has become more sophisticated over the years and has proved effective in eradicating or controlling cancer
- Most people receive their treatment as outpatients, which enables them to have some degree of normal life in between treatment cycles. It permits greater contact with their main source of support – family and friends; however, dealing with the side-effects of chemotherapy alone at home can be frightening and distressing
- This chapter has focused on chemotherapy as a treatment for certain cancer conditions and focuses on some of the more problematic side-effects. It is not possible to cover all side-effects in detail

- The key to successful management of chemotherapy is to prepare the person in advance of treatment starting, so they know what to expect, and forestall some of the worse side-effects through the use of prophylactic medication

- When side-effects occur, assessment is required to identify the cause and treat those which can be treated. If this is not possible, then it does mean that doses need to be adjusted or the person should have a break from chemotherapy to recover

Chapter | **27** |

Immunotherapy

Laureen Hemming

INTRODUCTION

Immunotherapy has developed from molecular biology.[1] Research into the manipulation of genes in the cells of the body was primarily undertaken to determine the possibility of treating hereditary conditions, infertility and to control tissue rejection during transplants of livers and kidneys. This was because, although the transplant surgery was successful, transplants subsequently failed because the host's body rejected the new tissue. The body has a very efficient immune surveillance system to protect it; we are bombarded with cancer causing agents thousands of times each day[2] but we do not all get cancer. The main thinking behind immunotherapy is that if we could enhance the workings of this system, maybe it could deal with cancer cells which have overcome the immune system and eradicate them.

However, immunotherapy is not a new concept. The idea of using the body's own immune system is said to date back to the late 1800s, when an American surgeon, William Coley, noted that a patient with erysipelas (a streptococcal bacterial infection) went into remission from cancer following the infection. William Coley went on to inject small amounts of streptococcal bacteria into bone tumours, the idea being that the infection would stimulate the body's immune system into action and it would target the cancer cells, causing them to die, which is called

apoptosis.[3] It had also been noted that people with active tuberculosis rarely developed cancer, which led to the use of the bacille Calmette–Guerin (BCG) vaccine being used to treat bladder cancers.

People who have had several severe infections, such as pneumonia, *Staphylococcus aureus* infections or who have had the BCG vaccine against tuberculosis or the yellow fever vaccine seem not to get malignant melanomas (skin cancers) because they have built up a protective immune system that recognises aberrant cells that will become carcinogenic, and kills them before they can replicate.[5] Unfortunately, as yet, treatment of people with melanomas with BCG vaccine does not always yield significant results. It has been proposed[5] that our current trend of living in very hygienic environments means that children are not exposed to substances that help us develop a useful immune system that protects us from disease and cancer. This may also help explain why more children are developing asthma and other allergic conditions, reaffirming the old wives' tale that everyone needs to eat a speck of dirt to survive.

Immunotherapy, which is treatment using biologically derived products either from cloning cells of mice or using human cells, or a mixture of the two, is one of a variety of biological therapies now used in the treatment of cancer. The other biological therapies sometimes referred to as biotechnology therapies are:

- Monoclonal antibodies that are produced artificially, which lock onto specific protein receptors excreted by the cancer cells and work in several ways:
  - They make the cancer cells responsive to attack from the body's own immune cells which then destroy them, or
  - They make the cancer cells resistant to enzymes that would enable the cells to grow.

An example is rituximab used to treat non-Hodgkin lymphomas; another is trastuzumab (Herceptin) used in certain types of breast cancer. Monoclonal antibodies do not cause infection so are unlike vaccines.[6]

- Vaccines, such as the human papilloma virus (HPV) vaccine, are given to prevent the development of cervical cancer. Vaccines are not all viral; some are currently being developed from tumour cells for reinjecting into the body. The cells are harvested and a vaccine is made from them, which is then injected into the body. This stimulates the immune system into producing antibodies which destroy the foreign material, i.e. the cancer.
- Anti-angiogenesis agents prevent the cancer cells under the influence of certain cytokines (soluble proteins) forming and developing blood capillaries, which will carry nutrients into the cancer and enable it to grow.

Sometimes these therapies are used on their own, but more often are combined with chemotherapy and radiotherapy, and are often used to combat the side-effects of chemotherapy, which allows for higher doses of chemotherapy to be used.[7] They aim to work more specifically than chemotherapy and are targeted to specific molecules in the cells and are principally used to treat solid cancer tumours such as cancers of the breast, colon, lung, prostate and kidney.[3]

Immunotherapy works by targeting the cells during the cell cycle of regeneration (see Chapter 26, Chemotherapy) and locking onto specific receptor sites on cell membranes. The receptor sites are protein molecules that react with specific agents (e.g. immunoglobulins) to set up a chain of further chemical reactions within the cell, which enable the cell to grow and multiply, or check for deviations and mutations, which if present, result in cell death (apoptosis).

PHYSIOLOGY OF THE IMMUNE RESPONSE

The body's immune system can differentiate between what is the body's true self and what is foreign, i.e. non-self. It detects bacteria that have been ingested, cells that have mutated and foreign proteins, as in transplanted organs, and sets up a chain of reactions to rid the body of what it considers harmful and dangerous to the body's continued survival. The immune system comprises of lymph glands, nodes and lymphatic tissue, white blood cells, lymphocytes, antibodies, cytokines (protein molecules).

There are three types of lymphocytes:

- T cells, which attack foreign proteins, tumour cells and cells containing viruses providing what is termed as cell mediated immunity. T cells change into four subtypes of cells:
  - Helper cells
  - Suppressor cells
  - Cytotoxic cells
  - Memory cells

- T cells are activated by an antigen which locks onto a specific receptor on its surface. It then results in a chain of responses; helper cells produce interleukins which mark the damaged cell for destruction which is then undertaken by the cytotoxic cells. Suppressor cells deactivate B cells when no more T cells are needed.
- B cells produce antibodies and proteins called immunoglobulins that target bacterial infections and provide humoral immunity; that is the building blocks to fight infection are within the plasma and interstitial fluids in the body. When B cells come into contact with an antigen, they produce antibodies, which destroy the antigens and stimulate the production of T cells. B cells retain a memory of the antigen it has encountered so that when it meets it again, the response is very quick.
- Natural killer cells provide immunosurveillance by checking the body tissue for foreign proteins, which they then surround and engulf, thus destroying it.

Some lymphocytes can live for a long time in the body, which is why exposure to certain bacterial substances can result in a lifetime of immunity, and the disease only occurs once. It is this immunity which leads to the old wives' tale mentioned above. Some diseases can recur, but the action of the antibodies means subsequent infections are not as severe as the first exposure, which is why it is better to get chicken pox as a child rather than in adulthood, where the condition is more serious. Lymphocytes are produced in the bone marrow and the thymus gland, some, like the B cells, stay in lymph tissue until required. The immune system becomes less effective as we age, which is one of the reasons why many cancers develop in the older population.[8]

Within the cells of the body (lymphocytes, in particular) and cancer cells, soluble proteins called cytokines are produced as a result of reaction within the cell and the cell membrane; they are cell messengers that sit on the cell surface and attract other protein molecules and lymphocytes, which then enter the cell and set up a chain reaction, which can lead to cells mutating or apoptosis. There are over 80 different cytokines,[9] which work in different ways; some stimulate the immune response while others dampen it down; others trigger the production of proteins that respond to a chemical stimulus depending on their concentrations – the more concentrated they are, the stronger the signal the emit. They are part of the body's normal response to inflammation controlling the function of the cells and tissues. During the cell cycle of regeneration, there are five stages and the cell only proceeds through each stage to regenerate if the splitting of the DNA strands and subsequent regrouping occurs without problems being detected by these enzymes and protein molecules, some referred to as kinases. When problems are detected, they initiate cell death (apoptosis). One such protein is called p53; this protein is missing in many cancers (40%), but not all. The main groups of cytokines are:

- Interleukins, 20 different types have been identified, Il-1 and Il-2 are the main ones, which stimulate lymphocytes stored in lymph tissue to migrate into the blood stream
- Interferons, which consist of three types, α, β and γ; they are produced in response to a viral infection
- Tumour necrosis factors
- Colony-stimulating factors
- Growth factors
- Angiogenic factors

When an infection occurs or in response to other changes such as mutations of cells that are regenerating, as in cancer, the body's proinflammatory process is triggered, stimulating cytokines to release interleukins and tumour necrosis factor, which act as cell messengers to stimulate the production of anti-inflammatory cytokines. In other words, there is a build up of a chemical soup warning surrounding tissues of danger before other chemicals or enzymes and protein molecules build up to deal with the problem; this is called a biofeedback loop.

Cancer cells can also produce cytokines that work on adjacent cells making the local cellular environment receptive to tumour growth. As the cancer grows, certain cytokines (tyrosine kinases) enable the development of blood vessels, which draw nutrients and oxygen into the centre of the tumour, thus allowing further growth. Many tumours contain a cytokine called granulocyte colony stimulating factor.

While a great deal is known about cytokines, no one has identified a single cytokine that is present in all cancers. It is thought that cytokines have a role to play in the following complications of cancer:

- Cachexia, which is a syndrome that can develop in some cancers where the person loses weight quickly, despite eating normally. As the cancer grows, the cytokines work in various ways; they suppress the release of glucose stored as glycogen in the liver, so that the body uses muscle protein as its source of energy, resulting in muscle loss and weakness. They also depress the sensors in the hypothalamus which signal when we are hungry, and thus depress appetite so the person no longer wants to eat, which is called anorexia
- Asthenia (muscle weakness) and chronic fatigue, tumour necrosis factor is known to produce muscle soreness
- Pain intensity particularly bone pain is attributed to cytokine action[9]

The main principle of immunotherapy is to harness and use cytokines to influence an inflammatory response that will weaken and destroy the cancer cells.

TREATMENT USING CYTOKINES

Interferon-alpha (α)

Interferon-α is used to treat:[10]

- Hairy cell leukaemia
- Multiple myeloma
- Cutaneous T cell lymphoma
- Malignant melanoma
- Carcinoid tumours
- Chronic myeloid leukaemia
- Non-Hodgkin lymphoma
- Renal cell carcinoma
- Kaposi sarcoma

Interferon-α stops tumour growth by making affected cells more responsive to an attack by the immune system, stops the cytokine's influence in the formation of a blood supply and makes tumour cells less aggressive. Interferons also slow down the cell cycle of replication acting specifically on the G_0 phase and are said to be tumoristatic because the cells do not go on to divide; this is opposed to being tumoricidal, which is killing the cell. It is usually given as a subcutaneous injection, but can be given intramuscularly or intravenously.[11]

The side-effects of interferon are similar to those experienced when fighting infection. The symptoms are described as 'flu like', with raised temperature, shivering, aches, fatigue and lethargy. Usually symptoms are mild and disappear once treatment has stopped. An antipyretic such as paracetamol can be given prophylactically to pre-empt the symptoms occurring.

Interleukin 2

Interleukin 2 is used to treat:

- Renal cell cancers
- Myeloid leukaemia
- Kaposi sarcoma
- Metastatic malignant melanoma
- Non-Hodgkin lymphomas

Interleukin 2 is very toxic and because of this, its use is limited. Like interferon-α, it produces 'flu like' symptoms but can also produce angina (heart pain), severe hypotension (low blood pressure), respiratory distress and multiorgan failure.[10]

Tumour necrosis factor

Tumour necrosis factor (TNF) is used to treat:

- Melanoma
- Sarcoma

Like interleukin 2, TNF is very toxic, producing severe side-effects, which means the preparation is used under drug trial condition, as it is as yet, an experimental treatment.[10]

Haemopoietic growth factors

Haemopoietic growth factors, of which there are three different types:

- Erythropoietin
- Granulocyte colony stimulating factor (G-CSF)
- Granulocyte macrophage colony stimulating factor (GM-CSF)

These are used when the bone marrow activity is suppressed by chemotherapy, as they influence the production of blood cells and counteract anaemia. They reduce the risk of the person developing neutropenia, which could result in the chemotherapy treatment being stopped for a short while. Their use means that higher doses of chemotherapy can be given and are thus an adjuvant treatment to chemotherapy.

OTHER TREATMENTS

Monoclonal antibodies

Monoclonal antibodies such as Rituximab are formed from a mixture of murine (mouse) and human immunoglobulins and are used to treat non-Hodgkin lymphoma; a neoplasm of the B and T cells in conjunction with chemotherapy. Rituximab, when used with the combination therapy of cyclophosphamide vincristine and prednisolone (CVP), is at least twice as effective as just using CVP alone. These antibodies target specific antigens (CD20) that sit on the surface of large B cell lymphomas. When the two combine, they attract natural killer cells (lymphocytes in the immune system), which then release perforin (a small protein), which enters the targeted cell and causes apoptosis.[6]

Rituximab is usually given with other chemotherapy agents intravenously but can be given singly (monotherapy). To pre-empt side-effects, the person receiving the treatment is given a premedication which consists of an antipyretic (e.g. paracetamol to keep the temperature down) and an antihistamine, usually chlorphenamine. The rate that the infusion is given is important. It should not be given too quickly as it can cause a reaction referred to as a cytokine release syndrome, which has been described as being similar to the onset of 'flu' and a mild rash. Cytokine release syndrome is more prominent following the first dose, as this is when most cells are targeted and destroyed reducing the tumour burden. Subsequent treatments affect fewer cells resulting in less cytokines being released.

The symptoms are graded 1–4, with 1 and 2 being a mild reaction, occurring about 2 hours after treatment; and 3 and 4 being more severe. Grade 2 differs from grade 1 in that the rash is itchy and the person may experience breathlessness. The treatment can be recommenced and given over a longer period. The more severe reactions are the same as an allergic reaction resulting in a low blood pressure, breathlessness, bronchospasm, which leads to a lack of sufficient oxygen intake and respiratory distress. This reaction usually occurs within minutes of the transfusion starting and affects about 10% of patients and constitutes a medical emergency.

When a severe reaction occurs, the infusion needs to be stopped immediately and the person needs treating with bronchodilators and oxygen therapy. Blood samples are taken for a full investigation of urea, electrolyte and haemoglobin levels. The reaction can cause thrombocytopenia (a decrease in the platelets which affects the blood clotting system) and hypocalcaemia (low calcium levels which result in a rash which looks like small red pin pricks).

Half of the people who experience such an allergic reaction can have the treatment recommenced without any further reactions occurring.

While the treatment infusion is in progress, the nurse needs to monitor the person's vital signs (temperature, pulse and blood pressure) every 15 minutes initially, for at least the first hour the infusion is in progress. If the person does not show any signs of a reaction, the recordings can then be made every half hour.

Radioimmunotherapy

Radioimmunotherapy is the attachment of a radioactive atom to the monoclonal antibody (rituximab); the agent is called ibritumomab tiuxetan (Zevelin). The addition of the radioactive atom means that the monoclonal antibody enters into the B cell lymphocyte once it has attached to the CD20 protein sitting on the cell surface, and its action can spread to adjacent cells, thus being more effective. This is a treatment for relapsed cases of non-Hodgkin lymphoma. It is given intravenously in outpatients as two treatments, 1 week apart. The radioactive ingredient is so small that the person is not a threat to their family and friends, however, the patient needs to wear a condom for sexual activity and women should avoid becoming pregnant during the treatment period.[12]

Tyrosine kinase inhibitors

Tyrosine kinase enzymes are needed for the formation of small capillaries (angiogenesis) within the tumour, which allows the tumour to receive nutrients and keep growing. Tyrosine kinase inhibitors, such as sorafenib, an oral drug, stop this process and are used to treat primary liver cancer.[13] Other antiangiogenesis drugs are sunitinib and bevacizumab, which are used in the treatment of renal cell cancers that are resistant to chemotherapy and radiotherapy.

Compared with interferon-α treatment, sunitinab seems to have a better result in renal cell cancers, resulting in an extra 2-year survival time, thus leading to its recommendation by NICE. Sunitinib 50 mg is taken as oral medication once a day for 4 weeks, followed by a 2-week gap and can be given with another drug, pazopanib 800 mg or on its own.[15]

The side-effects of these drugs are fatigue, nausea with or without vomiting, diarrhoea and hypertension (raised blood pressure). Once treatment stops, the side-effects disappear and while treatment continues an antiemetic can be taken to manage the nausea, and anti-diarrhoeal drugs can be given to manage the diarrhoea.

Bevacizumab is a monoclonal antibody which stops the vascular endothelial growth factor (VEGF) from working and initiating a capillary network in the tumour. VEGF is mainly active when fetuses are growing and, in adults, it is usually only present when needed for wound healing so its effect on other parts of the body is minimal, unlike chemotherapy agents, which affect normal and abnormal cells alike. It is used in combination with paclitaxel or docetaxel (taxanes used to treat breast cancer). It is also used to treat colorectal[16] and renal cell cancers.[17]

The side-effect profile is complicated, as it is given with chemotherapy (see Chapter 26, Chemotherapy, for details). In addition, bevacizumab causes hypertension, proteinuria (bleeding in the bladder and passed in the urine), epistaxis (nose bleeds) and thromboemboli (blood clots). It can also affect the heart, leading to heart failure.

CONDITIONS THAT CAN DEVELOP AFTER TREATMENT

Tumour lysis syndrome occurs when a large number of cells are destroyed at one time. These cells flood into the blood stream resulting in an alteration of the electrolytes (calcium, potassium and phosphates) and the formation of uric acid crystals in the fine tubules of the kidneys, which causes acute renal failure. It is especially significant in patients with a high tumour burden. If a high tumour burden is suspected, an intravenous infusion is set-up before treatment starts and allopurinol or rasburicase (drugs used to treat gout) is given.

Cardiac arrhythmias (heart flutters or fibrillation) can also occur in people who have had rituximab treatment, so people with a history of heart disease need careful monitoring.

VACCINATIONS

The UK has recently introduced a vaccination programme for all girls aged over 13 years against the strains of human papilloma virus (HPV) type 16 and 18, which is implicated in 70% of cervical cancers.[18] Unfortunately, it does not protect against all cervical cancers.[19] Cervical cancer represents the second most common cancer affecting women worldwide and has received wide media coverage since the celebrity Jade Goody died of the disease. While this programme does not directly target cancer cells, it has a role in the prevention of future cancers and therefore could be classified as immunotherapy, as it promotes immune protection.

Other vaccinations being used are *Mycobacterium vaccae* to treat adencarcinomas of the lung and, although still experimental, results suggest that some people can live for an extra 4 months.[4]

KEY POINTS

- Although immunotherapy is heralded as a new approach to treating cancer and many of the treatments are still part of planned clinical trials, it has a history spreading back to the 1800s when observations by clinicians prompted experimentation

- Some treatments have in the past only yielded modest cure rates; however, when combined with chemotherapy or radiotherapy, the results are more successful and offer hope to people with cancer

- The immune system is extremely complicated and scientific discoveries are still needed to put all the jigsaw puzzle pieces into place

- Like chemotherapy, immunotherapy is not for the faint-hearted, as it still has its share of adverse reactions, which have been detailed above

- The person receiving immunotherapy requires accurate information before consenting to the treatment and close monitoring during treatment by appropriately qualified staff

Section | 8 |

Performance and ethico-legal aspects of care

Section

8

Performance and ethico-legal aspects of care

Chapter | 28 |

Performance measures – measuring care

Martin Vosper

INTRODUCTION

It is probably true (but also probably unfair) to say that the typical medical imaging or radiotherapy department would not rank 'number one' in the minds of most healthcare workers within a 'top 10' chart of the most 'caring' localities in a hospital. To some health professionals in other fields, imaging and radiotherapy offer vital but technical support services, through which their patients pass, benefited but emotionally unmoved. There may be a perception in the eyes of doctors and nurses that these departments are driven by numerical measures of performance, such as the optimum X-ray image or radiotherapy target volume, rather than by the patient's question: 'Just how will all this affect me?' I can recall a staff comment (many years ago I am glad to say) that there were 'several spines and a couple of skulls' sitting in the X-ray waiting area. More recently, an imaging services manager told me that other staff in the hospital regarded medical imaging as 'semi-compassionate', and that he was fighting hard to challenge this description in his locality.

This chapter is about care measurement, and we may ask: 'How can care be measured?' Traditional measures of performance in medical imaging and radiotherapy have largely been based on quality assurance testing, perhaps within a cycle of audit. These have gathered quantifiable data, such as patient waiting times, radiation doses, image quality or tumour responses. More recently, many departments have introduced patient satisfaction surveys and patient feedback mechanisms to their everyday practice. These have revealed that patients are interested in many facets of their hospital visit – the friendliness and communicativeness of staff, good information, cleanliness and facilities, in addition to waiting times and clinical results. In essence, the patient's concept of 'care' can sometimes differ from the health professional's. Being responsive to patients' wishes is in-keeping with 'patient focus' or 'putting patients first', recognising that patients are not passive recipients of healthcare but knowledgeable clients or consumers with a capacity for choice and an independent voice. Choice is increasingly present (practicality permitting) as independent healthcare providers enter markets previously occupied solely by state healthcare provision, or as choices are offered between state hospitals. The commercial and business sector in countries worldwide has long recognised the importance of good customer care and feedback in maintaining market share and profitability. However, in 2012, the business case for providing the best quality of care is complicated by a worldwide economic recession, in which cash resources are scarce. Many imaging or radiotherapy managers face financial cuts (including staffing) coupled with demands for patient waiting time targets, diagnostic or treatment targets and 'profitability' to be met. This reality could result in a production line mentality in which numerical throughput is paramount and health services staff not only have limited time available for being 'caring' – communicating, reassuring, advising, assisting, but also have limited time in which to monitor quality data relating to healthcare performance.

The recognition that 'care quality' is as important as 'care quantity' in healthcare provision has resulted in an increasing number of mechanisms for quality reporting, appraisal and accreditation. Results are viewable online by patients, referrers and funding bodies. This chapter will consider the nature of 'care performance' data in medical imaging and radiotherapy, together with its assessment.

USE OF HEALTHCARE PERFORMANCE INDICATORS

Quantitative indicators have long been used as measures of performance in healthcare. The development of healthcare statistics occurred largely in response to a newfound interest in population health and survival in the 1800s, recognising that improved health could lessen 'avoidable deaths' and improve national productivity. Florence Nightingale, working in the Crimean War during the 1850s, was one of the earliest healthcare statisticians, in that she documented how her alteration of healthcare practices affected the survival of soldiers. The World Health Organization (WHO) has played a leading role in advocating the use of comparative indicators since the 1970s, in the face of regional and local variations in mortality and morbidity. For example, variations in longevity related to hunger and poverty, or in survival rates for common forms of cancer are well known and publicised. There is a pressing need for radiology to provide a timely diagnosis and staging of cancer and for radiotherapy to provide cancer treatment. Although full and accurate data are vital for examining variations in healthcare performance and providing central allocation of resources to areas of need, some authorities have questioned whether excessive data collection might detract from frontline patient care when healthcare staffing is short.

Quality indicators in healthcare tend to be quantitative (numerical) and are intended to satisfy demands from healthcare authorities, patients and staff, who want to know about the 'results' of diagnosis and treatment. Questions such as: 'What works best for my condition?'; 'How is my hospital performing?' and 'Is it cost-effective?', are common. It is important to note however that quality is often relative rather than absolute and that indicators may or may not be direct measures of performance.

The following terms are commonly used in connection with healthcare quality indicators:

Safety – the extent to which healthcare procedures are free from accidents, side-effects, complications or harms

Effectiveness – the accuracy or success of a diagnostic or therapeutic technique

Efficiency – the amount of effort, cost, waste or skill involved in achieving a desired healthcare result

Equity – the extent to which patients' experience of healthcare is 'fair', with equality of access, opportunity and quality

Acceptability – whether healthcare meets the wishes of patients, or is free from distress or discomfort

Responsiveness – the extent to which diagnosis or treatment is provided appropriately or 'in good time' (given the patient's needs or wishes)

Accessibility – whether healthcare services and information are available to patients who need them

Adequacy – whether healthcare services are sufficient in quantity and quality

Examples of readily quantifiable measures in healthcare might include:

- Patient waiting times for diagnosis or treatment
- Success rates (and complication rates) for procedures
- Incidence rates and survival rates for common medical conditions such as stroke, coronary artery disease or cancer
- Numbers and costs of diagnostic or therapeutic procedures
- Disease detection rates within national screening programmes (such as X-ray mammography)
- Results of local satisfaction surveys (aimed at patients and referring clinicians)

Health status questionnaires such as the Short Form 36 Item Health Survey (SF-36) are standardised tools and are used a lot in research for recording the patient's own perception of their health and wellbeing. They are particularly useful, e.g. in recording the extent to which a patient's perceived health status is affected by treatments or medical imaging tests. Medical imaging test results are not a goal in themselves but only the first stage in the healthcare process – they may bring about alterations in treatment or clinical management that can benefit patients. However, it is true that some patients may feel 'uplifted' simply by the fact that they have received an X-ray or an MRI scan.

It is possible to measure healthcare outcomes in terms of the patient's altered heath status, using concepts such as 'Quality Adjusted Life Years' (QALYs) and 'Disability Adjusted Life Years' (DALYs). These measures help to record the effect of health interventions, such as diagnosis or therapy, on the number of extra 'healthy life years' enjoyed by patients as a result of the intervention. Expressed in such terms, a single year of productive life with full mobility and freedom from pain might be equivalent to several years of disabled or painful existence. Although they may be helpful measures when the costs and benefits of treatments are considered, particularly in a climate of healthcare rationing, many clinicians feel uncomfortable about calculating whether patients should receive treatment or not on the basis of QALYs or DALYs.

QUALITY INDICATORS IN MEDICAL IMAGING AND RADIOTHERAPY

In medical imaging, as in some aspects of radiotherapy, performance monitoring has historically been based on audits of numerical data. Examples of audit may include:

- Radiographic image quality – resolution (line pairs per millimetre), contrast and signal to noise ratio, measured using test objects
- Image reporting accuracy – diagnostic sensitivity (% of cases with disease correctly identified) and specificity (% of cases without disease correctly excluded)
- Image reporting 'turn-around' times before receipt by the referrer
- Image reject analysis – percentage of non-diagnostic images and reasons for inadequacy
- Radiation exposures – as measured by dose area product meters in comparison with national diagnostic reference levels and also as measured by exposure indices on digital images in comparison with manufacturers' recommendations
- Contrast media and drug usage
- Adverse reactions and procedural complications
- Waiting times.

A proper implementation of a clinical audit requires that all stages of the audit cycle are actioned. These are:

1. Identification of problems
2. Suggesting solutions
3. Implementing solutions
4. Re-audit

This cycle can also be termed a 'quality improvement process'. Some healthcare 'audits' seem to stop at stage 1, simply recording situations or levels of performance without making any actions based upon them. Ongoing 'quality assurance' can be applied after the re-audit stage of the cycle, since the aim is then to maintain the now improved situation after solutions have been applied.

In radiotherapy, any assessment of 'performance' will necessarily be broad-based and mindful of the needs of patients with cancer. Indicators need to recognise a wide range of care quality domains:

Structure – resources, environment, facilities, staffing, cleanliness
Process – referral speed, assessment, treatment waiting time, treatment planning, treatment methods, radiation doses, treatment doses, fractionation regimes
Outcomes – success rate, survival, recurrence, patient satisfaction
Physical – radiation side-effects, skin reactions, pain, nausea, altered body function, weight loss
Psychological – depression, anxiety, altered self-image, support mechanisms

Care delivery – consultation, information, communication, continuity, discussion, planning, documentation
Spiritual and cultural – spiritual care, closure, sensitivity to cultural needs, interpretation and language.

The range of quality domains reflects the holistic nature of cancer care, the therapeutic process, as well as the long-term contact with and follow-up of patients.

Developments such as conformal radiotherapy and intensity modulated radiotherapy have brought about a greater integration with medical imaging methods and increased the complexity of treatments. The large number of treatment options further increases the need for quality monitoring and control.

Technical performance monitoring in radiotherapy may include:

- Portal verification of accuracy of patient set-up
- Treatment fields per planned treatment volume
- Treatment planning with CT and contouring of volumes of interest
- Radiation testing and dosimetry
- Equipment maintenance and downtime.

Both in medical imaging and radiotherapy, patients may be asked to complete satisfaction surveys or provide feedback comments. Feedback can be provided by means of electronic 'touch screens' or using traditional paper forms. Surveys can usefully explore patient attitudes to the appearance and friendliness of staff, staff–patient communication, clarity and availability of information, cleanliness, waiting room facilities, changing room facilities, waiting times, the procedures themselves and any positive or negative aspects of the experience. There is a shortage of qualitative research regarding patients' lived experiences and perceptions of medical imaging and radiotherapy.

QUALITY REGULATORY AGENCIES

Many countries have national regulatory agencies which oversee care and safety standards in health provision. For example, in England, the Care Quality Commission (CQC) has an overarching role for ensuring that healthcare satisfies the performance categories listed above. Lord Darzi, in his 2008 *NHS Next Stage Review*, noted that 'if quality is at the heart of everything we do, it must be understood from the perspective of patients'. In keeping with this philosophy, Lord Darzi called for more patient empowerment and choice, together with clinical accountability based on improved patient information and safety. Patient experience would be enhanced via attention to dignity and respect as well as to treatment effectiveness and improved diagnostics. The *Review* listed seven steps: bringing clarity to quality; measuring quality; publishing quality performance; recognising and rewarding quality; raising standards; safeguarding quality and staying ahead. An expressed goal was that all health providers should develop their own quality frameworks, combining national indicators with those relevant to their local circumstances.

The Care Quality Commission (CQC) was established in 2009 to be the independent regulator of healthcare quality in England, with powers to provide information and ensure compliance with registration requirements. It operates a system of assessment and inspection, which regularly reviews all available information and intelligence held about providers. There are 28 CQC outcomes, each reflecting a specific regulation, 16 of which are core and relate most directly to the quality and safety of care. The CQC undertakes specific inspections of compliance with the Ionising Radiation (Medical Exposure) Regulations 2000 within imaging and radiotherapy departments. It also has broader enforcement responsibilities within the Health and Social Care Act 2008 (Regulated Activities) Regulations 2010 and the Care Quality Commission (Registration) Regulations 2009. These general activities relate to: respect, dignity and patient experience; consent; safety; cooperation with other health providers; safeguarding; infection control; management of medicines; suitability of premises; suitability of equipment; staffing; quality monitoring; complaints and training and management.

Expert advisory bodies such as the UK National Institute for Health and Clinical Excellence (NICE) are not regulatory agencies as such, but publish guidelines which are aimed at helping healthcare staff to provide care that is both high quality and good value for money. Such bodies aim to disseminate the findings of evidence-based practice to a wider audience, ensuring that healthcare performance indicators such as safety, effectiveness, efficiency and equity are met.

ACCREDITATION STANDARDS

In recent years, a number of countries worldwide have introduced quality accreditation standards for medical imaging and radiotherapy. Such schemes recognise that accredited departments have been successful when measured against benchmarked standards and are thus entitled to advertise this attainment to patients and referrers. Although the standards are variable, they may contain requirements for safety, patient care, facilities, staff training, protocols, procedures and performance. Standards usually consist of a model of 'best practice', against which individual performance can be compared. Standards do not guarantee quality but they are a means of ensuring that proper procedures and protocols are in place and being correctly adhered to. They should be of direct benefit to patients, as they often have a 'customer care' focus and aim to improve service quality while maintaining the privacy, dignity and safety of patients. In general, accreditation has been voluntary rather than compulsory, although it is often

envisaged that possession of accreditation will not only certify quality of care but also offer 'reward' in the form of competitive advantages. It is also important to remember that death or injury due to medical errors is a recognised problem worldwide and that accreditation standards are designed to minimise such errors. The establishment of set standards should help to reduce variations in care quality, which have been referred to as a 'postcode lottery' in the UK for example. Market forces and also the costs of litigation claims have particularly driven accreditation schemes in the USA and these trends are now appearing in other health economies.

An internationally recognised system of accreditation standards is provided by the International Standards Organisation (ISO). Within Europe, adoption of mechanisms for radiology services accreditation has been heterogeneous, with some degree of national Government control. There has been consideration of common European technical requirements for imaging, e.g. in mammography, together with some limited use of ISO 9001:2001 as a universal quality standard. Certification of total quality management via ISO 9001 has been preferred at some sites due to its focus on reproducible technical standards and international recognition. The ISO standards are based on the principles of getting things 'right first time' and 'fit for purpose'. Target levels are designed to be realistic and achievable and may be discussed with them. There is an emphasis on the systematic undertaking and recording of procedures. The ISO standards require that management take responsibility for quality and implement quality systems. There is strong emphasis on testing, inspection, document control, purchasing, handling, servicing and audit. However, some authorities have commented that the ISO standards are mainly aimed at commercial manufacturing and have too small a human quality element for the healthcare sector. The ISO standards would normally be applied to all areas of the hospital, and not just medical imaging or radiotherapy in isolation.

In the USA, the Joint Commission on Accreditation of Healthcare Organizations (JCAHO) was developed as an over-arching regulatory body, initially to provide self-regulation but latterly in response to financial motives, since hospitals needed to satisfy standards in order to attract Medicaid revenue. The JCAHO has undertaken a lot of work on clinical outcome indicators and measures of good practice. The American College of Radiologists (ACR) realised in the 1960s that government interest in healthcare economics and quality standards was likely to intensify. The ACR standards, of which there are 80, were introduced in 1990 and encompass all aspects of medical imaging and radiotherapy, including procedures, communication and education. Draft standards are circulated widely for feedback, including to clinicians outside the field of radiology. The purpose of the ACR standards is to set out reasonable principles of practice that, if followed, will produce high quality radiology care.

In the USA, development of imaging accreditation schemes based on the ACR standards has ranged from individual programmes for specialities such as ultrasound and MRI to a single 'umbrella' accreditation programme, with re-accreditation at 3-year intervals. Although historically, imaging accreditation was a voluntary process embarked on in order to receive recognition for quality, in recent years it has become a mandatory requirement for organisations wishing to receive payment from medical insurance agencies. The market demand for accreditation was introduced into an already very competitive 'buyer's market', in which payers sought to minimise their costs while requiring high service quality. As a result, many healthcare providers were forced to operate on very low profit margins, aggravated by the high staff salary costs spent in maintaining accreditation.

In Australia, the Medical Imaging Accreditation Scheme (DIAS) was introduced in 2008. From that year on, radiology services had to be carried out within an accredited practice in order to be eligible for Medicare benefits. Practices registering by 2008 were permitted 12 months of 'deemed accredited' status before being required to demonstrate that they could meet entry level standards. Just less than half of the radiology practices participating in the scheme were independent, while the rest were in state-funded hospitals or general medical units (equivalent to UK GP-run units). Australian radiology services were able to choose their preferred accreditation agency from four alternatives. The accreditors involved in the scheme were: the Australian Council on Healthcare Standards, Health and Disability Auditing Australia, the National Association of Testing Authorities Australia and Quality in Practice. This multi-accreditor model was viewed positively by radiology managers, as a means of improving choice and reducing fees. The initial choice of accreditor was driven by a range of issues. For smaller businesses, 'provision of useful information' and 'recommendations' were the key motivators, while for larger businesses, pro-activity and price were important selection criteria. Many radiology decision-makers believed that DIAS should aim for best practice rather than minimum standards. However, opinions were divided on whether compliance with standards should be assessed by desk-audit or on-site audit. Many managers who supported the use of assessment by peers would be 'put off' if this increased the cost of the audit process.

The Pan American Health Organization (PAHO) has developed a basic radiology accreditation programme that can be adopted by any developing country. The process involves peer review of imaging equipment, staff qualifications, quality control, image quality and radiation dose, and carries a 3-year accreditation period.

The UK Imaging Services Accreditation Scheme (ISAS) was introduced in 2009. There are 31 ISAS standards in total, grouped within four domains: clinical; facilities, resources and workforce; patient experience; and safety. The 31 standards are further subdivided into nearly 200 criteria. It is expected that accredited departments should provide three types of evidence, namely policy documentation, policy implementation and policy monitoring. Successful accreditation is achieved via the online submission of documentary evidence and an on-site assessment visit by peers and lay assessors. As with the ISO standards, clinical departments work towards realistic targets and improvements, which are determined in conjunction with the assessing agency. Ongoing performance enhancement is expected, once baseline levels have been established.

KEY POINTS

- The measurement of performance has often focused on scientific measures in medical imaging and radiotherapy, via auditing. Examples are radiation doses, diagnostic sensitivity and specificity, image quality and radiotherapy treatment verification

- However, modern performance indicators recognise the importance of all aspects of health service provision, which impact on patients. These include communication, comfort, dignity, acceptability and safety, in addition to service effectiveness and efficiency

- Care quality monitoring recognises the rights and perspectives of patients as service users and seeks patient feedback, as well as measures of patient health outcome, within the range of available performance measures

- The quality of service provision (which includes consideration of care quality) is monitored by external regulatory agencies within healthcare systems

- Accreditation of imaging or radiotherapy services against set standards by external bodies is aimed to drive up care quality, to ensure verifiable levels of care for patients and to provide services with recognition for achievement

Chapter | **29** |

Ethical and legal considerations in professional practice

Aarthi Ramlaul, Tracey A. Gregory

INTRODUCTION

It is a common belief that ethics is a philosophical analysis of the way people ought to behave towards each other. Ethics actually encompass not only what should be done but also what must be done, and has an important part to play in a healthcare practitioners' professional and personal life. Medical imaging and radiotherapy practitioners must abide by ethical standards and principles in their everyday practice. These ethical standards are set out and governed by our professional and regulatory bodies.

The healthcare system today is dependent upon the ability of the workforce to deliver care to the patients in a manner which is sensitive to their needs and expectations. Both medical imaging and radiotherapy practitioners are key members of the healthcare team and recent government policies and their supporting legislation are continually identifying areas of priority and the skills necessary to deliver these priorities effectively.[1] It is therefore essential that practitioners understand the issues related to these developments and the changes which have taken place regarding the legal and governance issues. The public at large must have confidence in healthcare professionals and be assured of their competence, accountability and responsibilities. Where healthcare is concerned, areas of competence and ethics are increasingly being scrutinised, as higher expectations are held by both the government and public alike.[1]

Without a doubt, the chief duty of practitioners has always been that of having proper regard to the welfare of their patients. Training and education have therefore been focused on the clinical and technical aspects of the role. However, in recent years the needs have increasingly involved issues relating to law and its relevance to practitioners and their patients. Practitioners must be aware of and be able to act within the limits of their experience and knowledge and to do this; they must have an understanding of the legal framework within which they practise.[1]

The aim is not to make lawyers of health professionals, but to highlight the importance of knowing those laws that are relevant to their practice so that both they and their patient are protected. Ignorance of the law is no defence as professional practice requires that practitioners have a good understanding of the way in which the law both restricts and enables them to perform safely and professionally.[1]

In addition, practitioners must work according to the policies, regulations and procedures as set out by their employer. It is therefore essential to ensure that all new staff go through a period of induction and orientation and that this includes the local policies and procedures.

WHAT IS MEANT BY ETHICS?

Ethics simply means distinguishing between right and wrong; what is good or bad; or what ought or ought not to be done in a given instance. How we base our judgement in deciding what is right or wrong depends on our personal moral sense, values and beliefs. Our moral sense, values and beliefs are influenced by our cultural and family background, religious beliefs, political views and prejudices.

Many years ago, ethics was not taught formally in medical training, as it was thought that medical students would imbibe this ethos through working alongside more senior practitioners, and in so doing would pick up what was right and what was wrong. In contrast to this, teaching of ethics today aims to help foster an ability to make rational, moral decisions rather than simply to do things as they have been done in the past. The study of ethics is the study of moral behaviour.

> **!** For practitioners, there are two distinct ethical pathways – one involves moral conduct and behaviour from the practitioner themselves, i.e. how they communicate, dress etc.; and the other is in using their integrity and judgement in a manner which ensures that the right decision has been made for the patient.

Radiography has evolved over the years into a dynamic imaging profession which uses the latest technologies to diagnose and treat diseases; thus optimising the best management of the patient. The profession requires knowledge and skills in evaluation and decision-making, as competence in carrying out a range of radiographic examinations, forms a vital part of their role. The other requirement lies in providing high quality of care to the patient.

The role and scope of radiography practice has developed over the years. With practitioners taking on an extended role, there is the medico-legal responsibility of being accountable for one's action. In addition, the public is demanding greater accountability from government agencies and professional services including the National Health Service (NHS) and given the current climate of change, debates often feature the key word, 'accountability'.

Because of this transition in practice, practitioners are faced with ethical issues on a daily basis. These issues, although mostly minor in nature, require skilful handling and managing. Practitioners need to be able to make those decisions in a professional, methodical manner, in keeping the Codes of Conduct and Ethics, and the Standards of Proficiency as set out by the Society and College of Radiographers (SCoR) and the Health & Care Professions Council (HCPC) respectively.

Practitioners have a responsibility towards their patients in that their decisions have to be 'right' for the patient. The practitioner's personal moral qualities, i.e. their sense

of responsibility can enhance their performance of duties and decision-making, however, their moral outlook does not always blend harmoniously with their practice or performance of duties. They may act morally because it is required for them to carry out their duty but may not necessarily be moral in themselves.

> **!** Within radiography, patient care can be performed ethically or unethically depending on the professional standards the practitioners have set for themselves.

Ethical decision-making requires the ability of practitioners to recognise the presence of an ethical issue and to know the appropriate ethical action to take in order to justify a moral outcome.

The ability to be able to respond appropriately to moral issues requires one to develop moral sensitivity, moral reasoning, moral motivation and moral character, which need explanation. Moral sensitivity can be described as a 'sense' that requires interpreting an individual's verbal and non-verbal behaviours and needs and responding to them in an appropriate manner. Moral sensitivity is influenced by one's upbringing, culture, religion, education and life experiences; which ultimately affect the way in which we perceive the information we handle.

Moral reasoning is the process of drawing conclusions from evidence as well as the ability to determine what moral action is to be taken in a given situation. It may involve deciding between conflicting ideals, values or goals in order to decide how one will react; or what action one may take in order to resolve a conflict of values. This cognitive process may involve intuition and emotion, whereby one formulates and justifies an ethically defensible course of action to achieve an ideal moral outcome.

Moral motivation is described as a genuine desire to achieve good moral outcomes. This involves a sense of moral responsibility and integrity, as well as a commitment to achieving moral ends. It often involves a perspective of one being fair, honourable, morally competent and self-respecting. Moral character is described as one who has perseverance, strength of conviction and courage to enable them to carry out a moral action they have deemed imperative.

Learning about ethics and the standards required in radiographic professional practice helps the practitioner develop their own set of moral values, which in turn contribute to ethical behaviour and moral responsibility. The regulatory frameworks can sometimes give health professionals a false sense of security regarding responsibility. This might lead to the thinking that the guidelines alone are enough to do the job and forget that it is the practitioner who has the final moral responsibility to the patient.

> **!** The codes of conduct for professional practice are not directly enforced in a court of law but may be used as evidence in cases where reasonable professional standards of practice have not been followed.

Why is an understanding of ethics important to our practice?

Ethics are the rules of human conduct and in our lives as practitioners, it is the rules for professional conduct. Doing what is ethical according to those rules is doing what is right. As practitioners, we need to understand that. Moral principles instil within us a sense of doing the right thing for the good of all. Healthcare professionals need to study ethics in order to know what is right or wrong and how to protect the vulnerable in society. Medical advancements present ethical dilemmas and healthcare professionals need to know how to handle them as they arise. The challenge for us as practitioners is to be able to meet the demands of our code of professional conduct and statutory obligation to the Health & Care Professions Council in order to meet the expectation of the public at large.

> **!** Having a code of professional conduct is a hallmark of a profession because it signifies high principles of professional behaviour and willingness by the profession to control its own conduct, thereby instilling public confidence (SCoR, 2008).

In terms of ethical behaviour and the expectation to be professional, it is necessary to ask, '*What does it mean to be professional?* From the patient perspective, characteristics and attributes of a healthcare professional are as follows:

- Competent, whereby the practitioner must undertake CPD
- Committed, whereby they are reliable and work hard in the best interest of the patient
- They maintain confidentiality, thereby instilling trustworthiness into their role. In some instances, confidentiality will not be possible
- They are altruistic in nature displaying an image of selflessness and having a 'heart of gold'
- They possess integrity and honesty
- They have a good grounding in morality and ethics, whereby they are valued in society, of good standing and not judgemental
- They possess good communication skills

- Are caring and sensitive to patient needs
- Are serious in their work
- They hold a 'social contract', whereby they display similar behaviour outside of work
- They are law abiding and upstanding citizens
- Maintain a professional appearance, i.e. neatly attired to inspire trust in patients.

From an employer perspective, a professional should be:

- Responsible to the profession by following the professional codes of conduct; upholding the requirements for practice and the reputation of the profession
- Responsible to society sharing the ethos that 'patients come first'
- Must be competent in the practise of their profession
- Must undertake self-regulation and maintain fitness to practise
- Must be accountable, whereby you take responsibility for your own actions or decisions
- Must be a team worker
- Must exercise autonomy
- Must adhere to legal requirements and policies, e.g. confidentiality and informed consent
- Prioritise work and is not money orientated
- Must know own limitations of practice
- Must be an effective communicator.

Professionals are governed by codes of ethics, and have commitment to competence, integrity. Morality, altruism and promotion of public and good. They are accountable to all service users and to society.

Why do we have a code of conduct?

As practitioners we have to work to:

- Predefined professional standards and maintain them
- Maintain health and safety
- Reduce risks by undertaking appropriate risk assessments of, e.g. the equipment we use
- Ensure effective communication with patients and clinical colleagues
- Maintain confidentiality
- Be accountable for our practice
- Ensure that service users are supplied with information before they are able to give consent in an informed manner
- Continuously improve our knowledge base and skills
- Embrace advancing practice and role developments as necessary and appropriate.

Code of Conduct and Ethics

The Code of Conduct and Ethics from the Society and College of Radiographers[2] (SCoR) are given below. The guidance has been deliberately included in its entirety and uses the term 'radiographer' as opposed to 'practitioner', as given throughout our text. This document outlines the principles and precepts required for a professional working in the wide field of what is encompassed within the generic term 'radiography'. It provides advice and guidance and requires professionals to apply the principles to the various situations in which they practice; and in their personal lives, in order to maintain the widest public trust and confidence in the profession.

Radiographers are advised that this document is not an alternative but is an adjunct to the current Health & Care Professions Council (HCPC) Standards of Conduct, Performance and Ethics[3] and must be used in conjunction with it and all other relevant HCPC publications.

While this document addresses the profession of radiography and radiographers, most aspects contained within it are pertinent to members of the wider radiography workforce (e.g. student radiographers, assistant practitioners, trainee assistant practitioners and support workers). It is incumbent on this wider workforce to ensure that they apply these same principles and precepts within their own scope of practice to ensure the public's trust in radiography service provision and thus also in the profession of radiography.

Legal framework in which radiographers practice

Under the Health Professions Order[4] (2001) the terms 'radiographer', 'diagnostic radiographer' and 'therapeutic radiographer' are protected titles and can only be used by persons who have successfully completed an approved course leading to a diploma or degree in radiography and who are registered with the HCPC. Title protection is one way of assisting the public in the identification of those individuals who are not only registered with the regulatory body and subsequently accountable for the delivery of a wide range of radiographic services, but also meet the established standards of the profession. It is permissible for the term 'student radiographer' to be used, as long as it refers to an individual who is at the time following a recognised degree course, which leads to eligibility for full HCPC registration as a radiographer.

Individuals using any of the protected titles relevant to radiography in all clinical specialities (educational, research, managerial or industrial employment) must comply at all times with the current legislation and laws in their country of practice, with current best practice and with their employer's reasonable policies and procedures.

Complaints, professional conduct and fitness to practise

The HCPC, as the professional regulatory body, handles complaints concerning the professional conduct or fitness to practise of registrants. The Society of Radiographers is the body that handles complaints or considers matters of fitness to practise concerning members of the Society who are not regulated by the HCPC.

The HCPC and the SCoR will take into account adherence or otherwise to this code, by radiographers and the wider radiography workforce, in the event of any complaint received. (See: The Health & Care Professions Council-Fitness to Practise Proceedings below.)

Expectations

The Society and College of Radiographers expect members of the profession to, at all times, conduct themselves in a manner that will maintain public trust and confidence in the profession as a whole. The reputation of the profession must never be put into jeopardy through the actions or behaviours of either its members or the wider radiography workforce. In addition, individual members of the whole of the radiography workforce have a right to expect to be treated with respect and to be free from threats, violence or verbal abuse.

While this document addresses the ethical requirements of radiographers and, by implication, the radiography workforce, it is also intended to enable the public to know what to expect from the provision of radiography services and, as such, this document should be widely available.

Best practice

At the heart of best practice is a commitment to the health and safety of all service users: to integrity and honesty; to professional competence; to continuing self-development and to the development and maintenance of high standards of ethics and behaviour.

This document consists of four major areas of standards of ethical behaviour which underpin and sustain professional and personal conduct:

1. Scope of Professional Practice
2. Relationships with Service Users
3. Relationships with Professional Staff
4. Personal and Professional Standards

which are further informed by the following five philosophical precepts of:

1. Autonomy (respect for persons)
2. Beneficence (doing good)
3. Non-maleficence (not doing/preventing harm)
4. Justice (fair treatment of persons/environment)
5. Trustworthiness

(See: Tools for ethical decision-making, below.)

Note

The HCPC uses the term 'service users' to refer to anyone who uses or is affected by the services of registrants and will thus be applicable to all radiography registrants in whichever field they practise. The term 'service users' has therefore been adopted for this present publication.

In this document, the following terms are used:

'You must' is used as an overriding principle or duty. 'You should' is used where the principle or duty may not apply in all circumstances or where there are factors outside your control affecting your ability to comply.

This document replaces Statements for Professional Conduct 2, which was issued by The College of Radiographers in March 2002 and re-issued with minor amendments in September 2004.

1. Scope of professional practice

As a member of the radiography workforce you must practice in a safe and competent manner within your own scope of practice based on education, competency, knowledge, extent of experience and registration.[6]

Professional indemnity insurance is available through membership of The Society of Radiographers. There may be circumstances when public liability insurance is required, this would only be applicable for unusual conditions, for example, radiographers working as independent practitioners. You must seek to further the profession of radiography and to maintain public confidence in the profession.

1.1. Scope of practice of radiography All radiographers have a responsibility towards users of your services and a unique individual responsibility for the optimisation of any ionising or non-ionising radiation dose to individuals and to the genetic inheritance of the public at large. You are required to abide by current legislation and healthcare policy.

1.2. Individual scope of practice You must consider the requirements of your individual scope of practice and seek to develop and maintain your abilities, to recognise the limits of your competence and to practice within them. You must monitor your practice and any protocols you work within using evidence from audit findings and from the relevant research in order to develop best practice.

You will always be accountable for your actions, your omissions and your behaviours and need to be able to justify any decisions you take within your scope of practice. You should recognise any deficiencies you may have and take appropriate action to rectify them.

1.3. Development of the profession You should endeavour to ensure that the profession of radiography continues to develop in all fields and specialities and look for opportunities where development is possible. With this in mind you should seek out and work with others in pursuit of this goal, bearing in mind that your main responsibilities are always to service users.

1.4. Individual role development Opportunities for individual role development lie within the career progression framework. You must engage in educational planning relevant to your needs and the needs of the service arising from clinical practice. You should seek to become a reflective, self-directed learner; able to appraise recent relevant research and to discuss and review the evidence base with colleagues in a variety of situations. You should encourage colleagues and other members of the radiography workforce in their role development.

1.5. Competence and continuing professional development You must develop and maintain high standards of competency in skills, knowledge, acquired attitudes and behaviour and must work within current legislative and employers' frameworks.

You should actively engage in learning in a constant process of development through the integration of Continuing Professional Development (CPD) in your day to day practice. CPD is a requirement for registrants and therefore must be a planned activity which is evidenced.

Registrants must follow the HCPC guidelines in Your guide to our standards for continuing professional development.

1.6. Clinical supervision/teaching You should be willing to be involved in the supervision, teaching, training, appraising and assessing of student radiographers, assistant practitioners and trainees. You also have a professional obligation towards the teaching and training of other healthcare professionals (HCPs) in some practice areas, e.g. radiographers may be involved in mentoring nurses or midwives in ultrasound training. When involved in any such activities, you need to develop the skills, attitudes and practices of a caring and competent teacher/trainer. You should be objective and honest when supervising, appraising, evaluating or assessing the performance of others as service users will be at risk if you describe as competent someone who has not yet met or maintained a satisfactory standard of practice.

1.7. Professional liability insurance There are inherent risks arising from the wide practice of radiography so it is important that you have adequate insurance to cover these risks. Usually insurance coverage is vicariously undertaken by your employer as long as you practise within your own scope otherwise the vicarious liability of the employer may be negated. The SCoR, through its annual subscription, covers personal liability insurance for those members working in the UK or who are travelling and temporarily working abroad in all countries with the exception of the USA and Canada.

Radiographers undertaking imaging outside any recognised care management framework, e.g. social ultrasound scans arising from self-referrals are advised to obtain additional professional indemnity provision.

Radiographers who practise as independent practitioners must ensure that they have adequate vicarious, personal and third party liability insurance.

For further advice see SCoR documents Statements on Ultrasound Referrals and Professional Insurance Arrangement; and Professional Indemnity Insurance Statement.

2. Relationships with service users

You have moral and legal obligations to service users and a duty of care to all.

You should demonstrate respect for individual dignity, belief, culture and autonomy through a commitment to the principles of consent and confidentiality. You must neither engage in, nor condone, behaviour that causes physical, emotional or psychological distress or damage to anyone.

2.1. Provision of good care to service users You must ensure equality of care to all with no discrimination (gender, age, disability, ethnic origin, race, religion, beliefs, marital status, economic status, lifestyle, sexual orientation). You should strive for a consistency of care at all times and in all situations.

You must not be judgemental of any service users and ensure that children and other vulnerable groups are protected.

You must recognise the limits of your competence, consider the provision of appropriate health educational advice and, when deemed appropriate, consult with and take advice from colleagues. You should make good use of resources available to you and at all times optimise exposure to radiation.

2.2. Professional boundaries You should, if practicable, avoid providing imaging or radiotherapy services to anyone with whom you have a close personal relationship.

In order to maintain professional boundaries, you must not use your position to enter into relationships that may exploit service users sexually, emotionally, socially, financially or in any other manner.

You must use your professional judgement as to whether it may be prudent to involve a chaperone for a particular situation involving a service user. Wherever possible, it is good practice to offer the patient the presence of a chaperone during certain intimate procedures (e.g. transrectal or transvaginal examinations) whether or not you are the same gender as the patient.

Considerations of chaperoning should be annexed to patient consent for examinations and it is advisable to ensure that the patient agrees with, and understands the role of, staff that might be present during intimate examinations.

Conversations with service users which include references to sex, politics or religion should be avoided.

2.3. Communication You should introduce yourself by full name and job title to any user of your service and ask individuals how they wish to be addressed (e.g. you must not use first or given names without initially gaining permission).

You must listen and respect service users' views, communicate clearly, openly and effectively and be conscious of their ability to make decisions for themselves.

You should identify individuals with communication difficulties and make adjustments to accommodate their particular problems (e.g. if there are language difficulties you should use interpreters not family members wherever possible).

In addition, you should develop sensitivity to the different cultural needs of patients.

Good communication with vulnerable people such as the elderly or special needs patients is imperative; you must always listen carefully to them and respect their views.

2.4. Children You have a professional and personal duty to safeguard and protect children and therefore should follow the SCoR guidelines in The Child and The Law: the roles and responsibilities of the radiographer.

2.5. Consent You must satisfy yourself that the appropriate informed consent has been gained prior to undertaking any examination or procedure and follow the SCoR guidelines in Consent to imaging and radiotherapy treatment examinations: an ethical perspective and good practice guide for the radiography workforce.[6]

2.6. Confidentiality You must not share the medical or personal details of a patient/client with anyone except those healthcare professionals who are integral to the well being of the patient. Consent of the patient should be gained before sharing information with relatives, carers or whoever may accompany the patient.

You must neither misuse electronic mail nor discuss patients or their illnesses in a public place. Local policies and procedures should be followed with regard to the leaving of messages on telephone answering systems.

Service user confidence is imperative and you need to follow the SCoR guidelines in Consent to imaging and radiotherapy treatment examinations: an ethical perspective and good practice guide for the radiography workforce[6] and the HCPC guidelines in Confidentiality: guidance for registrants.[7]

2.7. Infection control You must ensure that you understand and follow the principles and practice of infection control and that you minimise the risks of cross infection. You should seek to advise service users and students on how to avoid cross infection and report instances where cross infection may arise from activities you have witnessed.

You should follow the SCoR guidelines in Healthcare Associated Infections: practical guidance and advice.

3. Relationships with professional staff

You are obliged to cooperate with carers, other healthcare professionals, hospital staff and social care professionals. You should seek to understand and respect their responsibilities, needs, skills and working practices to ensure the best interests of all service users and avoid inappropriate criticism of them.

3.1. Collaborative practice/collegiality Frequently, you may work as part of a multi-professional team and you need to respect the skills, knowledge and contributions of colleagues from other professions and other team members. You should communicate openly and effectively with team members, acknowledge their individual roles and avoid inappropriate criticism of them.

3.2. Responsibility for peer behaviour

Radiographers and the wider radiography workforce have responsibilities within the work environment to ensure the health and safety of service users and should seek to avert any inappropriate activity of colleagues or others. If you have a patient-safety concern, you must ensure you are aware of the procedures for 'whistle blowing' and must report serious breaches of behaviour and malpractice.

The Public Interest Disclosure Act (PIDA) 1998 which came into force in July 1999 encourages people to raise concerns about malpractice in the workplace and will help ensure that the organisation responds by addressing the message rather than the messenger and resist the temptation to cover up serious malpractice.

You are covered by the Act and employing authorities will have a written policy outlining the Act and provide processes and stages for the reporting of suspected malpractice.

Malpractice includes, amongst other things, negligence, incompetence, breach of contract, unprofessional behaviour, danger to health and safety or the environment and the cover up of any such issues.[8]

Should you have a reasonable belief that a malpractice has occurred, is occurring or is likely to occur, you must approach a manager or senior professional with your concerns and follow the employing authority's procedures. Concerns you may have about staffing levels which may compromise patient safety must also be reported.

You should not use 'whistle blowing' procedures to resolve a personal or business dispute. You are encouraged to contact the SCoR and the Health & Care Professions Council (HCPC) for guidance about any malpractice concerns.

3.3. Referrals

Radiographers may accept requests for clinical imaging from named, non-medically qualified, registered healthcare professionals who are acting in the capacity of referrer under IR(ME)R, provided that an up to date list of individuals entitled to act as a referrer is established, maintained and made available to radiographers by the employer. The referrer is required to have an understanding of IR(ME)R through appropriate training and experience. Further information is available from Clinical imaging requests from non-medically qualified professionals (RCN, SCoR 2007). Where an individual undergoes an exposure following an invitation to attend an authorised national screening programme, there is no requirement for a named referrer.

In the role of IR(ME)R practitioner, radiographers must take the responsibility for the justification of a medical exposure and should refuse the referral if the procedure cannot be justified. Where and when appropriate, the radiographer should propose the use of a procedure involving non-ionising radiation.

3.4. Delegation

If you delegate clinical procedures (e.g. radiographers delegating to students or assistant practitioners), you must satisfy yourself that that person is competent to carry out the procedure; you will retain ultimate responsibility for the manner in which the delegated task is performed. You must provide supervision commensurate with the level of competence of the person to whom the procedure is delegated.

4. Personal and professional standards

You must conduct yourself with honour and dignity and demonstrate trustworthiness and integrity in both your personal and professional life in order to maintain the widest public trust and confidence in the profession.

4.1. Personal conduct and deportment

You should support the health and wellbeing of yourself, your colleagues and your service users. You must carry out all activities conscientiously and treat all persons with whom you come into contact with respect and dignity irrespective of their gender, age, disability, ethnic origin, race, religion, beliefs, marital status, economic status, lifestyle, sexual orientation or political viewpoint.

4.2. Further employment

It is not appropriate to have any other employment outside radiography or in any other capacity within your place of employment, if that employment conflicts and compromises your role in the radiography workforce or brings the profession into disrepute.

4.3. Personal health

You must look after your own personal physical, emotional and psychological health and avoid any contact or involvement with service users if you are ill, emotionally distressed or on medication which may affect your performance or judgement. If you identify the need for help related to your own personal health you should feel able to ask for it without fear of discrimination. You must follow the requirements of the employing authority with regard to the need to disclose any illness and/or disease which you develop which potentially places others, including service users, at risk (e.g. if you have an infection which could harm others).

You should be aware of any risks which may lead to work related disorders and ensure that these are minimised. It is your responsibility to ensure that equipment and the working environment are appropriate to minimise such risks and to inform management if these are considered to be unsuitable.

4.4. Personal ethics

You shall not be required to become involved in any professional activity which you believe to be unsafe, illegal, unethical or detrimental to any service user.

4.5. Conscientious objection

You must report in writing to your employing authority, at the earliest date in your employment, any conscientious objection that may be relevant to your professional practice. You should explore with them ways in which you can avoid placing an unreasonable burden on colleagues because of this. Your right to conscientious objection does not exempt you from providing service users with full, unbiased information, e.g. prior to prenatal screening or testing.[8]

You do not have the right to refuse to take part in any emergency treatment.

4.6. Respect for the law You must keep within the law of the country where you live in all your professional and personal practices.

Radiographers are required to inform the HCPC if they have received a police caution or have been charged with, or found guilty of, a criminal offence; this applies even if outside the country where they live or work.

If asked to act as a witness in a formal inquiry or litigation process related to an employment situation, you must make clear the limits of your knowledge and competence.

4.7. Integrity in research You should either conduct research or be involved in research or its dissemination in order to further the evidence base of the profession. You must protect the interests and confidentiality of patients and ensure that you do not distort or misuse clinical and research findings.

4.8. Providing/publishing information related to services Radiographers who provide independent professional services can advertise but must ensure that any advertising is factual, legal, decent, honest and truthful and does not misrepresent the services on offer.

If you do provide independent professional services you must be honest in the financial arrangements with individuals informing them of any fees/charges at the earliest time and informing them if the NHS is able to provide the same service free of charge.

You must not accept commission from third parties for recommending, when practising, the purchase of goods or services related to your professional status.

4.9. Public accountability and respect for the environment (sustainability) The radiography workforce has a responsibility to society, to taxpayers, to the wider community and to the environment. You should demonstrate due regard for the sustainable management of resources at your disposal and should use resources as responsibly and efficiently as is practicable.

4.10. Record keeping The radiography workforce is required to write reports and complete forms and other documents for a variety of tasks (e.g. curriculum vitae, radiological reports, student supervision, travel claims, locum or out of hours work) in professional and personal circumstances. You must carry out these tasks using integrity and honesty and ensure that records are protected from loss, damage, tampering or inappropriate access. You must comply with the current Data Protection Act. You should adhere to any pertinent standards related to record keeping as in Standards for the Reporting and Interpretation of Imaging Investigations.

4.11. Uniform/work-based clothing You should wear appropriate uniform or work-based clothing which meets the need to inspire confidence in your patients and to afford protection against cross infection risks and other health and safety considerations. Your employing authority will determine the nature of your work-based clothing which will also take into account the cultural and religious requirements of members of staff. You should follow advice given in Guidance on protective clothing/uniforms worn in clinical imaging and radiotherapy and oncology departments.

Tools for ethical decision-making

Although medical practice is based on facts and grounded in scientific evidence, the examining of these facts requires articulate thinking, balance and judgement. These are informed by ethical considerations. At the point where service delivery occurs, the ethics input must be seamlessly blended with scientific facts. In order to enable this holistic competence, practitioners must have an understanding of the basic principles of ethics and how these may apply in practice.

> ! Practitioners must be able to think critically about ethical issues in practice and be able to reflect on their own beliefs and values.

There are five main ethical considerations[8] in professionalism, which are philosophical principles, as follows, and each will be considered in turn:

- Autonomy
- Non-maleficence
- Beneficence
- Justice
- Trustworthiness

Autonomy

The principle of *autonomy* means that individuals have the basic right to self-determine and should be permitted to make decisions regarding their bodies, particularly their health diagnosis and treatment. Autonomy is not all or nothing as very few of us are able to make fully autonomous decisions. There may be issues understanding the choices available to us. The more complex the choice, the more difficult it is to understand and hence, less likely to make an autonomous decision. The practitioner may be placed in the midst of a conflict between a physician's order to undergo a procedure or examination and the patient's wish to refuse. It is imperative that the practitioner act as an advocate for the patient thereby assuming, in this instance, an intermediary role between the physician and the patient. Informed consent plays a vital role in enabling the patient to exercise his autonomy.

Non-maleficence

Non-maleficence means 'to do no harm'. There is no specific action associated with this principle other than ask that one not harm the other. Non-maleficence is a professional obligation which encourages respect for the patient. This principle may pose a problem when a patient refuses to undergo a procedure or have treatment and the practitioner is aware that forgoing the procedure or treatment may bring the patient harm. In this instance choosing to do nothing may cause harm to the patient but going ahead with the procedure or treatment without the patient's consent will not only violate the patient's autonomy but also bring about emotional harm.

Beneficence

Beneficence means to 'prevent harm' or 'do good'. When a patient is unable to make an autonomous choice, the practitioner has a duty of beneficence. Beneficence usually relies on an objective view of what would be the best option for the patient. This principle may require the practitioner to intercede with the referring clinician for the patient's wellbeing. Beneficence promotes trust between practitioner and patient and is likely to enhance the care of the patient. For example, when a physician's order for a procedure is contrary to the patient's wishes, then the practitioner may have to intercede by speaking with the referring physician or other appropriate personnel. This is seen particularly with patients who are Jehovah's Witnesses, where blood or blood products will be refused.

Justice

The principle of *justice* refers to being treated in a fair manner. The moral obligation is to treat any claims from patients fairly and equally. Equality is at the heart of justice, however patients can be treated unjustly even if they are treated equally. As practitioners we have to be mindful of imposing our personal or professional views about the justice of others. We need to be able to recognise the competing moral concerns, e.g. right to equal healthcare to all those who need it; right to a fair distribution of resources when treating everybody is not an option; to allow patients as much choice as possible in selecting their healthcare, and so on.

Trustworthiness

Lastly, patients expect practitioners to be faithful to their expectations. This is known as fidelity. It is an expectation of the patient that the practitioner will meet their basic needs, including their need for modesty and privacy; be competent in the practice of their profession; work according to the relevant hospital's policies and regulations; abide by the agreements made by the patient, i.e. consent and refusal; and work according to the code of professional conduct as set out by their statutory and regulatory bodies.

Practitioners have to set aside their own preconceived ideas about a patient's age, gender, sexual orientation, race, social class and provide a service that treats all patients equally and fairly. Failing to set aside these ideas may force a practitioner to make a decision based on stereotypical biases rather than uphold the principle of justice. We all have natural preferences that may result in discriminatory treatment if we are not fully aware of them. Ask yourself: 'Which patients are you most comfortable with? Men or women? Those of your own race? Young people? Under 70? Middle class? Do you feel greater compassion for a patient with a heart problem than one with a sexually transmitted disease?

Framework for ethical decision-making

1. Identify the problem (sometimes you may become aware of a problem even before you fully identify it)
2. Identify the most logical solution (with most problems, there is almost always a logical solution that arises almost instantaneously as soon as you have identified the problem)
3. Identify alternate solutions (it is good practice to consider all possible solutions before making your decision; therefore note a full range of alternate solutions to the problem)
4. Choose the best solution (choosing the solution may force you to question your choice or cause doubts to arise in your mind. You must have a clear rationale for making the choice you did. This will require critical thinking based on a balance of judgement from medical evidence and ethical principles)
5. Defend your choice by grounding it in a seamless rendition of medical evidence and ethical principles (this may be done at step 4).

LEGAL CONSIDERATIONS IN PROFESSIONAL PRACTICE

The Health & Care Professions Council Standards of Proficiency[5] state that 'registrant radiographers must be able to practise within the legal and ethical boundaries of their profession'. While it is not expected that healthcare professionals are fully conversant with medical law, it is important that they have an understanding of the key areas of legislation and the regulatory frameworks that govern their practice. Practitioners should also understand how legislation and regulation apply to their everyday working practice; indeed, an understanding of the legal and regulatory context of their practice can support healthcare professionals in the delivery of high quality healthcare in a manner that is safe, effective and professional, and also serves to protect patients, colleagues and indeed themselves.

It is also important that practitioners understand the rights to which patients are entitled. Rights are legal entitlements protected by law. The NHS Constitution sets out the rights to which patients are entitled. The Handbook to the NHS Constitution details the legal basis of each of the rights.

Not all of the rights are directly related to the work of a medical imaging practitioner; those that are will be noted in each of the relevant sections below.

Registrant practitioners are expected to practise in accordance with the HCPC Standards of Proficiency[5] and the Standards of Conduct, Performance and Ethics.[3] Elements of these standards relate to certain aspects of medical law. These will be discussed in turn.

Confidentiality

All practitioners have a duty to maintain confidentiality of information they obtain from or about a patient. This is clearly laid out for practitioners in The Standards of Proficiency and the Standards of Conduct, Performance and Ethics:

- 'Registrant radiographers must understand the importance of and be able to maintain confidentiality'
- 'A registrant must respect the confidentiality of service users'.

The NHS Constitution states that patients have the right to privacy and confidentiality and to expect the NHS to keep their confidential information safe and secure.

A practitioner who breaches confidentiality will have acted illegally on the basis of a number of legal obligations – statute, tort law (negligence) and contract of employment.

Statute

There are two statutes that practitioners should be aware of with regard to confidentiality.[8] These are the Human Rights Act 1998 and the Data Protection Act 1998.

The Human Rights Act 1998 came into force in England and Wales in 2000. This Act enables citizens to bring an action in a court of law to enforce their rights laid out in the European Convention on Human Rights. The Human Rights Act 1998 enables an action to be brought by a person who claims that a public authority (such as an NHS Trust) has acted in a way that is incompatible with a convention right. A breach of confidentiality by a practitioner could be seen to contravene Article 8 of the Human Rights Act 1998, which states that everyone has a right to respect for private and family life (Human Rights Act 1998).

The Data Protection Act 1998 makes provision for the regulation of the processing of information relating to individuals, including the obtaining, holding, use or disclosure of such information (Data Protection Act 1998). Under the Data Protection Act 1998 a practitioner breaching confidentiality would be improperly using or disclosing information about the patient.

Tort law (negligence)

It is also important to consider confidentiality in light of tort law. A breach of confidentiality could amount to negligence on the part of the practitioner. This could result in the patient bringing an action against the employer of the practitioner on the basis of its vicarious liability for the actions of its employees.

Contract of employment

Practitioners are also required by their contract of employment to maintain confidentiality with regard to patient information. Improper use or disclosure of patient information could result in the employer taking action through disciplinary procedures.

It is important to note that there are exceptions to the duty of confidentiality. These are:

- Consent of the patient
- Disclosure in the clinical care or in the interests of the patient
- Court order or pre-trial disclosure
- Statutory duty to disclose
- Disclosure in the public interest.

With regard to confidentiality and the exceptions to this duty, both the SCoR and the HCPC offer guidance with regard to confidentiality and the exceptions to this duty. The SCOR Code of Conduct and Ethics state that:

> *You must not share the medical or personal details of a patient/client with anyone except those healthcare professionals who are integral to the well being of the patient. Consent of the patient should be gained before sharing information with relatives, carers or whoever may accompany the patient.*

The HCPC has produced information for registrants with regard to confidentiality. This document offers detailed guidance to registrants based on the following key principles:
You should:

- Take all reasonable steps to keep information about service users safe
- Get the service user's informed consent if you are passing on their information, and get express consent, in writing, if you are using the information for reasons which are not related to providing care or services for the service user
- Only disclose identifiable information if it is absolutely necessary, and, when it is necessary, only disclose the minimum amount necessary

- Tell service users when you have disclosed their information (if this is practical and possible)
- Keep appropriate records of disclosure
- Keep up-to-date with relevant law and good practice
- If appropriate, ask for advice from colleagues, professional bodies, unions, legal professionals or us
- Make your own informed decisions about disclosure and be able to justify them.

Consent

The DoH (2001) states that 'patients have a fundamental legal and ethical right to determine what happens to their own bodies'. Valid consent to treatment is therefore absolutely central in all forms of healthcare, from providing personal care to undertaking major surgery.

> **!** Seeking consent is also a matter of common courtesy between health professionals and patients.

The Standards of Proficiency state that registrant practitioners must 'understand the importance of and be able to obtain informed consent'. The Standards of Conduct Performance and Ethics state that as a registrant 'you must get informed consent to give treatment (except in an emergency)'.

There are two aspects of the law relating to consent. One is the act of the patient giving consent and the other is the duty of the radiographer to provide sufficient information on the procedure/examination prior to the patient giving consent. If a practitioner were to examine or treat a patient without consent, this can lead to the patient suing for trespass to the person; a failure on the part of the practitioner to provide sufficient information could be regarded as an act of negligence.

Practitioners need to create a balance between right and duty.

> **!** From the patients' perspective, informed consent appears to be a 'right'; while from the practitioners' viewpoint; it is a duty or obligation. Informed consent is an important patient right. This means that all patients should be given an equal opportunity at receiving information and consenting to their examinations/treatment.

Trespass to a person occurs when a patient has not given consent and either apprehends a touching of his person (assault) or is actually touched (battery). The individual who has suffered the trespass can sue for compensation in the civil courts; however, they must prove the touching or the apprehension of the touching, and that it was a (potentially) direct interference with his person.

In order for consent to be valid, the following factors are key:

- The person must be competent
- The person has to be sufficiently informed
- The person is not subject to coercion or influence.

Where a person is a competent adult, only they may consent to treatment or examination. While this text will not consider in depth those adults who lack capacity, it is important to mention how they can be treated when unable to consent. Patients who lack mental capacity, and are therefore unable to consent, may be treated if it is in their best interests under The Mental Capacity Act 2005. A relative may not consent for them; however, if treatment is deemed in their best interests, then they can be treated.

With regard to competence, children may consent to examination or treatment.

> **!** Children who are 16 or 17 may give consent in the same way as an adult; children below the age of 16 may give consent if they have 'Gillick competence', i.e. they have sufficient understanding and intelligence to fully understand the examination or treatment.

The NHS Constitution states that patients have the right to refuse or accept treatment and that they should not be given any physical examination or treatment unless they have given valid consent. Furthermore, patients also have the right to be given information about their treatment in advance, including any significant risks.

The SCoR Code of Conduct and Ethics makes a clear statement about consent.

> *'You must satisfy yourself that the appropriate informed consent has been gained prior to undertaking any examination or procedure and follow the SCoR guidelines in Consent to imaging and radiotherapy treatment examinations: an ethical perspective and good practice guide for the radiography workforce' (see 2.5 in Code of Conduct and Ethics, above)*

To provide an overview of the responsibilities of the radiographer with regard to consent and information giving, part of the executive summary for the SCoR guidelines in Consent to imaging and radiotherapy treatment examinations has been reproduced below. Readers are advised to consult the full SCoR document for further information:

Valid and legal consent (sections 5 and 6)

- Consent is ensuring the patient is aware of the purpose and nature of any procedure to be carried out. The practitioner must ensure that the patient is fully aware of his/her options, including alternatives, the right to refuse and the consequences of refusal. The practitioner is advised to always seek the patient's explicit verbal affirmation to proceed.
- Practitioners must distinguish between patient compliance and implied consent, both signalled through behaviour, as implied consent requires that the patient is provided with sufficient information on which to proceed with the examination or treatment.
- The practitioner should provide the patient with a limited amount of relevant and accurate information in a form that the individual practitioner deems the particular patient is able to grasp and thus understand. The amount will depend on the nature of the examination and whether there are any *significant* risks attached to the procedure.
- The practitioner should ask the patient to confirm in his or her own words their understanding of the procedure and whether they agree to continue.
- Practitioners should be aware of the circumstances and procedures requiring written consent and liaise with the appropriate medical or dental practitioner if delegated the task of obtaining consent in these instances.

Information giving (sections 7 and 8)

- Patients are entitled to know that they will receive a dose of radiation and should be informed of the benefits of the procedure.
- Some patients, on being made aware that radiation is involved in their examination, may ask pertinent questions about potential risks to themselves or future offspring. Practitioners should respond in an appropriate way using their own judgement to decide on the ability of the patient to understand a risk–benefit approach.
- Practitioners should respond to queries by avoiding the use of the term 'safe' in favour of terms that describe a radiation risk as being very low or acceptable compared with other risks in society. (Refer to broad levels of risk for common X-ray examinations and isotope scans, Appendix 4 of the ScoR document).
- In the case of procedures such as some CT examinations, certain nuclear medicine examinations, interventional procedures, or radiotherapy treatment, patients should be informed of any significant radiation dosage and the inherent risks of radiation.
- Information about other possible non-radiation linked side effects arising from any diagnostic or therapeutic procedure, should be part of an agreed departmental policy and made known to all radiographers working in the field.
- Practitioners should be cognisant of the potential harm that information on risk could cause.

Consent and children (section 9)

- If a child is not capable of understanding the nature of the procedure to be undertaken, the child's parent or guardian should be asked for their consent to proceed.
- Practitioners should be aware of the issues surrounding consent for procedures and consent to disclosure where children are involved. (Refer also to: 'The child and the law: roles and responsibilities of the radiographer', SCoR.)

Data protection

Data protection has briefly been considered when looking at the issue of confidentiality. However, this does need to be explored a little further in view of how it applies to practitioners working in clinical practice.

According to the HCPC Standards of Conduct, Performance and Ethics, radiographers 'must keep accurate records'. Examples of how this applies to practice would be:

- Ensuring that X-ray images have the correct patient details and anatomical markers
- Ensuring that any information that is recorded about an examination (such as the radiation dose) is correct.

The importance of accurate records with regard to patient treatment and management is obvious; incorrect records may lead to incorrect treatment or management. However, it is also important to realise that X-ray images and documentation associated with them form part of a patient's records. The NHS Constitution states that a patient has a right of access to their own healthcare records. The source of this right is the Data Protection Act 1998, which states that patients have the right to gain access to information held about them.

The Health & Care Professions Council – Fitness to Practise Proceedings

The Health & Care Professions Council was set up to protect the public. As a regulator, the HCPC maintains a register of those professionals who meet the Standards of Proficiency and the Standards of Conduct, Performance and Ethics. Should a registrant fall below these standards, then the HCPC can take action.

A professional who is fit to practise possesses the knowledge and skills, and acts in a manner that is appropriate to practice their profession safely and effectively; however, there are occasions when a professional's fitness to practise is impaired and that there are some concerns over whether they can practise safely and effectively. Such cases are investigated, which can result in sanctions being applied to the scope of practice of the individual.

When a complaint is received by the HCPC, the Investigating Committee Panel considers the allegation and decides whether there is a case to answer. The Investigating Committee Panel can decide that (a), there is no case to answer; (b) there is a case to answer (meaning that the case will proceed to a final hearing or (c) there is no case to answer (the evidence available will not be able to establish that the registrant's fitness to practise is impaired).

If the allegation is considered to be serious enough to suggest that a registrant may cause harm to themselves or others, an interim order may be applied for; this can either prevent the registrant from practising or can place limits on their practice until the case is heard.

Within the context of this chapter, and the legal issues considered, it is important to appreciate the types of cases that have resulted in 'case to answer' decisions and progress to a final hearing. Such cases include:

- Breach of service user confidentiality
- Failure to maintain adequate service user records
- Falsifying service user records.

Final hearings are usually held in public and the registrant is encouraged to attend; hearings can be heard in the absence of the registrant.

Allegations relating to misconduct (under which the above examples would fall) are heard by panels of the Conduct and Competence Committee. Sanctions that can be applied are:

- A caution
- Application of conditions of practice
- Suspension
- Striking off.

KEY POINTS

- Ethics means distinguishing between right and wrong; what is good or bad; or what ought or ought not to be done in a given instance
- Practitioners must be aware of and be able to act within the limits of their experience and knowledge and to do this, they must have an understanding of the legal framework within which they practice

- Ethical decision-making requires the ability of radiographers to recognise the presence of an ethical issue and to know the appropriate ethical action to take in order to justify a moral outcome
- In addition to following the necessary regulations set out by our statutory and regulatory bodies, practitioners must work according to the policies, regulations and procedures, as set out by their employer. It is therefore essential to ensure that all new staff go through a period of induction and orientation and that this includes the local policies and procedures
- The five main ethical considerations and philosophical principles in professionalism are autonomy, non-maleficence, beneficence, justice and trustworthiness
- Practitioners should have an understanding of the legal context within which they work to be able to comprehend how the law both enables them and restricts them in their role
- Practitioners have a duty to maintain confidentiality of information they obtain from or about a patient
- Valid consent to treatment is absolutely central in all forms of healthcare, from providing personal care to undertaking major surgery. Seeking consent is also a matter of common courtesy between health professionals and patients
- Practitioners should keep accurate records of patients' management and treatment information
- Fitness to practise referrals will be made in cases where professional practice falls below the required standards

The Code of Conduct and Ethics has been reprinted with kind permission of the Society and College of Radiographers, UK.

Glossary

Adjuvant   A therapy given in addition to the main or primary treatment

Agonist   In pharmacology, a substance that binds to a cell receptor and triggers a response

Allergy   A hypersensitivity reaction to a particular substance

Analgesia   Reduction of pain

Antagonist   In pharmacology, a substance that blocks or opposes the action of an agonist

Altruism   A principle of concern or regard for the needs of others before one's own

Anaphylaxis   Extreme hypersensitivity to a foreign substance, involving constriction of the airways and movement of fluid from the blood plasma into body tissues

Anaphylactoid reaction   A mild body reaction to a contrast agent or other foreign substance, characterised by skin flushing, rash, nausea and vomiting responses

Antibody   A component of the specific immune system, produced by the body to target antigens

Antigen   An agent which causes the body to produce antibodies within the specific immune response

Antimicrobial   To kill or suppress microorganisms

Antisepsis   Destruction of pathogenic microorganisms that cause infection

Attitude   The way in which a person views something or tends to behave towards something

Autism   A developmental disorder characterised by severe deficits in social interaction and communication and by abnormal behaviour patterns

Bariatric   Overweight or obese

Behaviour   Manner of acting or controlling oneself

Benign   Having little or no harmful or detrimental effect

Biocide   A physical or chemical agent that kills all living organisms

Bioreductive agents   Drugs that become cytotoxic agents by chemical reduction in the presence of low oxygen levels or reducing compounds

Bipolar disorder   A mood disorder that involves alternating episodes of elation and depression

Blood pool agents   Compounds that remain longer in the bloodstream, due to binding to cells or proteins

Brachytherapy   A radiotherapy treatment that employs a radioactive source or sources placed within the patient

Bradycardia   An abnormal slowing of the heart beat, typically to less than 50 beats per minute

Cataract   A partial or complete opacity of the crystalline lens of the eye

Cleaning   A process using detergent or an enzymatic soaking solution that will remove foreign matter, such as dirt or microorganisms, from an object

Commensal   An organism that lives on or within another organism, and derives benefit without harming the host

Compliance   To act according to accepted standards

Computed radiography (CR)   An X-ray technique in which a digital image is processed from a latent image obtained in a cassette

Computed tomography (CT)   An X-ray technique in which a sectional imaging slice is obtained in a patient, via a rotation of the X-ray tube around the patient

Confidentiality   Discretion, keeping information secret

Consent   To give permission, or agree/accept

Contrast agent or medium   A chemical or physical substance given to patients within diagnostic imaging procedures to increase signal differences (contrast) between different tissues

Culture   A form or stage of civilisation, or the behaviours and beliefs of a particular social, ethnic or age group

Cytotoxic   "Cell killing", agents that kill body cells (aimed at cancers)

Decibel (dB)   A logarithmic scale of audible sound intensity

Decontamination   The physical or chemical process that will remove, inactivate or destroy pathogens in order to make the object incapable of transmitting infectious particles. The process could include cleaning, disinfection or sterilisation

Dementia   A state of mental deterioration involving reduction in memory, judgement, awareness and concentration

Deterministic effect A damaging effect of radiation involving whole tissues rather than single cells. Only occurs above a dose threshold and increases in severity with increasing dose

Digital radiography A technique in which a digital image is obtained electronically without requiring any latent image processing

Dimer With respect to contrast media, a molecule that contains two linked benzene rings

Disinfectant A chemical agent that destroys most pathogens but may not kill bacterial spores

Disinfection A chemical or physical process that destroys pathogens

DNA Deoxyribonucleic acid. A large molecule found in cell nuclei, containing the genetic code and heavily involved in cell division. It is vulnerable to radiation damage.

Empathy A deep emotional understanding of another person's feelings or problems

Erythema A deterministic effect of radiation damage at large doses, involving skin reddening and fibrosis

Ethnicity A group of human beings whose members identify with each other on the basis of common cultural, linguistic, or religious characteristics

External beam radiotherapy A radiotherapy treatment that employs a beam of X-rays or gamma rays arising from a source external to the patient

Ferromagnetic A substance (such as iron) that experiences a powerful force when placed in a magnetic field

Fibrillation An uncontrolled spasm in heart muscle

Fractionation A radiotherapy technique in which a course of radiation treatment is divided into parts or "fractions" over a period of time, in order to reduce adverse side effects and increase tumour cell killing

Geriatric Relating to old age, the elderly. Now replaced by the term "elderly" for healthcare use

Glaucoma A disease of the eye in which the pressure of fluid inside the eyeball is abnormally high, caused by obstructed outflow of the fluid. The increased pressure can damage the optic nerve and lead to partial or complete loss of vision

Healthcare associated infection (HCAI) HCAIs can affect any part of the body, including the urinary system (urinary tract infection), the lungs (pneumonia or respiratory tract infection), the skin, surgical wounds (surgical site infection), the digestive (gastrointestinal) system and even the bloodstream (bacteraemia)

Histamines A substance secreted by the body's immune system during allergic reactions to counteract the allergens

Holistic To take into account the whole picture rather than component parts

Hypertension An abnormal increase in blood pressure that is consistently above 140 mm systolic and 90 mm diastolic

Hypotension An abnormal decrease in blood pressure that is below 90 mm systolic and 60 mm diastolic

Infarction Loss of blood supply to an area of body tissue, resulting in tissue death

Infection Invasion by and multiplication of pathogenic microorganisms in a bodily part or tissue, which may produce subsequent tissue injury and progress to overt disease through a variety of cellular or toxic mechanisms

Interventional procedure A clinical procedure (including imaging) in which treatment takes place

Ionising Removal of electrons from atoms and molecules, forming charged ions and involving the breakage of chemical bonds. Caused by ionising radiations such as X-rays and gamma rays.

Justification With regard to ionising radiation exposures, a principle that likely benefit must exceed risk

Ligand An ion or molecule that binds to a metal within a chemical compound

Limitation With regard to ionising radiation exposures, a principle that exposures must be kept within socially and legally acceptable dose limits

Linear accelerator (LINAC) The device most commonly used for external beam X-radiation radiotherapy treatments for patients with cancer

Magnetic resonance imaging (MRI) A technique in which sectional images of slices in patients are obtained by the excitation and relaxation of hydrogen nuclei, using powerful magnetic fields and radio waves

Malignant Uncontrollable, rapidly spreading with a tendency to be destructive. In the case of cancer, malignant cells are poorly differentiated, rapidly dividing and spread by local invasion or metastasis

Magnetic resonance imaging (MRI) A technique that obtains sectional images (slices) in patients, via the excitation and relaxation of hydrogen nuclei, when exposed to powerful magnetic fields and radio waves

Mitosis Cell division in all body cells except those involved in the sexual reproduction process

Monoclonal Antibodies or cells derived from a single ancestral cell

Monomer With respect to contrast media, a molecule that contains a single benzene ring

Morbidity The frequency with which a particular disease occurs, or causes harm

Mortality rate The rate of deaths in an area in relation to the population or a particular disease

Mutation A possible effect of ionising radiations and some chemicals, involving permanent abnormal changes in form, affecting cells or individuals

Neoplasia "New growth" ie tumour

Nosocomial Infections resulting from medical care or treatment in hospital (in- or outpatient), nursing homes or even the patient's own home

Oedema   An abnormal increase in extracellular fluid within body tissues, associated with tumours, trauma, tissue death, infection and anaphylaxis

Oncology   A branch of medical practice that involves the study and treatment of cancers

Oncogene   A gene that contributes to abnormal increased cell division in cancer

Optimal   The most desirable possibility under given restrictions or conditions

Optimisation   With regard to ionising radiation exposures, a principle that exposure levels must be minimised whilst still providing sufficient quality of diagnosis or treatment

Osmolality   The concentration of a fluid, measured in terms of numbers of dissolved particles per kilogram of solute. A high osmolar compound causes osmotoxity when introduced into the body, specifically due to movement of water from body tissues to blood plasma and effects on the kidneys

Osmolarity   The concentration of a fluid, measured in terms of numbers of dissolved particles per litre of solution. A high osmolar compound causes osmotoxity when introduced into the body, specifically due to movement of water from body tissues to blood plasma and effects on the kidneys

Paediatric   Relating to children, the very young

Palliative   A remedy that relieves pain without providing a cure

Pathogen   A bacterium, virus or other microorganism that can cause disease

Phobia   An anxiety disorder involving an irrational fear e.g. of a situation or object

Planning (or planned) target volume (PTV)   The volume of tissue deliberately irradiated in radiotherapy, to include the whole volume of the tumour and a margin surrounding it

Positron   A positively charged electron, not found naturally but produced when some artificial radioactive isotopes decay

Positron emission tomography (PET)   A sectional imaging technique used in nuclear medicine. It employs man-made positron-emitting radioactive isotopes introduced into patients. These emit very high energy gamma rays. A fixed ring of gamma ray detectors surrounds the patient.

Privacy   The quality of being secluded from the presence or view of others

Radionuclide   A radioactive atomic nucleus, which may emit particles and gamma rays. Used in nuclear medicine and some types of radiotherapy

Resistance   The capacity of an organism to defend itself against a disease

Simulation   In radiotherapy, the external beam treatment is simulated before delivery in order to achieve an accurate set-up, position the body and plan the radiation dose delivered to the tumour

Single photon emission computed tomography (SPECT)   A sectional imaging technique used in nuclear medicine. It employs radioactive isotopes introduced into patients. These emit gamma rays. A "gamma camera" rotates around the patient.

Somatic effects   Effects of radiation which appear in the exposed individual and not in his or her offspring

Sterilant   An agent that destroys all viable forms of microbial life

Stochastic effect   A damaging effect of radiation that is governed by chance and is not inevitable. The risk of the effect increases with dose. Includes cancer induction and genetic damage.

Sterilisation   A chemical or physical process that destroys or removes all microbial life, including bacterial spores

Tachycardia   An abnormal speeding up of the heart beat, typically to more than 100 beats per minute at rest in adults

Targeting   The use of drugs or contrast agents that attach specifically to certain types of cells or tissues

Telemedicine   The use of various telecommunications by physicians and medical institutions that provide healthcare to their patients through electronic or digital means

Tesla (T)   A unit of magnetic flux density (often referred to popularly as magnetic "field strength")

Tumour suppressor gene   A protective gene that when fully functional prevents abnormal increased cell division

Trimester   A period of three months. In pregnancy, the developing child is most vulnerable to radiation and chemical effects during the first trimester

Ultrasound   High frequency sound above the audible range in humans, used medically for diagnostic imaging scans and therapeutic purposes

Vertigo   Dizzyness

Virulence   The capacity of a microorganism for causing a disease

Bibliography

Chapter 9

Allisy-Roberts, P., Williams, J., 2008. Farr's physics for medical imaging, second ed. Elsevier, Edinburgh.

Brusin, J.H., 2007. Radiation protection. Radiol. Technol. 78 (5), 378–392.

Bushong, S.C., 2008. Radiologic science for technologists; physics, biology and protection, nineth ed. Elsevier, St Louis.

Dal Masso L, Bossetti C, La Vecchia C et-al. Risk factors for thyroid cancer: an epidemiological review focused on nutritional factors. Cancer Causes Control; 20(1):75–86.

Department of Health, 1999. Ionising Radiation Regulations. (S.I. 1999/3232) HMSO, London.

Department of Health, 2000. Ionising radiation (Medical Exposure) Regulations. (S.I. 2000/1059) HMSO, London.

Environment Agency, 2002. Radioactive substances regulation process management. Interim guidance on 'best practicable means' for non-nuclear users of radioactive substances. Environment Agency, London.

Furlow, B., 2011. Radiation protection in pediatric imaging. Radiol. Technol. 82 (5), 421–439.

Graham, D.T., Cloke, P., Vosper, M., 2011. Principles and applications of radiological physics, sixth ed. Churchill Livingstone Elsevier, Edinburgh.

Health and Safety Executive, 1974. Health and Safety at Work Act. HMSO, London.

International Commission on Radiological Protection, 1991. ICRP 1990 Recommendations of the International Commission on Radiological Protection. vol. 21, nos 1–3 (ICRP Publication No 60) Pergamon Press, Oxford.

National Radiological Protection Board and Royal College of Radiologists, 1990. Patient dose reduction in diagnostic radiology. vol. 1, no. 3 NRPB.

Royal College of Radiologists. Making the best use of clinical radiology services: referral guidelines, sixth ed. London: Royal College of Radiologists.

United Nations Scientific Committee on the effect of atomic radiation, 2008. Report to the General Assembly Scientific Annexes A and B Sources and effects of ionising radiation. United Nations Scientific Committee on the effects of atomic radiation. vol. 1. United Nations, New York.

Chapter 10
MRI

De Wilde, J., Rivers, A., Price, D., 2005. A review of the current use of magnetic resonance imaging in pregnancy and safety implications for the fetus. Prog. Biophys. Mol. Biol. 87, 335–353.

Department of Health, 2007. Medicines and Healthcare Products Regulatory Agency. Safety guidelines for magnetic resonance imaging equipment in clinical use Device Bulletin, 3.

Feychting, M., 2005. Health effects of static magnetic fields – a review of the epidemiological evidence. Prog. Biophys. Mol. Biol. 87, 241–246.

Formica, D., Silvestri, S., 2004. Biological effects of exposure to magnetic resonance imaging: an overview. Biomed. Eng. Online 3, 11.

International Commission on Non-Ionising Radiation Protection, 2009. Amendment to the ICNIRP 'Statement on medical magnetic resonance (MR) procedures: protection of patients'. Health Phys. 97 (3), 259–261.

National Radiological Protection Board, 2003. Health effects from radiofrequency magnetic fields: Report of an Independent Advisory Group on Non-Ionising Radiation. Documents of the NRPB 14 (2).

Shellock, F., Crues, J., 2004. MR Procedures: biologic effects, safety and patient care. Radiology 232, 635–652.

Ultrasound

British Medical Ultrasound Society, 2009. Guidelines for the safe use of diagnostic ultrasound equipment: Basic and detailed guidelines. BMUS, London.

Duck, F., 2008. Hazards, risks and safety of diagnostic ultrasound. Med. Eng. Phys. 30, 1138–1348.

Health Protection Agency, 2010. Health effects of exposure to ultrasound and infrasound. Report of an Independent Advisory Group on Non-ionising Radiation. February 2010 Documents of the HPA: Radiation, Chemical and Environmental Hazards, .

Martin, K., 2010. The acoustic safety of new ultrasound technologies. Ultrasound 18, 110–118.

Salveson, K., 2002. Epidemiology of diagnostic ultrasound exposure during pregnancy – European committee for medical ultrasound safety tutorial. Eur. J. Ultrasound 15, 165–171.

Ter Haar, G., 2011. Ultrasonic imaging: safety considerations. Interface Focus 1, 686–697.

United Kingdom Association of Ultrasonographers, 2008. Guidelines for Professional Working Standards: Ultrasound Practice. UKAS, London.

Chapter 11

Bellin, M.F., Jakobsen, J.A., Tomassin, I., et al., 2002. Contrast medium extravasation injury: guidelines for prevention and management. Eur. Radiol. 12 (11), 2807–2812.

European Society for Urogenital Radiology, 2008. ESUR Guidelines on Contrast Media. ESUR, Vienna.

Forsberg, F., Merton, D.A., Liu, J.B., et al., 1998. Clinical applications of ultrasound contrast agents. Ultrasonics 36 (1–5), 695–701.

Levey, A.S., Eckhardt, K.U., Tsukamoto, Y., et al., 2005. Definition and classification of chronic kidney disease: a position statement from Kidney Disease: Improving Global Outcomes (KDIGO). Kidney Int. 67 (6), 2089–2100.

Mehran, R., Nikolsky, E., 2006. Contrast-induced nephropathy: definition, epidemiology, and patients at risk. Kidney Int. Suppl. Apr (100), S11–S15.

Newman, J., 2007. Breastfeeding and radiologic procedures. Can. Fam. Physician 53 (4), 630–631.

Qin, S., Caskey, C.F., Ferrara, K.W., 2009. Ultrasound contrast microbubbles in imaging and therapy: physical principles and engineering. Phys. Med. Biol. 54 (6), R27–R57.

Raffa, R., 2006. Pharmacological aspects of successful long-term analgesia. Clin. Rheumatol. 25 (Suppl 1), S9–S15.

Singh, J., Daftary, A., 2008. Iodinated contrast media and their adverse reactions. J. Nucl. Med. Technol. 36 (2), 69–77.

Webb, J.A.W., 2009. Prevention of acute reactions. In: Thomsen, H.S., Webb, J.A.W. (Eds.), Contrast Media Safety Issues and ESUR Guidelines, Springer-Verlag, Berlin, pp. 43–49.

Zinner, S.H., 2007. Antibiotic use: present and future. New Microbiol. 30 (3), 321–325.

Chapter 12

Bharadwaj, R., Yu, H., 2004. The spindle checkpoint, aneuploidy, and cancer. Oncogene 23 (11), 2016–2027.

Brito, D.A., Yang, Z., Rieder, C.L., 2008. Microtubules do not promote mitotic slippage when the spindle assembly checkpoint cannot be satisfied. J. Cell. Biol. 182 (4), 623–629.

Brown, J.M., 2007. Tumor hypoxia in cancer therapy. Methods Enzymol. 4435, 297–321.

Han-Chung, W., Chia-Ting, H., De-Kuan, C., 2008. Anti-angiogenic therapeutic drugs for treatment of human cancer. J. Cancer Mol. 4 (2), 37–45.

Luqmani, Y.A., 2005. Mechanisms of drug resistance in cancer chemotherapy. Med. Princ. Pract. 14 (Suppl 1), 35–48.

McKeown, S.R., Cowen, R.L., Williams, K.J., 2007. Bioreductive drugs: from concept to clinic. Clin. Oncol. (R. Coll. Radiol.) 19 (6), 427–442.

Peters, G.J., van der Wilt, C.L., van Moorsel, C.J., et al., 2000. Basis for effective combination cancer chemotherapy with antimetabolites. Pharmacol. Ther. 87 (2–3), 227–253.

Peterson, C., 2011. Drug therapy of cancer. Eur. J. Clin. Pharmacol. 67 (5), 437–447.

Sahasranaman, S., Howard, D., Roy, S., 2008. Clinical pharmacology and pharmacogenetics of thiopurines. Eur. J. Clin. Pharmacol. 64 (8), 753–767.

Takimoto, C.H., Calvo, E., 2008. Principles of oncologic pharmacotherapy. In: Pazdur, R., Wagman, L.D., Camphausen, K.A. (Eds.), Cancer management: a multidisciplinary approach, Eleventh ed. CMP Medica, Manhasset, NY.

Trigg, M.E., Higa, G.M., 2010. Chemotherapy-induced nausea and vomiting: antiemetic trials that impacted clinical practice. J. Oncol. Pharm. Pract. 16 (4), 233–244.

Chapter 13

Anon, 2006. New approaches to preventing xerostomia. J. Support Oncol. 4 (2) 88–88.

Bischoff, P., Altmeyer, A., Dumont, F., 2009. Radiosensitising agents for radiotherapy of cancer: advances in traditional and hypoxia targeted radiosensitisers. Expert Opin. Ther. Pat. 19 (5), 643–662.

Colyer, H., 2000. The role of the therapy treatment review radiographer. Radiography 6, 253–260.

Dale, R.G., Jones, B., Carabe-Fernandez, A., 2009. Why more needs to be known about RBE effects in modern radiotherapy. Appl. Radiat. Isot. 67, 387–392.

Diggelmann, K.V., Zytkovicz, A.E., Tuaine, J.M., et al., 2010. Mepilex Lite dressings for the management of radiation-induced erythema: a systematic inpatient controlled clinical trial. Br. J. Radiol. 83, 971–978.

Eddy, A., 2008. Advanced practice for therapy radiographers – a discussion paper. Radiography 14, 24–31.

Emami, B., Lyman, J., Brown, A., et al., 1991. Tolerance of normal tissue to therapeutic irradiation. Int. J. Radiat. Oncol. Biol. Phys. 21 (1), 109–122.

Faithful, S., Wells, M., 2003. Supportive care in radiotherapy. Churchill Livingstone, Edinburgh.

Fisch, M., Bruera, E., 2003. Handbook of advanced cancer care. Cambridge University Press.

Hanahan, D., Weinberg, R., 2011. Hallmarks of cancer: the next generation. Cell 144 (5), 646–674.

Hoskin, P.J., Rojas, A.M., Bentzen, S.M., et al., 2010. Radiotherapy with concurrent carbogen and nicotinamide in bladder carcinoma. J. Clin. Oncol. 28 (33), 4912–4918.

Lees, L., 2008. The role of the 'on treatment' review radiographer: what are the requirements? J. Radiother. Pract. 7, 113–131.

MacMillan, 2008. Macmillan study of the health and well-being of cancer survivors – follow-up survey of awareness of late effects and use of health services for ongoing health problems. Macmillan Cancer Support.

McLaren, D., 2003. Kidney, bladder, prostate, testis, urethra, penis. In: Bomford, C.K., Kunkler, I.H. (Eds.), Walter and Miller's textbook of radiotherapy, sixth ed. Churchill Livingstone, London, p. 487.

National Cancer Survivorship Initiative, NCSI, www.ncsi.org.uk

Pajonk, F., Vlashi, E., McBride, W.H., 2010. Radiation resistance of cancer stem cells: The 4 R's of radiobiology revisited. Stem Cells 28, 639–648.

Radiotherapy Action Group Exposure, RAGE, www.rageuk.org

Richardson, J., Smith, J.E., McIntyre, et al., 2005. Aloe vera for preventing radiation-induced skin reactions: a systematic literature review. Clin. Oncol. 17 (6), 478–484.

Rizza, L., D'Agostino, A., Girlando, A., et al., 2010. Evaluation of the effect of topical agents on radiation induced skin disease by reflectance spectrophotometry. J. Pharm. Pharmacol. 62 (6), 779–785.

Rosewall, T., Yan, J., Bayley, A.J., et al., 2009. Inter-professional variability in the assignment and recording of acute toxicity grade using the RTOG system during prostate radiotherapy. Radiother. Oncol. 90, 395–399.

Salvo, N., Barnes, E., van Draanen, J., et al., 2010. Prophylaxis and management of acute radiation-induced skin reactions: a systematic review of the literature. Curr. Oncol. 17 (4), 94–112.

Schlegel, W., Bortfeld, T., Grosu, A. (Eds.), 2006. New technologies in radiation oncology, Springer, Heidelberg.

Sirzen, F., Kjellen, E., Sorenson, et al., 2003. A systematic review of radiation therapy in non-small cell lung cancer. Acta. Oncol. 42 (5), 493–515.

Swamy, U., Ashmalla, H., Guirguis, A., 2009. A nationwide survey of radiation oncologists' management practices of radiation-induced skin reactions (RISK). J. Radiother. Pract. 8, 195–205.

Tabata, T., Katoh, M., Tokudome, S., et al., 2004. Bioactivation of capecitabine in human liver: involvement of the cytosolic enzyme on 5-deoxy-5-fluorourocytidine formation. Drug Metab. Dispos. 32 (7), 762–767.

Thomas, J., Beinhorn, C., Norton, D., et al., 2010. Managing radiation therapy side-effects with complimentary medicine. J. Soc. Integr. Oncol. 8 (2), 65–80.

Tobias, J., Hochhauser, D., 2005. Cancer and its management, sixth ed. Wiley-Blackwell, Oxford.

Witt, M.E., Haas, M., Marrinan, M.A., Brown, C.N., 2003. Understanding stereotactic radiosurgery for intracranial tumors, seed implants for prostate cancer, and intravascular brachytherapy for cardiac restenosis. Cancer Nurs. 26 (6), 494–502.

Yen, J., McLeod, H.L., 2007. Should DPS analysis be required prior to prescribing fluoropyrimidines? Eur. J. Cancer 43, 1011–1016.

Zachariah, B., Jacob, S.S., Gwede, C., et al., 2001. Effect of fractionated regional external beam radiotherapy on peripheral blood cell count. Int. J. Radiat. Oncol. Biol. Phys. 50 (2), 465–472.

Chapter 14

Ruszala, S., 2010. Moving and handling people: an illustrated guide. Clinical Skills Ltd, London.

Chapter 15

Hannigan, B., Moore, C., Quinn, D., 2009. Immunology, second ed. Scion, Bloxham.

Kitchen, G., 2007. Crash course: immunology and haematology, third ed. Elsevier, Oxford.

Sompayrac, L., 2008. How the immune system works, third ed. Wiley-Blackwell, Oxford.

Chapter 16

Department of Health. Health and Social Care Act, 2008. Code of Practice on the prevention and control of infections and related guidance. Department of Health, London.

National Institute for Health and Clinical Excellence (NICE), 2010. Infection control prevention of healthcare-associated infections in primary and community care, www.nice.org.uk.

World Health Organization, 2002. Prevention of hospital-acquired infections. A practical guide, second ed. Department of Communicable Disease, Surveillance and Response.

World Health Organization, 2009. WHO Guidelines on Hand Hygiene in Health Care. ISBN 978 92 4 159790 6.

Chapter 19

British Medical Ultrasound Society. Safety Guidelines 2009, www.bmus.org/policies-guides/BMUS-Safety-Guidelines-2009-revision-FINAL-Nov-2009.pdf.

Epstein, R., Street, R., 2011. The values and value of patient-centered care. Ann. Fam. Med. 9, 100–103.

Gibbs, V., Cole, D., Sassano, A., 2009. Ultrasound physics and technology: How, why and when. Churchill Livingstone, Edinburgh.

Society and College of Radiographers, 2006. Industry standards for the prevention of work related musculoskeletal disorders in sonography. Society of Radiographers, London.

Chapter 23

Adler, A., Carlton, R., 1999. Introduction to radiography and patient care, second ed. Saunders, Philadelphia.

Frush, D., 2006. Evidence-based principles and protocols for pediatric body multislice computed tomography. In: Knollman, F., Coakley, F. (Eds.), Multislice CT: Principles and protocols, Saunders Elsevier, Philadelphia.

Hurwitz, L., Yoshizumi, T., Reiman, R., et al., 2006. Radiation dose to the fetus from body MDCT during early gestation. Am. J. Roentgenol. 186, 871–876.

Kalra, M., Maher, M., Toth, T., et al., 2004. Strategies for CT radiation dose optimization. Radiology 230, 619–624.

McCollough, C., Bruesewitz, R., Kofler, J., 2006. CT dose reduction and dose management tools: Overview of available options. Radiographics 26, 503–512.

Paterson, A., Frush, D., 2007. Dose reduction in paediatric MDCT, general principles. Clin. Radiol. 62, 507–517.

Rogalla, P., 2006. Biopsies under computed tomography fluoroscopy control. In: Knollman, F., Coakley, F. (Eds.), Multislice CT: Principles and protocols, Saunders Elsevier, Philadelphia.

Smith, A., Dillon, P., Lau, B., et al., 2008. Radiation dose reduction strategy for CT protocols: successful implementation in neuroradiology. Radiology 247, 499–506.

Bibliography

Chapter 24

Faithful, S., Wells, M., 2003. Supportive care in radiotherapy. Churchill Livingstone, Edinburgh.

Fisch, M., Bruera, E., 2003. Handbook of advanced cancer care. Cambridge University Press.

Schlegel, W., Bortfeld, T., Grosu, A. (Eds.), 2006. New technologies in radiation oncology, Springer, Berlin.

Tobias, J., Hochhauser, D., 2005. Cancer and its management, sixth ed. Wiley-Blackwell, Oxford.

Chapter 25

Guedea, F., Venselaar, J., Hoskin, P., et al., 2010. Patterns of care for brachytherapy in Europe: updated results. Radiother. Oncol. 97 (3), 514–520.

Hoskin, P., Coyle, C., 2011. Radiotherapy in practice – brachytherapy, second ed. Oxford University Press, .

Royal College of Radiologists, 2007. The Role and development of brachytherapy services in the United Kingdom. the Royal College of Radiologists, London, www.rcr.ac.uk/publications.aspx?PageID=149&PublicationID=254.

Chapter 26

Barr, L., Cowan, R., Nicholson, M., 2004. Oncology, second ed. Churchill Livingstone, London.

Kelland, L.R., 2005. Cancer cell biology, drug action and resistance. In: Brighton, D., Wood, M. (Eds.), The Royal Marsden's Hospital Handbook of Cancer Chemotherapy, Churchill Livingstone, Edinburgh, pp. 3–17.

McIlfatrick, S., Sullivan, K., McKenna, H., et al., 2007. Patients' experiences of having chemotherapy in a day hospital setting. J. Adv. Nurs. 59 (3), 264–273.

Neal, A.J., Hoskins, P.J., 2003. Clinical oncology: Basic principles and practice, third ed. Arnold, Hodder Headline, London.

Saltmarsh, K., De Vries, K., 2008. The paradoxical image of chemotherapy: a phenomenological description of nurses' experiences of administering chemotherapy. Eur. J. Cancer Care (Engl). 17, 500–508.

Spence, R.A., Johnston, P.G., 2001. Oncology. Oxford University Press, Oxford.

Tadman, M., Roberts, D., 2007. Oxford handbook of cancer nursing.. Oxford University Press, Oxford.

Watson, M., Barrett, A., Spence, R., et al., 2006. Oncology, second ed. Oxford University Press, Oxford.

Chapter 27

Causer, L., 2005. Radioimmunotherapy in the treatment of non Hodgkin's lymphoma. Canc. Nurs. Pract. 4 (9), 27–33.

Copier, J., Dalgleish, A.G., Britten, C.M., et al., 2009. Improving efficacy of cancer immunotherapy. Eur. J. Cancer 45, 1424–1431.

Godfrey, H., 2004. Understanding the human body: biological perspectives for health care. Churchill Livingstone, Edinburgh.

Graham, A.H., 2009. Administering rituximab: infusion-related reactions and nursing implications. Canc. Nurs. Pract. 8 (2), 30–35.

Grange, J.M., Krone, B., Stanford, J.L., 2009. Immunotherapy for malignant melanoma – tracing Ariadne's thread through a labyrinth. Eur. J. Cancer 45, 2266–2273.

Hemminki, A., 2002. From molecular changes to customised therapy. Eur. J. Cancer 38, 33–338.

Tadman, M., Roberts, D., 2007. Oxford handbook of cancer nursing. Oxford University Press, Oxford.

Ward, U., 1995. Biological therapy in the treatment of cancer. Br. J. Nurs. 41 (15), 869–891.

Chapter 28

Cionini, L., Gardani, G., Gabriele, P., et al., 2007. Quality indicators in radiotherapy. Radiother. Oncol. 82, 191–200.

Gillies, A., 1997. Improving the quality of patient care. Wiley, Chichester.

Klazinga, N., Stronks, K., Delnoij, D., et al., 2001. Indicators without a cause. Reflections on the development and use of indicators in healthcare from a public health perspective. Int. J. Qual. Health Care 13 (6), 433–438.

Parsley, K., Corrigan, P., 1999. Quality improvement in healthcare: Putting evidence into practice, second ed. Stanley Thornes, Cheltenham.

Seow, H., Snyder, C., Mularski, R., et al., 2009. A framework for assessing quality indicators for cancer care at the end of life. J. Pain. Symptom Manage 38, 903–912.

References

Chapter 1

1. McGilton, K., Robinson, H.I., Roscart, V., 2006. Communication enhancement: nurse and patient satisfaction outcomes in a complex continuing care facility. Journal of Advanced Nursing 54 (1), 35.

2. Anderson, D., 2002. Dialogue and collaboration: A path for progress. SciPract Perspect 10 (1), 3.

3. Little, P., Everitt, H., Williamson, I., Wagner, G., Moore, M., Gould, C., et al., 2001. Preferences of patients for patient centred approach to consultation in primary care: Observational study. BMJ 322, 468–472.

4. McCormak, L.A., Treiman, K., Rupert, D., Williams-Piehota, P., Nadler, E., Arora, N.K., et al., 2011. Measuring patient-centered communication in cancer care: A literature review and the development of a systematic approach. Social Sciences and Medicine 72, 1085–1095.

5. Berwick, D.M., 2002. Escape fire. Lessons for the future of health care. The Commonwealth Fund, New York.

6. Nash, E.S., 1979. Medical student training in doctor-patient communication. SAMJ [cited 13 August 2011]; 22 December 1979:1118-1124. Available from http://archive.samj.org.za/1979%20VOL%20LVI%20Jul-Dec/Articles/12%20December/4.6%20MEDICAL%20STUDENT%20TRAINING%20IN%20DOCTOR-PATIENT%20COMMUNICATION,%20Eleanor%20S.Nash.pdf.

7. Jones, L., Woodhouse, D., Rowe, J., 2007. Effective nurse parent communication: a study of parents' perceptions in the NICU environment. Patient Education and Counseling 69 (1-3), 06–212.

8. Greenhill, N., Anderson, C., Avery, A., Pilnick, A., 2011. Analysis of pharmacist-patient communication using the Calgary-Cambridge guide. Patient Education and Counseling 83, 423–431.

9. Mullan, B.A., Kothe, E.J., 2010. Evaluating a nursing communication skills training course: The relationships between self-rated ability, satisfaction, and actual performance. Nurse Education in Practice 10, 374–378.

10. Vydelingnum, V., 2006. Nurses' experiences of caring for South Asian minority ethnic patients in a general hospital in England. Nursing Enquiry 13 (1), 23–32.

11. Watermeyer, J., Penn, C., 2009. Working across language and culture barriers: communication skills for pharmacists. University of Witwatersrand, Johannesburg.

12. Noordman, J., Verhaak, P., van Dulman, S., 2011. Web-enabled video-feedback: A method to reflect on the communication skills of experienced physicians. Patient Education and Counseling 82, 335–340.

13. Kosunen, E., 2008. Teaching a patient-centered approach and communication skills needs to be extended to clinical postgraduate training: A challenge to general practice. Scan J Primary Health Care 26, 1–2.

14. Cameron, K.A., Engel, K.G., McCarthy, D.M., Buckley, B.A., Kollar, L.M.M., Donlan, S.A., et al., 2010. Examining emergency department communication through a staff-based participatory research method: Identifying barriers and solutions to meaningful change. Annals of Emergency Medicine 56 (96), 614–622.

15. Crawford, P., Brown, B., 2011. Fast healthcare: Brief communication, traps and opportunities. Patient Education and Counseling 82, 3–10.

16. Beck, R., Daughridge, R., Sloane, P., 2002. Physician-patient communication in the primary care office: a systematic review. Journal of Am Board Fam Pract 15, 25–38.

17. Trummer, U.F., Mueller, U.O., Nowak, P., Stidl, T., Pelikan, J.M., 2006. Does physician-patient communication that aims at empowering patients improve clinical outcome? A case study. Patient Education and Counseling 61, 299–306.

18. Priebe, S., Dimic, S., Wildgrube, C., Jankovic, J., Cushing, A., McCabe, R., 2011. Good communication in psychiatry – a conceptual review. Article in press European Psychiatry (201). doi:10.1016/j.eurpsy.2010.07.010.

19. Street, R.L., Makoul, G., Aroroa, N.K., Epstein, R.M., 2009. How does communication heal? Pathways linking clinician-patient communication to health outcomes. Patient Education and Counseling 74, 295–301.

20. Collins, L.G., Schrimmer, A., Diamond, J., Burke, J., 2011. Evaluating verbal and non verbal communication skills, in an ethnogeriatric OSCE. Patient Education and Counseling 83, 58–16.

21. Jangland, Eva, Gunningberg, Lena, Carlsson, Maria, 2009. Patients' and relatives' complaints about

encounters and communication in health care: Evidence for quality improvement. Patient Education and Counseling 75 (2), 199–204. DOI:10.1016/j.pec.2008.10.007.

22. Tamblyn, R., Abrahamowicz, M., Dauphinee, D., Wenghofer, E., Jacques, A., Klass, D., Smee, S., et al., 2007. Physician scores on a national clinical skills examination as predictors of complaints to Medical Regulatory Authorities. JAMA 298 (9), 993–1001.

23. Pincock, S., 2004. Poor communication lies at heart of NHS complaints, says ombudsman. BMJ 328 (7430), 10, 3.

24. Kuzel, A.J., Woolf, S.H., Gilchrist, V.J., Engel, J.D., LaVeist, T.A., Vincent, C., et al., 2004. Patient reports of preventable problems and harms in primary health care. Ann Fam Med. 2.

25. Smith, I.J., 2005. The Joint Commission Guide to Improving Staff Communication. Joint Commission Resources, Oakbrook Terrace, IL.

26. Arora, V., Johnson, J., Lovinger, D., Humphrey, H.J., Meltzer, D.O., 2005. Communication failures in patient sign-out and suggestions for improvement: a critical incident analysis. QualSaf Health Care 14, 401–407.

27. Ooi, S.B., 1997. Emergency department complaints: a ten year review. Singapore Medical Journal 38, 102–107.

28. Neumann, M., Kreps, G., Visser, A., 2011. Methodological pluralism in health communication research. Patient Education and Counseling 82, 281–284.

29. Mowlana, H., Wilson, L.J., 1988. *Communication technology and development.* Paris, UNESCO [cited 1 August 2011]. Available from http://unesdoc.unesco.org/images/0008/000811/081109eo.pdf.

30. Ruxandra, R., Filimon, S., 2010. Improving communication between doctors and patients. *Annals of Faculty of Economics* [cited 1 August 2011]; 1(2):1137-1140. Available from http://anale.steconomiceuoradea.ro/volume/2010/n2/182.pdf.

31. Feldman-Stewart, D., Brundage, M.D., Tishelman, C.A., 2005. conceptual framework for patient-professional communication: An application to the cancer context. Psycho-oncology 14, 801–809.

32. Carlsson, L., Feldman-Stewart, D., Tishelman, C., Brundage, M., 2005. Patient-professional communication research in cancer: An integrative review of research methods in the context of a conceptual framework. Psycho-oncology 14, 812–828.

33. Weissman, G.V., 2011. Evaluating associate degree nursing students' self-efficacy in communication skills and attitudes in caring or the dying patients. Teaching and Learning in Nursing 6, 64–72.

34. Ruiz-Moral, R., Rodriguez, E.R., Perula de Torres, L.A., de la Torre, J., 2006. Physician- patient communication: A study on the observed behaviours of specialty physicians and the ways their patients perceive them. Patient Education and Counseling 64, 242–248.

35. Van den Brink_Muinen, A., Verhaak, P.F.M., Bensing, J.M., Bahrs, O., Deveugele, M., Gask, L., et al., 2000. Doctor-patient communication in different European health care systems: Relevance and performance from the patients' perspective. Patient Education and Counseling 39, 115–127.

36. Shannon, C., Weaver, W., 1949. The mathematical theory of communication.. University of Illinois Press, Urbana.

37. Jones, S.E., LeBaron, C.D., 2002. Research on the relationship between verbal and nonverbal communication: emerging interactions. J of Communication, 499–521 [cited 12 August 2011]. DOI:10.111/j.1460-2466.2002.tbo2559.x.

38. Arora, R., 2000. Message and framing and credibility: application in dental services. Health Mark Q 18, 29–44.

39. Van Weert, J.C.M., Jansen, J., Spreeuwenberg, P.M.M., van Dulamn, S., Bensing, J.M., 2010. Article in press. Effects of communication skills training and a question prompt sheet to improve communication with older cancer patients: A randomized controlled trial. Crit Rev Oncol / Hematol. DOI:10.1016/j.critrevonc.2010.10.010.

40. Van Staa, A.L., 2010. Unraveling triadic communication in hospital consultations with adolescents with chronic conditions: The added value of mixed methods research. Patient Education and Counseling 82, 455–464.

41. Wissow, L., Gadomski, A., Roter, D., Larson, S., Lewis, B., Brown, J., 2011. Aspects of mental health communication skills training that predict parent and child outcomes in pediatric primary care. Patient Education and Counseling 82, 226–232.

42. Mitchell, W., Sloper, P., 2011. Making choices in my life: Listening to the ideas and experiences of young people in the UK who communicate non-verbally. Children and Youth Services Review 33, 521–527.

43. Roter, D.L., 2011. Oral literacy demand of health care communication: Challenges and solutions. Nursing Outlook 59, 79–84.

44. Schouten, B.C., Meeuwesen, L., 2006. Cultural differences in medical communication: a review of the literature. Patient Education and Counseling 64, 21–34.

45. Cooper, L.A., Roter, D.L., Johnson, R.L., Ford, D.E., Steinwachs, D.M., Powe, N.R., 2003. Patient-centered communication, ratings of care and concordance of patient and physician race. American College of Physician 139 (11), 907–915 Available from http://www.upenn.edu/ldi/paper-cooper.pdf.

46. Jain, P., Krieger, J.L., 2011. Moving beyond the language barrier: The communication strategies used by international medical graduates in intercultural medical encounters. Patient Education and Counseling 84, 98–104.

47. Hack, T.F., Degner, L.F., Parker, P.A., 2005. The communication goals and needs of cancer patients: a review. Psycho-Oncology 14, 831–845.

48. Farin, E., Gramm, L., Koisol, D., 2011. Development of a questionnaire to assess communication preferences of

patients with chronic illness. Patient Education and Counseling 82, 81–88.

49. Williams, K.N., Herman, R.E., 2001. Linking resident behavior to dementia care communication: Effects of emotional tone. Behavior Therapy 42, 42–46.

50. Helitzer, D.L., NaLoue, M., Wilson, B., Urquieta de Hernandez, B., Warner, T., Roter, D., 2011. A randomized controlled trial of communication training with primary care providers to improve patient-centeredness and health risk communication. Patient Education and Counseling. 82, 21–29.

51. Myren, H., Ekeberg, O., Stokland, O., 2010. Article in press: Satisfaction with communication in ICU patients and relatives: Comparisons with medical staffs' expectations and the relationship with psychological distress. Patient Education and Counseling. DOI: 10.1016/j.pec.2010.11.005.

52. Ye, J., Rust, G., Fry-Johnson, Y., Strothers, H., 2010. E-mail in patient-provider communication: A systematic review. Patient Education and Counseling 80, 266–273.

53. Masters, K., 2008. For what purpose and reasons do doctors use the internet: a systematic review. Int J Med Inform 74, 4–16.

54. Danesi M. Messages, signs, and meanings. third ed. Toronto: Canadian Scholars' Press Inc.

55. Valsiner, J., Hiatti, F.L., 2001. Process structure of semiotic mediation in human development. Human Development [cited 12 August 2011]; Mar- Jun;44/2/3: 84-97. Available from http://lcho.ucsd.edu/mac/Mail/xmcamail.2006_10.di/att-0296/01_Process_structure_Valsiner.pdf.

56. Littlejohn, S.W., Foss, K.A., Theories of human communication. [cited 1 August 2011]; 2-13. Available from http://www.cengagebrain.com/shop/content/littlejohn95877_0495095877_02.01_chapter01.

57. Ekman, P., Friesen, W., 1981. The repertoire of nonverbal behavior: categories, origins, usage, and coding. In: Kindon, A. (Ed.), Nonverbal communication,

interaction and gesture, Mouton Publishers, The Hague.

58. Uko Iniobong, I., 2006. Verbal and nonverbal communication. An Encyclopaedia of the Arts 3 (1), 1–5.

59. Mehrabian Albert, 1971. Silent messages, first ed. Wadsworth, Belmont, CA.

60. Ambady, N., LaPlante, D., Nguyen, T., Rosenthal, R., Chaumeton, N., Levinson, W., 2002. Surgeons' tone of voice: A clue to malpractice history. Surgery 132.

61. Buck, R., VanLear, C.A., September, 2002. Verbal and nonverbal communication: distinguishing symbolic, spontaneous, and pseudo-spontaneous nonverbal behaviour. J of Com, 522–541.

62. Ozlem Alp, K., 2010. A comparison of sign and symbol (their contents and boundaries). Semiotica [cited 1 August 2011];182-1/4:1-13. DOI: 10.1515/semi.2010.048.

63. Wiener, M., Devoe, S., Rubinow, S., Geller, J., Nonverbal behaviour and non-verbal communication. Psychological Review 79(3):185–214

64. Cantor, R.M., 2000. Foundation of Roentgen semiotics. Semiotica [cited 1 August 2011]; 131:1-18. Available from http://www.roentgensemiotics.net/foundations.htm.

65. Rogers, C.R., Roethlisberger, F.J., 1991. Barriers and gateways to communication. HBR [cited 1 August 2011];Nov-Dec 1991;105-111. Available from http://www.deloitte.com/assests/Dcom-SouthAfrica/ Local%20Assests/Documents/Article.pdf.

66. Frank, L.K., 1961. Interprofessional communication. AJPH [cited 1 July 2011];51:12:1798-1804. Available from http://ajph.aphapublications.org/cgi/reprint/51/12/1798.pdf.

67. Berne, E., 1996. Games people play: The basic handbook of transactional analysis. Ballatine Books, New York.

68. Booth, L., 2007. Observations and reflections of communication in health care – could Transactional Analysis be used as an effective approach? Radiography 13, 135–141.

69. Henwood, S.M., Lister, J., 2007. NLP and coaching in health care: Developing expert practice. Wiley, Chichester.

Chapter 2

1. Reeves, P.J., 1999. Models of Care for Diagnostic Radiography and Their Use in the Education of Undergraduate and Postgraduate Students. PhD thesis. University of Wales, Bangor.

2. Lown, B.A., Roy, E., Gorman, P., Sasson, J.P., 2009. Womens' and Residents' Experiences of Communication in the Diagnostic Mammography Suite. Patient Education and Counselling 77, 328–337.

3. Hendry, J.A., 2011. A Qualitative Focus Group Study to Explore the Information, Support and Communication Needs of Women Receiving Adjuvant Radiotherapy for Breast Cancer. Journal of Radiotherapy in Practice 10, 103–115.

4. Johnson, J., 1999. "Living with Radiotherapy": The Experiences of Women with Breast Cancer. Journal of Radiotherapy in Practice 1, 17–25.

5. Menard, C., 2005. Management of Breast Cancer ... a Personal Perspective. When a Radiation Therapist becomes the Patient. CAMRT 36 (4), 45.

6. Reeves, P., 2006. The Pink Ribbon: Personal Experiences of the Breast Screening Service Synergy February.

7. Singh, K., Hodgson, D., 2010. How can the Multidisciplinary Team meet the Psychological Needs of Adolescents with Cancer? A Review of the Literature Journal of Radiotherapy in Practice, 1–10 (in press).

8. Bolderston, A., Lewis, D., Chai, M.J., 2010. The Concept of Caring: Perceptions of Radiation Therapists. Radiography 16, 198–208.

9. Hughes, J.H., Schemitzki, P., Byers, J., Likes, K., 1980. Trauma in Patients Influenced by Drugs and Alcohol. Ann Emerg Med 9 (1), 7–11.

10. Helpguide.org; Drug Abuse and Addiction. Last accessed 8/8/11 at http://helpguide.org/mental/drug_substance_abuse_addiction_signs_effects_treatment.htm

11. Halkett, G.K.B., McKay, J., Shaw, T., 2011. Improving Students' Confidence Levels in Communicating with Patients

and Introducing Students to the Importance of History Taking. Radiography 17, 55–60.

12. Taylor, C., Benger, J.R., 2004. Patient Satisfaction in Emergency Medicine. Emergency Medicine Journal 21, 528–532.

13. Wiman, E., Wikblad, K., Idvall, E., 2007. Trauma Patients' Encounters with the Team in the Emergency Department- A Qualitative Study. International Journal of Nursing Studies 44, 714–722.

14. Proctor, A., Morse, J.M., Khonsari, E.S., 1996. Sounds of Comfort in the Trauma Center: How Nurses Talk to Patients in Pain. Social Science & Medicine 42 (12), 1669–1680.

15. Culmer, P., 1995. Care of the Patient in Diagnostic Radiography, seventh ed. Blackwell Science, Oxford.

16. Sisson, R., 1990. Effects of Auditory Stimuli on Comatose Patients with Head Injury Heart And Lung 19 (4), 373–378.

17. Leigh, K., 2001. Communicating with. Unconscious Patients Nursing Times 97 (48), 35–39.

18. Child Development Institute. http://www.childdevelopmentinfo. com/development/piaget.shtml Last accessed 13/8/11

19. BTEC First Children's Care learning and Development http:// www.pearsonschoolsandfecolleges. co.uk/FEAndVocational/Childcare /BTEC/BTECFirstChildrensCareLea rningandDevelop/Samples/Sampl eMaterial/UCD%20Unit%201.pdf Last accessed 13/8/11

20. Boynes, S., Hardy, M., 2003. Paediatric Radiography. Blackwell Scientific, Oxford.

21. Howells, R., Lopez, T., 2008. Better Communication with Children and Patients Paediatrics & Child Health 18 (8), 381–385.

22. Chesson, R., Good, M., Hart, C.L., 2002. Will it Hurt? Patients' Experience of X-ray Examinations: A Pilot Study. Paediatric Radiology 32, 67–73.

23. Mathers, S., Anderson, H., McDonald, S., 2011. A survey of Imaging Services for Children in England, Wales and Scotland. Radiography 17, 20–27.

24. Pimm, P., Fitzgerald, E., Taylor, L., 1997. Caring for Children Undergoing Radiotherapy Radiography 3, 27–30.

25. Tonkin, A., Weldon, C., 2011. Letter to the Editor: A Survey of Imaging Services for Children in England, Wales and Scotland – The Role of the Play Specialist Radiography In press. DOI:10.1016/j. radi.2011.04.004.

26. Byczkowski, T.L., Kollar, L.M., Britto, M.T., 2010. Family Experiences With Outpatient Care: Do Adolescents and Parents Have the Same Perceptions? Journal of Adolescent Health 47, 92–98.

27. Teenage Cancer Trust website http://www.teenagecancertrust.org/ who-we-are/about-us/reflections- on-20-years/ Last accessed 23/8/11

28. Bull, S. (2006), Radiography and the ageing population Synergy, December 22–27

29. Reeves, P., 2006. Chronic Disease & Independence; a Case Study Radiography 12 (3), 235–257. DOI:10.1016/j.radi.2005.06.003.

30. McGhie, J., McClellan, M., 1997. Catering for the Needs of an Increasingly Elderly Population in Diagnostic Imaging. Radiography 3, 209–216.

31. Fowler, P., 1997. Attitudes towards the Older Adult Patient: A Study of the Influence that Radiographers have on Radiography Students. Radiography 3, 217–227.

32. We may be Fat but we're Healthier than Ever: How British Life expectancy has soared to 80 years http://www.dailymail.co.uk/health/ article-1367471/Were-healthier- How-British-life-expectancy- soared-past-U-S-80-years-old.html Last accessed 19/8/11

33. Hope, J., Neglect of the Elderly who die in NHS Hospitals. http:// www.dailymail.co.uk/news/article- 1328538/Shameful-neglect-elderly- die-NHS-hospitals.html November 2010. Last accessed 21/8/11.

34. Kada, S., 2009. Radiographers' Attitudes towards Persons with Dementia European Journal of Radiography 1, 163–168.

35. Lambrinou, E., Sourtzi, P., Kalokerinou, A., Lemonidu, C., 2009. Attitudes and Knowledge of the Greek Nursing Students towards Older People. Nurse Education Today 29, 617–622.

36. Hobbs, C., Dean, C.M., Higgs, J., Adamson, B., 2006. Physiotherapy Students' Attitudes Towards and Knowledge of Older People. Australian Journal of Physiotherapy 52, 115–119.

37. Koh, L.C., 2011. Student attitudes and educational support in caring for older people- A review of literature. Nurse Education in Practice. DOI:10.1016/j.nepr. 2011.04.007.

38. Coping with Aggressive Dementia http://medicsalertbracelets.com/ how-to-diffuse-anger-in- dementia-patients/ Last accessed 25/8/11

39. Mowbray, J., Mowbray, H., 2010. A Consideration of the Needs of the Adult Patient with Dementia Attending for Radiotherapy and its Impact on the Practical Consent Process. Journal of Radiotherapy in Practice 9, 107–116.

Acknowledgements go to radiotherapy colleagues at the Society of Radiographers and in centres nationwide who were kind enough to email me details of their practice with children.

Chapter 3

1. Office for Disability Issues, Disability Prevalence Factsheet. updated June 2010 available at http://odi.dwp.gov.uk/disability- statistics-and-research/disability- facts-and-figures.php accessed August 2011.

2. Equality Act, 2010. Public sector equality duty, what do I need to know? A quick start guide for public sector organisations. Government Equality Office available at http://www.homeoffic e.gov.uk/publications/equalities/ equality-act-publications/equality- act-guidance/equality-duty? view=Binary accessed July 2011.

3. Koprowska, J., 2010. Communication and interpersonal skills in social work. Learning Matters, Exeter.

4. Oliver, M., 1990. The politics of disablement. MacMillan, Basingstoke.

5. Strudwick, R., Mackay, S., Hicks, S., 2010. Guest Editorial Synergy April. Is diagnostic radiography a caring profession?

6. Koubel, G., Bungay, H. (Eds.), 2009. The challenge of person-centred care: An interprofessional perspective, Palgrave Macmillan, Basingstoke.

7. Office of Disability Issues (2011) available at http://odi.dwp.gov.uk/index.php accessed on June 2011.

8. Department of Health, 2003. The essence of care: Patient focussed benchmarks for health care practitioners. Department of Health, London.

9. Bungay, H., Sandys, R., 2009. Person-centred care: with dignity and respect. In: Koubel, G., Bungay, H. (Eds.), The challenge of person-centred care: An interprofessional perspective, Palgrave Macmillan, Basingstoke.

10. Department of Education and Employment (1995) The Disability and Discrimination Act available at http://www.legislation. gov.uk/ukpga/1995/50 accessed July 2011

11. Disability and Discrimination Act. http://www.legislation.gov.uk/uk pga/2005/.

12. Society of Radiographers, Code of Conduct and Ethics. www.sor.org.uk accessed July 2011.

13. Action on Hearing Loss, About deafness and hearing loss: statistics. http://www.actiononhe aringloss.org.uk/ accessed August 2011.

14. McAleer, M., 2006. Communicating effectively with deaf patients. Nursing Standard 20 (19), 51–54.

15. Reeves, D., Kokoruwe, B., 2005. Communication and communication support in primary care: A survey of Deaf patients. Audiological Medicine 3 (2), 95–107.

16. Royal National Institute for Deaf People (RNID), 2004. A Simple Cure. RNID, London.

17. Alzheimers Society, Top Tips for Nurses: Communication. available at http://www.alzheimers.org.uk/ site/scripts/documents_info.php? documentID=1211&categoryID= 200306&pageNumber=2.

18. The Stroke Association, 2009. Communication problems after stroke fact sheet 3 The Stroke Association. available at www.stroke.org.uk accessed July 2011.

19. Department of Health, 2001. Valuing people: A new strategy for learning disability for the 21st century. Department of Health, London.

20. Bradshaw, J., 2007. Between you and me: Developing communication in partnership with people with learning disabilities. In: Carnaby, S. (Ed.), (2007) Learning Disability Today, Pavilion Publishing, Brighton.

21. Williamson, A., 2004. Improving services for people with learning disabilities. Nursing Standard 18 (24), 43–51.

22. Mental Capacity Act, Code of Practice (2007), Department of Constitutional Affairs. available at http://www.publicguardian.gov.uk/ docs/mca-code-practice-0509.pdf.

Chapter 4

1. Hall, P., May 2005. Interprofessional teamwork: professional cultures as barriers. Journal of Interprofessional Care [cited 1 July 2011]; Supplement 1: 188 - 196 . DOI:10.1080/13561 820500081745.

2. Watermeyer, J., Penn, C., 2009. Working across language and culture barriers: communication skills for pharmacists. University of Witwatersrand, Johannesburg.

3. Robbins, S.P., 2002. Organizational behavior, tenth ed. Prentice-Hall, Englewood Cliffs.

4. Lingard, L., Espin, S., Rubin, B., et al., 2005. Getting teams to talk: development and pilot implementation or a checklist to promote interprofessional communication in OR. Qual Saf Health Care [cited 1 July 2011]; 14:304-346 . DOI:0.1136/q shc.2004.012377.

5. Leonard, M., Graham, S., Bonacum, D., 2004. The human factor: the critical importance of effective teamwork and communication in providing safe care. Qual Saf Health Care [cited 1 July 2011];13(Suppl 1): i85-i90. DOI:10.1136/q shc.2004.010033.

6. Weissman, G.V., 2011. Evaluating associate degree nursing students' self-efficacy in communication skills and attitudes in caring or the dying patients. Teaching and Learning in Nursing 6 (2), 64–72.

7. Thomas, E.J., Bryan, Sexton J, Helmreich, R.L., 2003. Discrepant attitudes about teamwork among critical care nurses and physicians. Crit Care Med [cited 1 July 2011];31:3:956. DOI:10.1097/ 01.ccm.000056183.89175.76 http://bmhlibrary.info/956.pdf.

8. Solet, D.J., Norvell, J.M., Gale, H.R., Frankel, R., 2005. Lost in translation: Challenges and opportunities in physician-to-physician communication during patient handoffs. Acad Med [cited 1 July 2011]; 80:1094-1099. Available from http://cms.feinberg. northwestern.edu/bin/u/h/Solet_ et_al_2005.pdf.

9. Schoop, M., Wastell, D.G., 1999. Effective multidisciplinary communication in healthcare: cooperative documentation systems. Method Inform Med [cited 1 July 2011];265-274. Available from http://www.schatteur.de/en/magazi ne/subject-areas/journals-a-z/meth ods/contents/archive/issue/715/ma nuscript/82.html.

10. West, E., 2001. Management matters: the link between hospital organization and quality patient care. Quality in Health Care [cited 1 July 2011];10:40-48. Available from http://www.ncbi.nlm.nih.gov/pmc/ articles/PMC1743422/pdf/v010p00 040.pdf.

11. Frank, L.K., 1961. Interprofessional communication. AJPH [cited 1 July 2011];51:12:1798-1804. Available from http://ajph.aphap ublications.org/cgi/reprint/51/12/ 1798.pdf.

12. Schoop, M., 1999. An empirical study of multidisciplinary communication in healthcare using a language-action perspective. , [cited 1 July 2011]. Available from http://scholar.goog

le.co.za/scholar?start=10&q=Schoo
p+M&hl=en&as_sdt=0,5.

13. Rafferty, A.M., Ball, J., Aiken, L.H.,
2001. Are team and professional
autonomy compatible, and do they
result in improved hospital care?
Quality in Health Care [cited 1
July 2011];10(Suppl II):ii32-ii37.
Available from http://www.ncbi.nl
m.nih.gov/pmc/articles/PMC1765
758/pdf/v010p0ii32.pdf.

14. Kubik-Huch, R.A., Klaghofer,
R., Römpler, M., Weber, A.,
Buddeberg-Fischer, 2010.
Workplace experience of
radiographers: impact of structural
and interpersonal interventions.
Eur Radiol [cited 1 July
2011];20:377-384 . DOI:10.1007/
s00330-009-1565-5.

15. Verhovesk, E.L., Bvington,
R.L., Deshkulkarni, S., 2010.
Perceptions of interprofessional
communication: impact on
patient care, occupational stress,
and job satisfaction. The Internet
Journal of Radiology [cited 1 July
2011] available from http://www.
ispub.com/journal/the_internet_
journal_of_radiology/volume_
12_number_2_6/article/perc
eptions-of-interprofessional-
communication-impact-on-
patient-care-occupational-stress-
and-job-satisfaction.html.

16. Aston, J., Shi, E., Bullǫt, H.,
Galway, R., Crisp, J., 2005.
Qualitative evaluation of regular
morning meetings aimed at
improving interdisciplinary
communication and patient
outcomes. International J of Nurs
practice [cited 1 July 2011];11:206-
213. https://www.cihc.ca/library/
bitstream/10296/376/1/AstonEtAl_
MorningMeetings_2005.pdf.

17. Jenkins, V.A., Fallowfield, L.F.,
Poole, K., 2001. Are members of
multidisciplinary teams in breast
cancer aware of each other's
informational roles? Quality
in Health Care [cited 7 August
2011];10:70-75. Available from
http://www.ncbi.nlm.nih.gov/pmc
/articles/PMC1757990/pdf/v010p
00070.pdf.

18. Martìn-Rodrìguez, L.S., Beaulieu,
M., D'Amour, D., Ferrada-Videla,
M., 2005. The determinants of
successful collaboration: a review
of theoretical and empirical studies

[cited 1 July 2011]; Suppl 1:132-147.
DOI:10.1080/13561820500082677.

19. Zwarenstein, M., Goldman, J.,
Reeves Scott. Interprofessional
collaboration, 2009. effects of
practice-based interventions on
professional practice and healthcare.
[Cochrane review]. The Cochrane
Library, Issue 4. Available at http://
www.thecochranelibrary.com.

20. Parsell, G., Bligh, J., 1999. The
development of a questionnaire
to assess the readiness of health
care students for interprofessional
learning (RIPLS). Medical
Education [cited 7 August 2011],
33, 095±100. Available from
http://www.med.monash.edu/srh/
mudrih/document_links/hsin/
development-questionnaire-
ripls.pdf.

21. Sullivan, E.J., Decker, P.J.,
2009. Effective leadership and
management in nursing, seventh
ed. Pearson Publishing, London.

22. Etheredge, H.R., 2011. An opinion
on radiography, ethics and law in
South Africa. The South African
Radiographer 49 (1), 9–12.

23. Philipp, R., Dodwell, P., 2005.
Improved communication between
doctors and with managers would
benefit professional integrity and
reduce the occupational medicine
workload. Occ Med [cited 30 July
2001];55: 40-47, DOI:10.1093/occ
med/kqh125.

24. Code of ethics –ISRRT, 2011.
The South African Radiographer
49 (1), 8.

25. Anthony, W.P., Perrewé, P.L.,
Kacmar, K.M., 1996. Strategic
human resource management,
second ed. Harcourt Brace & Co,
Orlando.

26. Jones, S.E., LeBaron, C.D., 2002.
Research on the relationship
between verbal and nonverbal
communication: emerging
interactions. J of Communication
[cited 12 August 2011];499-
521, DOI:10.111/j.1460-
2466.2002.tbo2559.

27. Bordia, P., 1997. Face-to-face
versus computer- mediated
communication: A synthesis
of the experimental literature.
The Journal of Business
Communication 34 (I), 99–120
[cited 12 August 2011].

28. Branger, P.J., van der Wouden,
J.C., Schudel, B.R., Verboog, E.,
Duisterhout, J.S., van der Lei, J.,
vanBemmel, J.H., 1992. Electronic
communication between providers
of primary and secondary care.
BMJ [cited 21 August 2011];305, 31
October 1992: 1068-1070. Available
from http://www.bmj.com/content/
305/6861/1068.full.pdf.

29. Shapiro, N.Z., Anderson, R.H.,
1985. Toward an ethics and
etiquette for electronic mail, [Cited
12 August 2011] Available from
http://www.rand.org/pubs/reports/
2007/R3283.pdf.

30. Albersheim, S., 2010. E-mail
communication in paediatrics:
Ethical and clinical considerations.
Paediatr Child Health [cited 21
August 2011]; March; 15(3):163-
165. Available from http://www.
ncbi.nlm.nih.gov/pmc/articles/
PMC2865955/.

31. Damian, D.E., Zowghi, D.,
2003. Requirement engineering
challenges in multi-site software
development organizations.
Requirements Engineering Journal
8, 149–160 [cited 21 August 2011].

32. Currell, R., Urquhart, C.,
Wainwright, P., Lewis, R.,
Telemedicine versus face to face
patient care: effects on professional
practice and health care outcomes
(Cochrane review). [cited 12
August 2011]; In The Cochrane
Library 2010, Issue 1. Available at
http://www.thecochranelibrary.
com

33. Chau, P.Y.K., Jen-Hwa Hu, P.,
2002. Investigating healthcare
professionals' decisions to
accept telemedicine technology:
an empirical test of competing
theories. Information
&Management [cited 12 August
2011]; 39: 297-311. Available from
http://etidweb.tamu.edu/faculty/
beasley/ENTC489/2011_Spring_
ENTC489/Chau-InfoManag-2002-
telemedicine_adoption.pdf.

Chapter 5

1. Andrews, M.A., Boyle, J., 2003.
Transcultural concepts in nursing
care, fourth ed. Lippincott,
Philadelphia.

2. Huff, M.H., Kline, M.V., 1999.
Promoting health in multicultural

populations. SAGE Publication, Thousand Oaks, CA.

3. Leininger, M.M., 1991. Culture, care, diversity and universality: A theory of nursing. National League of Nursing, New York.

4. Durham, W.H., 2008. COEVOLUTION: Gene, culture and human diversity. Stanford University Press, Stanford, California.

5. World Health Organization. What do we mean by "sex" and "gender"? Retrieved 10 November 2011, from http://www.who.int/gender/whatisgender/en/

6. Bruner, J., 1990. Acts of meaning. Harvard University Press, Cambridge, MA.

7. The College of Radiographers, 2002. Statements for professional conduct. College of Radiographers, London.

8. Health Professions Council. Standards of proficiency for radiographers. Retrieved 20 November 2011, from http://www.hpc-uk.org/assets/documents/10000DBstandards_of_proficiency_Radiographers.pdf

9. United Kingdom National Statistics. Retrieved 27 December 2011, from http://www.statistics.gov.uk/hub/population/ageing/older-people/index.html

10. Acas. The Equality Act. What's new for employers. Retrieved 23 December 2011, from http://www.acas.org.uk/training.

11. Matthews R., Cultural patterns of South Asian and Southeast Asian Americans. Intervention in School and Clinic: November 2000.

12. Ahmad, F., Gupta, A., Rawlins, J., Stewart, D.E., 2002. Preferences for gender of family physician among Canadian-European descent and South-Asian immigrant women. family Practice 19 (2), 146–153.

13. Casse, P., 1981. Training for the cross-cultural mind, second ed. The Society for Intercultural Education, Washington DC.

14. Bochner, S., 1982. Cultures in contact. Pergamon Press, Oxford.

15. Blais, K., 1984. Florida's task force on cultural diversity. The Florida Nurse 12.

16. Harris, P.R., Moran, R.T., 1987. Managing cultural differences, second ed. Gulf Publishing Co, Houston.

Chapter 6

1. Dryden, W., 1986. Individual Therapy in Britain. Harper & Row, London.

2. Pavlov, I.P., 1927. Lectures on Conditioned Reflexes. Liveright, New York.

3. Skinner, B.F., 1953. Science and Human Behaviour. Macmillan, New York.

4. Rogers, C.R., 1969. Freedom to Learn. Charles E. Merrill, Columbus, Ohio.

5. Rogers, C.R., 1980. A Way of Being. Houghton Mifflin, Boston.

6. Maslow AH. Motivation and Personality. New York: Harper & Row.

7. Lee, S., Tsang, A., Ruscio, A.M., Haro, J.M., Stein, D.J., Alonso, J., et al., 2009. Implications of modifying the duration requirement of generalized anxiety disorder in developed and developing countries. Psychol Med 39 (07), 1163.

8. Russell, G., 1999. Essential Psychology. Routledge, London.

9. Miller, N.E., 1941. The Frustration-aggression Hypothesis. Psychological Review 48 (4), 337.

10. Janis, I.L., Mann, L., 1979. Decision Making. Free Press, New York.

11. Yerkes, R.M., Dodson, D.J., 1908. The Relative Strength of Stimulus to Rapidity of Habit Formation. J Comp Nuero Psych 18, 459–482.

12. Carr, D.B., Goudas, L.C., 1999. Acute Pain. The Lancet 353, 2051–2058.

13. Hoffman, G.A., Harrington, A., Fields, H.L., 2005. Pain and the Placebo: What we have learned. Perspectives in Biology and Medicine 48 (2), 248–265.

14. Benedetti, F., 2006. Placebo Analgesia. Neurological Science 27, S100–S127.

15. Erikson, E.H., 1950. Childhood and Society. Norton, New York.

16. Piaget, J., 1954. The Construction of Reality in the Child. Basic books, New york.

17. Veldtman, G.R., Matley, S.L., Kendall, L., Quirk, J., Gibbs, J.L., Parsons, J.M., et al., 2000. Illness Understanding in Children and Adolescents With Heart Disease. Heart 84 (4), 395–397.

18. Donaldson, M., 1990. Children's Minds, second ed. Fontana, Glasgow.

19. Bowlby, J., 1981. Attachment and Loss. Penguin, Middlesex.

20. Saunders, A.N., 1994. Changing Nurse's Attitudes Toward Parenting in NICU. Pediatric Nursing 20 (4), 392–394.

21. Wandrak, R., 1998. Interpersonal Skills for Nurses & Health Care Professionals. Blackwell Sciences, Oxford.

22. Coleman, P.G., O'Hanlon, A., 2004. Ageing and Development. Arnold, London.

23. Ferri, C.P., Prince, M., Bravne, C., Brodaty, H., Fratiglioni, L., Ganguli, M., et al., 2005. Global prevalence of dementia: a Delphi consensus study. The Lancet 366, 2112–2117.

24. Walker, J., Payne, S., Smith, P., Jarrett, N., 2007. Psychology for Nurses and the Caring Professions, third ed. Open University Press, Maidenhead.

25. Meadows, S., 1993. The Child as Thinker. Routlegde, London.

Chapter 7

1. http://info.cancerresearchuk.org/cancerstats/incidence/prevalence/

2. http://www.nhs.uk/Livewell/cancer/Pages/Gettingyourresults.aspx)

3. http://www.statistics.gov.uk/pdfdir/can0711.pdf

4. Paraphrased from A W Frank At the Will of the Body: Reflection on Illness, 2001.

5. Buckman, R., 1996. Talking to patients about cancer. No excuse now for not doing it. BMJ 313, 699–700.

6. White, C., 2004. Meaning and its measurement in psychosocial oncology. Psychooncology 13 (7), 468–481.

7. Hegel, M., Collins, E., Kearing, S., Gillock, K., Moore, C., Ahles, T., 2008. Sensitivity and specificity of the Distress Thermometer for depression in newly

diagnosed breast cancer patients. Psychooncology 17 (6), 556–560.

8. http://www.informationprescript ion. info accessed 09.08.11)

9. www.gponeclick.com. Accessed 12.08.11

Chapter 8

1. NICE, 2004. Improving Supportive and Palliative Care for Adults With Cancer.

2. Department of Health. End of Life Care Strategy - promoting high quality care for all adults at the end of life. 2008.

3. Dunlop R., 2001 Specialist palliative care and non-malignant diseases. In: Addington-Hall, J., Higginson, I., (Eds.), Palliative Care for Non-cancer Patients; 189.

4. NCPC, 2011. National Council for Palliative Care. Available at http://www.ncpc.org.uk/ Accessed 08/18, 2011.

5. Health Select Committee, 2004. House of Commons Health Select Committee Report, 3.

6. Department of Health, 2003. Building on the Best: Choice, Responsiveness and Equality in the NHS.

7. DoH, 2011. End of Life Care for All – eLearning (e-ELCA). Available at http://www.endoflifecareforadults. nhs.uk/education-and-training/ eelca Accessed 08/18, 2011.

8. ACT, 2011. Association for Childrens Palliative Care. Available at www.act.org.uk Accessed 08/18, 2011.

9. Department of Health, 2007. Palliative Care Statistics for Children and Young Adults.

10. Gomes, B., Higginson, I., 2008. Where people die (1974-2030): past trends, future projections and implications for care. Palliative medicine 22, 33.

11. National Audit Office, 2008. End of Life Care.

12. Ncpc, NEoLCP, 2011. Commissioning End of Life Care: Act & Early.

Chapter 9

1. Allisy-Roberts, P., Williams, J., 2008. Farr's physics for medical imaging, second ed. Elsevier, Edinburgh.

2. Hall, E.J., 1997. Radiation: the two-edged sword: risks factors and protection. RSNA Refresher Course 320, Chicago.

3. Brusin, J.H., 2007. Radiation protection. Radiologic Technology 78 (5), 378–392.

4. Dal Masso, L., Bossetti, C., La Vecchia, C., Francceschi, S., Risk factors for thyroid cancer: an epidemiological review focused on nutritional factors, Cancer Causes Control; 20(1), 75–86.

5. The Health and Safety at Work Act. London, HMSO: 1974.

6. The Ionising Radiation Regulations. HMSO, London S.I. 1999/3232.

7. The Ionising Radiation (Medical Exposure) Regulations. HMSO, London S.I. 2000/1059.

8. The Royal College of Radiologists. Making the best use of clinical radiology services: referral guidelines, sixth ed. London; Royal College of Radiologists.

9. Environment Agency, 2002. Radioactive Substances Regulation Process Managemnt. Interim guidance on "best practicable means" for non-nuclear users of radioactive substances. Environment Agency, London.

10. International Commission on Radiological Protection. 1990 Recommendations of the international commission on radiological protection. vol. 21. Pergamon Press, Oxford nos 1–3. (ICRP Publication No 60).

11. National Radiological Protection Board and Royal College of Radiologists. Patient dose reduction in diagnostic radiology. vol, 1. NRPB, no. 3.

12. Bushong, S.C., 2008. Radiologic Science for Technologists; physics, biology and protection, nineth ed. Elsevier, St Louis.

13. Furlow, B., 2011. Radiation protection in pediatric imaging. Radiologic Technology 82 (5), 421–439.

14. United Nations Scientific Committe on the effect of atomic radiation, 2008. Sources and effects of ionising radiation. United Nations Scientific Committe on the effects of atomic radiation. Report to the General Assembly Scientific

Annexes A and B. Vol. 1. United Nations, New York.

Chapter 11

1. The Prescription only Medicines (Human Use) Amendment Order 2000. TSO, London. 2000.

2. Ott, D.J., Chen, Y.M., Gelfand, D.W., Wu, W.C., Munitz, H.A., 1986 May. Single-contrast vs double-contrast barium enema in the detection of colonic polyps. AJR Am J Roentgenol 146 (5), 993–996.

3. Coblentz, C.L., Frost, R.A., Molinaro, V., Stevenson, G.W., 1985 Oct. Pain after barium enema: effect of CO_2 and air on double-contrast study. Radiology 157 (1), 35–36.

4. Webb, J.A.W., 2009. Prevention of acute reactions. In: Thomsen, H.S., Webb JAW, J.A.W. (Eds.), Contrast Media Safety Issues and ESUR Guidelines, Springer-Verlag, Berlin, pp. 43–49.

5. European Society for Urogenital Radiology. ESUR Guidelines on Contrast Media. 2008.

6. Morcos, S.K., Thomsen, H.S., Webb, J.A., 1999. Contrast-media-induced nephrotoxicity: a consensus report. Contrast Media Safety Committee, European Society of Urogenital Radiology (ESUR). Eur Radiol 9 (8), 1602–1613.

7. Thomsen, H.S., Morcos, S.K., 2003 Aug. Contrast media and the kidney: European Society of Urogenital Radiology (ESUR) guidelines. Br J Radiol 76 (908), 513–518.

8. Mehran, R., Nikolsky, E., 2006 Apr. Contrast-induced nephropathy: definition, epidemiology, and patients at risk. Kidney Int Suppl (100), S11–S15.

9. Chalmers, N., Jackson, R.W., 1999 Jul. Comparison of iodixanol and iohexol in renal impairment. Br J Radiol 72 (859), 701–703.

10. Heinrich, M.C., Haberle, L., Muller, V., Bautz, W., Uder, M., 2009 Jan. Nephrotoxicity of iso-osmolar iodixanol compared with nonionic low-osmolar contrast media: meta-analysis of randomized controlled trials. Radiology 250 (1), 68–86.

11. Duncan, L., Heathcote, J., Djurdjev, O., Levin, A., 2001 May. Screening for renal disease using serum creatinine: who are we missing? Nephrol Dial Transplant 16 (5), 1042–1046.

12. Levey, A.S., Eckardt, K.U., Tsukamoto, Y., Levin, A., Coresh, J., Rossert, J., et al., 2005 Jun. Definition and classification of chronic kidney disease: a position statement from Kidney Disease: Improving Global Outcomes (KDIGO). Kidney Int 67 (6), 2089–2100.

13. McCullough, P.A., Wolyn, R., Rocher, L.L., Levin, R.N., O'Neill, W.W., 1997 Nov. Acute renal failure after coronary intervention: incidence, risk factors, and relationship to mortality. Am J Med 103 (5), 368–375.

14. Levey, A.S., Bosch, J.P., Lewis, J.B., Greene, T., Rogers, N., Roth, D., 1999 Mar 16. A more accurate method to estimate glomerular filtration rate from serum creatinine: a new prediction equation. Modification of Diet in Renal Disease Study Group. Ann Intern Med 130 (6), 461–470.

15. Cockcroft, D.W., Gault, M.H., 1976. Prediction of creatinine clearance from serum creatinine. Nephron 16 (1), 31–41.

16. Stein, J., 2011. Drugs offer no CIN protection. Renal & Urology News [serial on the Internet]. [cited 2011 31 August]; Jan: Available from http://www.renalandurologynews.com/drug-offers-no-cin-protection/article/194033.

17. McCartney, M.M., Gilbert, F.J., Murchison, L.E., Pearson, D., McHardy, K., Murray, A.D., 1999 Jan. Metformin and contrast media–a dangerous combination? Clin Radiol 54 (1), 29–33.

18. Bellin, M.F., Jakobsen, J.A., Tomassin, I., Thomsen, H.S., Morcos, S.K., Almen, T., et al., 2002 Nov. Contrast medium extravasation injury: guidelines for prevention and management. Eur Radiol 12 (11), 2807–2812.

19. Grand, A., Yeager, B., Wollstein, R., 2008 Fall. Compartment syndrome presenting as ischemia following extravasation of contrast material. Can J Plast Surg 16(3):173–174.

20. McCarthy, C.S., Becker, J.A., 1992 May. Multiple myeloma and contrast media. Radiology 183 (2), 519–521.

21. Webb, J.A., Thomsen, H.S., Morcos, S.K., 2005 Jun. The use of iodinated and gadolinium contrast media during pregnancy and lactation. Eur Radiol 15 (6), 1234–1240.

22. Atwell, T.D., Lteif, A.N., Brown, D.L., McCann, M., Townsend, J.E., Leroy, A.J., 2008 Jul. Neonatal thyroid function after administration of IV iodinated contrast agent to 21 pregnant patients. AJR Am J Roentgenol 191 (1), 268–271.

23. Newman, J., 2007 Apr. Breastfeeding and radiologic procedures. Can Fam Physician 53 (4), 630–631.

24. Singh, J., Daftary, A., 2008 Jun. Iodinated contrast media and their adverse reactions. J Nucl Med Technol 36 (2), 69–74 quiz 6–7.

25. Miller, S.H., 1997 Apr. Anaphylactoid reaction after oral administration of diatrizoate meglumine and diatrizoate sodium solution. AJR Am J Roentgenol 168 (4), 959–961.

26. Seymour, C.W., Pryor, J.P., Gupta, R., Schwab, C.W., 2004 Nov. Anaphylactoid reaction to oral contrast for computed tomography. J Trauma 57 (5), 1105–1107.

27. Qin, S., Caskey, C.F., Ferrara, K.W., 2009 Mar 21. Ultrasound contrast microbubbles in imaging and therapy: physical principles and engineering. Phys Med Biol 54 (6), R27–R57.

28. Dayton, P.A., Morgan, K.E., Klibanov, A.L., Brandenburger, G.H., Ferrara, K.W., 1999. Optical and acoustical observations of the effects of ultrasound on contrast agents. IEEE Trans Ultrason Ferroelectr Freq Control 46 (1), 220–232.

29. Forsberg, F., Merton, D.A., Liu, J.B., Needleman, L., Goldberg, B.B., 1998 Feb. Clinical applications of ultrasound contrast agents. Ultrasonics 36 (1-5), 695–701.

30. Morawski, A.M., Lanza, G.A., Wickline, S.A., 2005 Feb. Targeted contrast agents for magnetic resonance imaging and ultrasound.

Curr Opin Biotechnol 16 (1), 89–92.

31. Hauff, P., Reinhardt, M., Briel, A., Debus, N., Schirner, M., 2004 Jun. Molecular targeting of lymph nodes with L-selectin ligand-specific US contrast agent: a feasibility study in mice and dogs. Radiology 231 (3), 667–673.

32. Leong-Poi, H., Christiansen, J., Klibanov, A.L., Kaul, S., Lindner, J.R., 2003 Jan 28. Noninvasive assessment of angiogenesis by ultrasound and microbubbles targeted to alpha(v)-integrins. Circulation 107 (3), 455–460.

33. Schumann, P.A., Christiansen, J.P., Quigley, R.M., McCreery, T.P., Sweitzer, R.H., Unger, E.C., et al., 2002 Nov. Targeted-microbubble binding selectively to GPIIb IIIa receptors of platelet thrombi. Invest Radiol 37 (11), 587–593.

34. Ellegala, D.B., Leong-Poi, H., Carpenter, J.E., Klibanov, A.L., Kaul, S., Shaffrey, M.E., et al., 2003 Jul 22. Imaging tumor angiogenesis with contrast ultrasound and microbubbles targeted to alpha(v)beta3. Circulation 108 (3), 336–341.

35. Weller, G.E., Lu, E., Csikari, M.M., Klibanov, A.L., Fischer, D., Wagner, W.R., et al., 2003 Jul 15. Ultrasound imaging of acute cardiac transplant rejection with microbubbles targeted to intercellular adhesion molecule-1. Circulation 108 (2), 218–224.

36. Rinck, P.A., Muller, R.N., 1999. Field strength and dose dependence of contrast enhancement by gadolinium-based MR contrast agents. Eur Radiol 9 (5), 998–1004.

37. Noda, Y., Ogawa, Y., Nishioka, A., Inomata, T., Yoshida, S., Toki, T., et al., 1996 Sep-Oct. New barium paste mixture for helical (slip-ring) CT evaluation of the esophagus. J Comput Assist Tomogr 20 (5), 773–776.

38. Pavone, P., Cardone, G.P., Cisternino, S., Di Girolamo, M., Aytan, E., Passariello, R., 1992 Oct. Gadopentetate dimeglumine-barium paste for opacification of the esophageal lumen on MR images. AJR Am J Roentgenol 159 (4), 762–764.

39. Gulati, K., Shah, Z.K., Sainani, N., Uppot, R., Sahani, D.V., 2008 May. Gastrointestinal tract labeling for MDCT of abdomen: comparison of low density barium and low density barium in combination with water. Eur Radiol 18 (5), 868–873.

40. Zinner, S.H., 2007 Jul. Antibiotic use: present and future. New Microbiol 30 (3), 321–325.

41. Ceyhan, B., Karaaslan, Y., Caymaz, O., Oto, A., Oram, E., Oram, A., et al., 1990 Feb. Comparison of sublingual captopril and sublingual nifedipine in hypertensive emergencies. Jpn J Pharmacol 52 (2), 189–193.

42. Vaughan Williams, E.M., 1992 Nov. Classifying antiarrhythmic actions: by facts or speculation. J Clin Pharmacol 32 (11), 964–977.

43. Law, M.R., Wald, N.J., Rudnicka, A.R., 2003 Jun 28. Quantifying effect of statins on low density lipoprotein cholesterol, ischaemic heart disease, and stroke: systematic review and meta-analysis. BMJ 326 (7404), 1423.

44. Baigent, C., Blackwell, L., Collins, R., Emberson, J., Godwin, J., Peto, R., et al., 2009 May 30. Aspirin in the primary and secondary prevention of vascular disease: collaborative meta-analysis of individual participant data from randomised trials. Lancet 373 (9678), 1849–1860.

45. McKevitt, F.M., Randall, M.S., Cleveland, T.J., Gaines, P.A., Tan, K.T., Venables, G.S., 2005 May. The benefits of combined anti-platelet treatment in carotid artery stenting. Eur J Vasc Endovasc Surg 29 (5), 522–527.

46. World Health Organisation (WHO), 1996. Cancer pain relief, 2nd ed. World Health Organisation, Geneva.

47. Raffa, R., 2006. Pharmacological aspects of successful long-term analgesia. Clin Rheumatol 25 (Suppl. 1), S9–S15.

48. Katzen, B.T., Edwards, K.C., 1983 Jan. Nitrous-oxide analgesia for interventional radiologic procedures. AJR Am J Roentgenol 140 (1), 145–148.

49. Ramsay, M.A., Savege, T.M., Simpson, B.R., Goodwin, R., 1974 Jun 22. Controlled sedation with alphaxalone-alphadolone. Br Med J 2 (5920), 656–659.

50. Fink, A.M., Aylward, G.W., 1995 Mar. Buscopan and glaucoma: a survey of current practice. Clin Radiol 50 (3), 160–164.

51. Goei, R., Nix, M., Kessels, A.H., Ten Tusscher, M.P., 1995 Aug. Use of antispasmodic drugs in double contrast barium enema examination: glucagon or buscopan? Clin Radiol 50 (8), 553–557.

52. Asao, T., Kuwano, H., Ide, M., Hirayama, I., Nakamura, J.I., Fujita, K.I., et al., 2003 Apr. Spasmolytic effect of peppermint oil in barium during double-contrast barium enema compared with Buscopan. Clin Radiol 58 (4), 301–305.

Chapter 12

1. Takimoto, C.H., Calvo, E., 2008. Principles of Oncologic Pharmacotherapy. In: Pazdur, R., Wagman, L.D., Camphausen, K.A., Hoskins, W.J. (Eds.), eleventh ed. A Multidisciplinary Approach, Cancer Management.

2. Cruet-Hennequart, S., Glynn, M.T., Murillo, L.S., Coyne, S., Carty, M.P., 2008. Enhanced DNA-PK-mediated RPA2 hyperphosphorylation in DNA polymerase eta-deficient human cells treated with cisplatin and oxaliplatin. DNA Repair (Amst.) 7 (4), 582–596.

3. Peters, G.J., van der Wilt, C.L., van Moorsel, C.J., Kroep, J.R., Bergman, A.M., Ackland, S.P., 2000. Basis for effective combination cancer chemotherapy with antimetabolites. Pharmacol. Ther 87 (2-3), 227–253.

4. Longley, D.B., Harkin, D.P., Johnston, P.G., May 2003. 5-fluorouracil: mechanisms of action and clinical strategies. Nat. Rev. Cancer. 3 (5), 330–338.

5. Sahasranaman, S., Howard, D., Roy, S., August 2008. Clinical pharmacology and pharmacogenetics of thiopurines. Eur. J. Clin. Pharmacol 64 (8), 753–767.

6. Rajagopalan, P. T. Ravi, Zhang, Zhiquan, McCourt, Lynn, Dwyer, Mary, Benkovic, Stephen J., Hammes, Gordon G., 2002. Interaction of dihydrofolate reductase with methotrexate: Ensemble and single-molecule kinetics. Proceedings of the National Academy of Sciences 99 (21), 13481–13486.

7. Bharadwaj, R., Yu, H., 2004. The spindle checkpoint, aneuploidy, and cancer. Oncogene 23 (11), 2016–2027.

8. Brito, D.A., Yang, Z., Rieder, C.L., 2008. Microtubules do not promote mitotic slippage when the spindle assembly checkpoint cannot be satisfied. J. Cell Biol. 182 (4), 623–629.

9. Gordaliza, M., García, P.A., del Corral, J.M., Castro, M.A., Gómez-Zurita, M.A., 2004. Podophyllotoxin: distribution, sources, applications and new cytotoxic derivatives. Toxicon 44 (4), 441–459.

10. Jordan, V.C., 1993. Fourteenth Gaddum Memorial Lecture. A current view of tamoxifen for the treatment and prevention of breast cancer. Br J Pharmacol 110 (2), 507–517.

11. BIG Collaborative Group, Aug. 20, 2009. Letrozole Therapy Alone or in Sequence with Tamoxifen in Women with Breast Cancer. N Engl J Med. 361 (766).

12. Furr, B.J., 1996. The development of Casodex (bicalutamide): preclinical studies. Eur. Urol. 29 (Suppl 2), 83–95.

13. Toshihiko, Kotake, Usami, Michiyuki, Akaza, Hideyuki, et al., August 1999. Goserelin Acetate with or without Antiandrogen or Estrogen in the Treatment of Patients with Advanced Prostate Cancer: a Multicenter, Randomized, Controlled Trial in Japan. Japanese Journal of Clin. Oncol. 29 (11), 562–570.

14. Han-Chung, W., Chia-Ting, H., De-Kuan, C., 2008. Anti-angiogenic Therapeutic drugs for treatment of human cancer. J. Cancer. Mol. 4 (2), 37–45.

15. Shan, Y., Zhang, J., Liu, Z., Wang, M., Dong, Y., 2011. Developments of combretastatin A-4 derivatives as anticancer agents. Current Medicinal Chemistry 18 (4), 523–538.

16. Brown, J.M., 2007. Tumor hypoxia in cancer therapy. Methods in Enzymology 435, 297–321.

17. Reddy, S.B., Williamson, S.K., 2009. Tirapazamine: a novel agent

targeting hypoxic tumor cells. Expert Opinion on Investigational Drugs 18 (1), 77–87.

18. Papadopoulos, K.P., Goel, S., Beeram, M., Wong, A., Desai, K., Haigentz, M., Milian, M.L., Mani, S., Tolcher, A., Lalani, A.S., Sarantopoulos, J., 2008. A phase 1 open-label, accelerated dose-escalation study of the hypoxia-activated prodrug AQ4N in patients with advanced malignancies. Clinical Cancer Research 14 (21), 7110–7115.

19. McKeown, S.R., Cowen, R.L., Williams, K.J., 2007. Bioreductive drugs: from concept to clinic. Clinical Oncology (Royal College of Radiologists) 19 (6), 427–442.

20. Greenberg, J.I., Cheresh, D.A., 2009. VEGF as an inhibitor of tumor vessel maturation: implications for cancer therapy. Expert Opinion on Biological Therapy 9 (11), 1347–1356.

21. Waldner, M.J., Neurath, M.F., 2010. The molecular therapy of colorectal cancer. Molecular Aspects of Medicine 31 (2), 171–178.

22. Trigg, M.E., Higa, G.M., 2010. Chemotherapy-induced nausea and vomiting: antiemetic trials that impacted clinical practice. Journal of Oncology Pharmacy Practice 16 (4), 233–244, 2010 Dec.

23. Brydøy, M., Fosså, S.D., Dahl, O., Bjøro, T., 2007. Gonadal dysfunction and fertility problems in cancer survivors. Acta Oncol 46 (4), 480–489.

24. Luqmani, Y.A., 2005. Mechanisms of Drug Resistance in Cancer Chemotherapy. Med. Princ. Pract. 14 (Suppl. 1), 35–48.

Chapter 17

1. Health Protection Agency, 2007. Doses to patients from Radiographic and fluoroscopic x-ray imaging procedures in the U.K -2005 review HPA-RPD-029.

2. Strauss, K.J., Kaste, S.C., 2006. The ALARA (as low as reasonably achievable)concept in pediatric interventional and fluoroscopic imaging:striving to keep radiation doses as low as possible during fluoroscopy of pediatric patients-a White Paper executive summary. Radiology 240 (3), 621–622, 2006 Sept.

3. Mahadevappa, M., 2001. Fluoroscopy patient radiation exposure issues. Radiographics July-Aug 2001 volume 21 (issue 4), 1033–1045.

4. Department of Health, 2000. The NHS Plan;a plan for investment, a plan for reform DoH Crown copyright.

5. NHS Institute for innovation and improvement, 2008. Quality and service improvement tools NHS.

6. British National Formularly Edition 62 (2011) BMJ Publishing Group LTD and Royal Pharmaceutical Society of Great Britain

7. http://www.npsa.nhs.uk/nrls/alerts-and directives/rapidrr/reducing-risk-of-harm-from-oral-bowel-cleansing-solutions-(Accessed Aug 2011)

8. Consensus guidelines for the prescription and administration of oral bowel cleansing agents, 2009. The Association of coloproctology of Great Britain and Ireland for the Royal College of Surgeons, The British Society of Gastroenterology, The British Society of GI and abdominal radiology. The renal association and The Royal College of Radiologists.

9. Royal College of Radiologists, 2005. Standards for patient consent particular to Radiology The board of the faculty of Clinical Radiology RCR 2005.

10. Department of Health, 2011. Essence of care benchmarks for respect and dignity 2010 TSO (The stationary office).

Chapter 18

1. Dotter, C.T., Judkins, M.P., 1964 Nov. Transluminal Treatment of Arteriosclerotic Obstruction. Description of a New Technic and a Preliminary Report of Its Application. Circulation 30, 654–670.

2. AbuRahma, A.F., Robinson, P.A., Boland, J.P., Umstot, R.K., Clubb, E.A., Grandia, R.A., et al., 1993 Mar. Complications of arteriography in a recent series of 707 cases: factors affecting outcome. Ann Vasc Surg 7 (2), 122–129.

3. Roberts, R.J., Weerts, T.C., 1982 Feb. Cardiovascular responding

during anger and fear imagery. Psychol Rep 50 (1), 219–230.

4. Johnston, K.W., Rae, M., Hogg-Johnston, S.A., Colapinto, R.F., Walker, P.M., Baird, R.J., et al., 1987 Oct. 5-year results of a prospective study of percutaneous transluminal angioplasty. Ann Surg 206 (4), 403–413.

5. Thomson, K.R., 1997 Aug 2. Interventional radiology. Lancet 350 (9074), 354–358.

6. Wheatley, K., Ives, N., Gray, R., Kalra, P.A., Moss, J.G., Baigent, C., et al., 2009 Nov 12. Revascularization versus medical therapy for renal-artery stenosis. N Engl J Med 361 (20), 1953–1962.

7. North American Symptomatic Carotid Endarterectomy Trial Collaborators, 1991 Aug 15. Beneficial effect of carotid endarterectomy in symptomatic patients with high-grade carotid stenosis. N Engl J Med 325 (7), 445–453.

8. Barnett, H.J., Taylor, D.W., Eliasziw, M., Fox, A.J., Ferguson, G.G., Haynes, R.B., et al., 1998 Nov 12. Benefit of carotid endarterectomy in patients with symptomatic moderate or severe stenosis. North American Symptomatic Carotid Endarterectomy Trial Collaborators. N Engl J Med 339 (20), 1415–1425.

9. Brott, T.G., Hobson 2nd., R.W., Howard, G., Roubin, G.S., Clark, W.M., Brooks, W., et al., 2010 Jul 1. Stenting versus endarterectomy for treatment of carotid-artery stenosis. N Engl J Med 363 (1), 11–23.

10. Ederle, J., Dobson, J., Featherstone, R.L., Bonati, L.H., van der Worp, H.B., de Borst, G.J., et al., 2010 Mar 20. Carotid artery stenting compared with endarterectomy in patients with symptomatic carotid stenosis (International Carotid Stenting Study): an interim analysis of a randomised controlled trial. Lancet 375 (9719), 985–997.

11. Axisa, B., Fishwick, G., Bolia, A., Thompson, M.M., London, N.J., Bell, P.R., et al., 2002 Jan. Complications following peripheral angioplasty. Ann R Coll Surg Engl 84 (1), 39–42.

12. Duda, S.H., Bosiers, M., Lammer, J., Scheinert, D., Zeller, T., Oliva, V., et al., 2006 Dec. Drug-eluting and bare nitinol stents for the treatment of atherosclerotic lesions in the superficial femoral artery: long-term results from the SIROCCO trial. J Endovasc Ther 13 (6), 701–710.

13. Bosiers, M., Cagiannos, C., Deloose, K., Verbist, J., Peeters, P., 2008. Drug-eluting stents in the management of peripheral arterial disease. Vasc Health Risk Manag 4 (3), 553–559.

14. Dake, M., 2011. The Zilver PTX randomized trial of paclitaxel-eluting stents for femoropopliteal disease: 24-month update. 7th Leipzig Interventional Cource (LINC); 19–22 January 2011, Leipzig, Germany.

15. National Institue for Healthcare and Clinical Excellence, 2002. Guidance on the use of ultrasound locating devices for placing central venous catheters. TAG49. National Institue for Healthcare and Clinical Excellence, London.

16. Mirza, A.N., Fornage, B.D., Sneige, N., Kuerer, H.M., Newman, L.A., Ames, F.C., et al., 2001 Mar-Apr. Radiofrequency ablation of solid tumors. Cancer J 7 (2), 95–102.

17. Moss, J.G., Cooper, K.G., Khaund, A., Murray, L.S., Murray, G.D., Wu, O., et al., 2011 Jul. Randomised comparison of uterine artery embolisation (UAE) with surgical treatment in patients with symptomatic uterine fibroids (REST trial): 5-year results. BJOG 118 (8), 936–944.

18. Gervais, D.A., Hahn, P.F., O'Neill, M.J., Mueller, P.R., 2002 Mar. Percutaneous abscess drainage in Crohn disease: technical success and short- and long-term outcomes during 14 years. Radiology 222 (3), 645–651.

19. Kim, Y.J., Han, J.K., Lee, J.M., Kim, S.H., Lee, K.H., Park, S.H., et al., 2006 May. Percutaneous drainage of postoperative abdominal abscess with limited accessibility: preexisting surgical drains as alternative access route. Radiology 239 (2), 591–598.

20. Chio, A., Galletti, R., Finocchiaro, C., Righi, D., Ruffino, M.A., Calvo, A., et al., 2004 Apr. Percutaneous radiological gastrostomy: a safe and effective method of nutritional tube placement in advanced ALS. J Neurol Neurosurg Psychiatry 75 (4), 645–647.

21. Lee, S.H., 2001 Oct. The role of oesophageal stenting in the non-surgical management of oesophageal strictures. Br J Radiol 74 (886), 891–900.

22. Mehta, S., Hindmarsh, A., Cheong, E., Cockburn, J., Saada, J., Tighe, R., et al., 2006 Feb. Prospective randomized trial of laparoscopic gastrojejunostomy versus duodenal stenting for malignant gastric outflow obstruction. Surg Endosc 20 (2), 239–242.

23. Jeurnink, S.M., Polinder, S., Steyerberg, E.W., Kuipers, E.J., Siersema, P.D., 2010 May. Cost comparison of gastrojejunostomy versus duodenal stent placement for malignant gastric outlet obstruction. J Gastroenterol 45 (5), 537–543.

24. van Hooft, J.E., Bemelman, W.A., Oldenburg, B., Marinelli, A.W., Holzik, M.F., Grubben, M.J., et al., 2011 Apr. Colonic stenting versus emergency surgery for acute left-sided malignant colonic obstruction: a multicentre randomised trial. Lancet Oncol 12 (4), 344–352.

25. National Institute for Healthcare and Clinical Excellence, 2003. Percutaneous vertebroplasty. IPG012. National Institue for Healthcare and Clinical Excellence, London.

Chapter 19

1. Epstein, R.M., Street, R.L. 2011. "The Values and Value of Patient-Centered Care" Annals of Family Medicine 9:100–103.

2. Gibbs, V., Cole, D., Sassano, A. 2009 Ultrasound Physics and Technology How, Why and When Churchill Livingstone

3. http://www.bmus.org/policies-guides/BMUS-Safety-Guidelines-2009-revision-FINAL-Nov-2009.pdf

4. Industry Standards for the Prevention of Work Related Musculoskeletal Disorders in Sonography 2006. ScOR.

5. American College of Radiology http://www.acr.org/secondarymaincategories/quality_safety(guidelines)breast/us_guided_breast.aspx. acr.org (2009) Accessed July 2011

6. Nizard, J "Amniocentesis: technique and education" Current Opinion in Obstetrics and Gynaecology 2010;vol. 22; issue.

7. FASP "Amniocentesis and Chorionic Villus Sampling Policy Standards and Protocols 2008"

8. Bates, J.A. Abdominal Ultrasound How Why and When. London Churchill Livingstone, 1999

9. http://www.nhs.uk/choiceintheNHS/Yourchoices/hospitalchoice/Pages/Choosingahospital.aspx

10. http://ratings2005.healthcarecommission.org.uk/Trust/Indicator/indicatorDescriptionShort.asp?indicatorId1007

11. http://www.rcr.ac.uk/content.aspx?PageID-323

12. http://guidance.nice.org.uk/nicemedia/live/12018/41316/41316.pdf

13. Darzi. A, 2008 "High Quality Care For All" NHS Next Stage Review Final Report "DOH http://www.dh.gov.uk/prod_consum_dh/groups/dh_digitalassets/@dh/@en/documents/digitalasset/dh_085826.pdf Accessed 25/08/11

14. http://www.bmus.org/policies-guides/SoR-Professional-Working-Standards-guidelines.pdf

Chapter 20

1. http://www.radiologyinfo.org/en/info.cfm?pg=gennuclear Accessed 9/5/2011.

2. http://www.molecularimagingcenter.org/index.cfm?PageID=7083 Accessed 09-05-2011

3. http://rpop.iaea.org/RPOP/RPoP/Content/InformationFor/Patients/patient-information-nuclear-medicine/index.htm Accessed 24-6-2011

4. http://rpop.iaea.org/RPOP/RPoP/Content/Documents/Whitepapers/patient-information.pdf Accessed 24-6-2011

5. http://rpop.iaea.org/RPOP/RPoP/Content/InformationFor/HealthProfessionals/3_NuclearMedicine/DiagnosticNuclearMedicine/index.htm Accessed 15-6-2011

6. Understanding Your Nuclear Medicine. http://www.nuclearimaging.com.auNMPET_InfoGuide.pdf Accessed 18-7-2011

7. Procedure Guidelines and Patient Information – Nuclear Medicine Department, IALCH. 2010.

8. Donohoe, K.J., Brown, M.L., Collier, B.D., Carretta, R.F., Henkin, R.E., O'Mara, R.E., Royal, H.D., 2003. Society of Nuclear Medicine Procedure Guideline for Bone Scintigraphy 3.0. http://www.snm.org/index.cfm?PageID=772 Accessed 2-11-2006.

9. Delbeke, D., Coleman, R.E., Guiberteau, M.J., Brown, M.L., Royal, H.D., Siegel, B.A., Townsend, D.W., Berland, L.L., Parker, J.A., Hubner, K., Stabin, M.G., Zubal, G., Kachelriess, M., Cronin, V., Holbrook, S., 2006. Procedure Guideline for Tumor Imaging with 18F-FDG PET/CT 1.0. http://www.snm.org/index.cfm?PageID=772 Accessed 02-11-2006.

10. Silberstein, E.B., Alavi, A., Balon, H.R., Becker, D.V., Brill, D.R., Clarke, S.E.M., Divgi, C., Goldsmith, S.J., Lull, R.J., Meier, D.A., Royal, H.D., Siegel, J.A., Waxman, A.D., 2005. Society of Nuclear Medicine Procedure Guideline for Therapy of Thyroid Disease with Iodine-131 (Sodium Iodide). 2.0. Society of Nuclear Medicine Procedure Guidelines Manual http://www.snm.org/index.cfm?PageID=772 Accessed 10-8-2011.

11. The SNM Practice Guideline for Somatostatin Receptor Scintigraphy 2.0. 2011. http://www.snm.org/index.cfm?PageID=772 Accessed 2-8-2011.

12. Becker, D.V., Charkes, N.D., Hurley, J.R., McDougall, I.R., Price, D.C., Royal, H.D., Sarkar, S.D., Dworkin, H.J., 1999. Society of Nuclear Medicine Procedure Guideline for Thyroid Scintigraphy 2.0. 1999. http://www.snm.org/index.cfm?PageID=772 Accessed 3-11-2006.

13. Greenspan, B.S., Brown, M.L., Dillehay, G.L., McBiles, M., Sandler, M.P., Seabold, J.E., Sisson, J.C., 2004. The Society of Nuclear Medicine Procedure Guideline for Parathyroid Scintigraphy 3.0. 2004. http://www.snm.org/index.cfm?PageID=772 Accessed 3-11-2006.

14. Strauss, H.W., Miller, D.D., Wittry, M.D., Cerqueira, M.D., Garcia, E.V., Iskandrian, A.S., Schelbert, H.R., Wackers, F.J., Balon, H.R., Lang, O., Machac, J., September 2008. Society of Nuclear Medicine Procedure Guideline for Myocardial Perfusion Imaging. 3.3. 2008. Journal of Nuclear Medicine Technology Vol. 36 (3)http://www.snm.org/index.cfm?PageID=772 Accessed 10-7-2011.

15. SNM Practice Guideline for Lung Scintigraphy V4.0. 2011. http://www.snm.org/index.cfm?PageID=772 Accessed 2-8-2011.

16. Shulkin, B.L., Mandell, G.A., Cooper, J.A., Leonard, J.C., Majd, M., Parisi, M.T., Sfakianakis, G.N., Balon, H.R., Donohoe, K.J., 2008. Procedure Guideline for Diuretic Renography in Children 3.0. 2008. http://www.snm.org/index.cfm?PageID=772 Accessed 10-7-2011.

17. Mandell, G.A., Eggli, D.F., Gilday, D.L., Heyman, S., Leonard, J.C., Miller, J.H., Nadel, H.R., Piepsz, A., Treves, S.T., 2003. Society of Nuclear Medicine Procedure Guideline for Renal Cortical Scintigraphy in Children 3.0. 2003. http://www.snm.org/index.cfm?PageID=772 Accessed 3-11-2006.

18. The SNM Procedure Guideline For Hepatobiliary Scintigraphy 4.0. 2010. http://www.snm.org/index.cfm?PageID=772 Accessed 21-7-2011.

19. Royal, H.D., Brown, M.L., Drum, D.E., Nagle, C.E., Sylvester, J.M., Ziessman, H.A., 2003. Society of Nuclear Medicine P rocedure Guideline for Hepatic and Splenic Imaging 3.0. http://www.snm.org/index.cfm?PageID=772 Accessed 3-11-2006.

20. Donohoe, K.J., Maurer, A.H., Ziessman, H.A., Urbain, J.C., Royal, H.D., Martin-Comin, J., 2009. Procedure Guideline for Adult Solid-Meal Gastric-Emptying Study 3.0. http://www.snm.org/index.cfm?PageID=772 Accessed 10-7-2011.

21. Ford, P.V., Bartold, S.P., Fink-Bennett, D.M., Jolles, P.R., Lull, R.J., Maurer, A.H., Seabold,

J.E., 1999. Society of Nuclear Medicine Procedure Guideline for Gastrointestinal Bleeding and Meckel's Diverticulum Scintigraphy 1.0. http://www.snm.org/index.cfm?PageID=772 Accessed 3-11-2006.

22. Juni, J.E., Waxman, A.D., Devous, M.D., Tikofsky, R.S., Ichise, M., Van Heertum, R.L., Carretta, R.F., Chen, C.C., 2009. Procedure Guideline for Brain Perfusion SPECT Using 99mTc radiopharmaceuticals 3.0. http://www.snm.org/index.cfm?PageID=772 Accessed 10-7-2011.

23. Waxman, A.D., Herholz, K., Lewis, D.H., Herscovitch, P., Minoshima, S., Ichise, M., Drzezga, A.E., Devous, M.D., Mountz, J.M., 2009. Society of Nuclear Medicine Procedure Guideline for FDG PET Brain Imaging 1.0. http://www.snm.org/index.cfm?PageID=772 Accessed 10-7-2011.

24. Referrer Guide to Nuclear Medicine. http//www.uclh.nhs.ukOurServicesServiceA-ZIMAGINGNUCDocumentsReferrerguide. Accessed 1-8-2011

25. PET-CT Scanning https://rpop.iaea.orgRPOPRPoPContentInformationForHealthProfessionals6_OtherClinicalSpecialitiesPETCTscan.htm. Accessed 15-6-2011

26. Information about your Nuclear Medicine Therapy, 2009. NM Therapy Patient Leaflet [1]. http//www.anzapnm.org.au Accessed 21-7-2011.

27. Society of Nuclear Medicine Performance and Responsibility Guidelines for NMT - Revision 2003. Society of Nuclear Medicine Procedure Guidelines Manual August 2003. http://interactive.snm.org/docs/pg_ch16_0803.pdf Accessed 10-6-2011.

28. Calculate Your Radiation Dose. http://www.epa.gov/radiation/understand/calculate.html. Accessed 19-8-2011

29. Peer, F.I., 2009. A balancing act: potential benefits versus possible risks of radiation exposure. 2009. The South African Radiographer Vol. 47 (2)http://www.sar.org.za/index.php/sar/article/viewArticle/147 Accessed 10-01-2010.

Chapter 21

1. Gowland, P., 2005. Present and future magnetic resonance sources of exposure to static fields. Progress in Biophysics and Molecular Biology 87, 175–183.

2. Society & Radiographers, 2007. Safety in Magnetic Resonance Imaging. SOR, London.

3. Shellock, F., Woods, T., Crues, J., 2009. MRI Labeling Information for Implants and Devices: Explanation of Terminology. Radiology 253, 26–30.

4. Chaljub, G., Kramer, L., Johnson, R., Johnson Jr., R., Singh, H., Crow, W., 2001. Projectile cylinder accidents resulting from the presence of ferromagnetic nitrous oxide or oxygen tanks in the MR suite. American Journal of Roentgenology 177 (1), 27–30.

5. Medicines and Healthcare products Regsitration Agency, 2002. Guidelines for magnetic resonance equipment in clinical use. MHRA, London.

6. Shellock, F., 2011. Reference Manual for Magnetic Resonance Safety, Implants, and Devices, Edition. Biomedical Research Publishing Company, Los Angeles, CA.

7. Farrelly, C., Davarpanah, A., Brennan, S., Sampson, M., Eustace, 2010. Imaging of soft tissues adjacent to orthopedic hardware: comparison of 3-T and 1.5-T MRI. American Journal Roentgenology 194 (1), 60–64.

8. Jarvik, J., Ramsey, G., 2000. Radiographic screening for orbital foreign bodies prior to MR imaging: Is it worth it? American Journal of Neuroradiology 21, 245.

9. Seidenwurm, D., McDonnell, C., Raghavan, N., Breslau, J., 2000. Cost utility analysis of radiographic screening for an orbital foreign body before MR imaging. American Journal of Neuroradiology 21 (2), 426–433.

10. Hall, D.A., 2009. Acoustic, psychophysical, and neuroimaging measurements of the effectiveness of active cancellation during auditory functional magnetic resonance imaging. Journal of the Acoustical Society of America 125, 347–359.

11. Moelker, A., Maas, R., Pattynama, P., 2004. Verbal communication in MR environments: Effect of MR system acoustic noise on speech understanding. Radiology 232, 107–113.

12. Thorpe, S., Salkovskis, P., Dittner, A., 2008. Claustrophobia in MRI: the role of cognitions. Magnetic Resonance Imaging 26, 1081–1088.

13. Dempsey, M., Condon, B., 2001. Thermal injuries associated with MRI. Clinical Radiology 56, 457–465.

14. Dewey, M., Schink, T., Dewey, C., 2007. Claustrophobia during Magnetic Resonance Imaging: Cohort Study in Over 55,000 Patient. Journal of Magnetic Resonance Imaging 26, 1322–1327.

15. Harris, L., Robinson, J., Menzies, R., 2001. Evidence for fear restriction and fear of suffocation as components of claustrophobia. Behavior Research & Therapy 37, 155–159.

16. Bigsley, J., Griffiths, P., Prydderch, A., Romanowski, C., Lidiard, H., Hoggard, N., 2010; Neurolinguistic programming used to reduce the need for anaesthesia in claustrophobic patients undergoing MRI. 83:113–117.

17. Reeves, M., Brandreth, M., Whitby, E., Hart, A., Paley, M., Griffiths, P., Stevens, J., 2010. Neonatal cochlear function: measurement after exposure to acoustic noise during in utero MR imaging. Radiology 257 (3), 802–809.

Chapter 22

1. Lee, L., Stickland, V., Wilson, R., Evans, A., 2002. Fundamentals of Mammography, second ed. Churchill Livingstone, Edinburgh.

2. Eklund, G.W., Cardenosa, G., 1992. The art of mammographic positioning. Radiologic Clinics of North America 30 (1), 21–53.

3. Poulos, A., Llewellyn, G., 2005. Mammography discomfort: A holistic perspective derived from women's experiences. Radiography 11 (1), 17–25.

4. Law, J., Faulkner, K., Young, K.C., 2007 Apr. Risk factors for induction of breast cancer by X-rays and their implications for breast screening. British Journal of Radiology 80 (952), 261–266.

5. Law, J., Faulkner, K., 2002 Nov. Two-view screening and extending the age range: the balance of benefit and risk. British Journal of Radiology 75 (899), 889–894.

6. de Gelder, R., Draisma, G., Heijnsdijk, E.A.M., de Koning, H.J., 2011 Mar 29. Population-based mammography screening below age 50: balancing radiation-induced vs prevented breast cancer deaths. British Journal of Cancer. [Research Support, Non-U.S. Gov't] 104 (7), 1214–1220.

7. McParland, B.J., 2000. Image quality and dose in film-screen magnification mammography. British Journal of Radiology 73 (874), 1068–1077.

8. Helvie, M.A., Chan, H.P., Adler, D.D., Boyd, P.G., 1994. Breast thickness in routine mammograms: Effect on image quality and radiation dose. American Journal of Roentgenology 163 (6), 1371–1374.

9. Davey, B., 2007. Pain during mammography: possible risk factors and ways to alleviate pain. Radiography 13 (3), 229–234.

10. Kornguth, P.J., Keefe, F.J., Conaway, M.R., 1996 Aug. Pain during mammography: characteristics and relationship to demographic and medical variables. Pain. [Clinical Trial] 66 (2-3), 187–194.

11. Hafslund, B., 2000. Mammography and the experience of pain and anxiety. Radiography 6 (4), 269–272.

12. Van Goethem, M., Mortelmans, D., Bruyninckx, E., Verslegers, I., Biltjes, I., Van Hove, E., et al., 2003 Oct. Influence of the radiographer on the pain felt during mammography. European Radiology 13 (10), 2384–2389.

13. Elwood, M., McNoe, B., Smith, I., Bandaranayake, M., Adam, H., Doyle, T.C.A., 1998. Once is enough - Why some women do not continue to participate in a breast cancer screening programme. New Zealand Medical Journal 111 (1066), 180–183.

14. Drossaert, C.H.C., Boer, H., Seydel, E.R., 2002. Monitoring women's experiences during three rounds of breast cancer screening: Results from a longitudinal study. Journal of Medical Screening 9 (4), 168–175.

15. Miller, D., Livingstone, V., Herbison, G.P., 2008. Interventions for relieving the pain and discomfort of screening mammography. Cochrane Database of Systematic Reviews (1).

16. Cawson, J.N., Malara, F.A., 2004. False-positive breast screening to fat necrosis following mammography. Australasian Radiology 48 (2), 217–219.

17. Roelke, M., Rubinstein, V.J., Kamath, S., Krauser, D., Ngarmukos, T., Parsonnet, V., 1999. Pacemaker interference with screening mammography. PACE - Pacing and Clinical Electrophysiology 22 (7), 1106–1107.

18. Sherman, M.M., 2005. Damage to pacemaker lead during mammography [7]. New England Journal of Medicine 353 (17), 1865.

19. Brown, S.L., Todd, J.F., Luu, H.M.D., 2004. Breast implant adverse events during mammography: Reports to the Food and Drug Administration. Journal of Women's Health 13 (4), 371–378.

20. Board of the Faculty of Clinical Radiology, 2003. Guidance on Screening and Symptomatic Breast Imaging, Second Edition. Royal College of Radiologists, London.

21. Keemers-Gels, M.E., Groenendijk, R.P., van den Heuvel, J.H., Boetes, C., Peer, P.G., Wobbes, T.H., 2000 Apr. Pain experienced by women attending breast cancer screening. Breast Cancer Research & Treatment 60 (3), 235–240.

22. Brett, J., Austoker, J., Ong, G., 1998. Do women who undergo further investigation for breast screening suffer adverse psychological consequences? A multi-centre follow-up study comparing different breast screening result groups five months after their last breast screening appointment. Journal of Public Health Medicine 20 (4), 396–403.

23. Ong, G., Austoker, J., 1997. Recalling women for further investigation of breast screening: Women's experiences at the clinic and afterwards. Journal of Public Health Medicine 19 (1), 29–36.

24. Beral, V., Alexander, M., Duffy, S., Ellis, I.O., Given-Wilson, R., Holmberg, L., et al., 2011. The number of women who would need to be screened regularly by mammography to prevent one death from breast cancer. Journal of Medical Screening 18 (4), 210–212.

25. Duffy, S.W., Tabar, L., Olsen, A.H., Vitak, B., Allgood, P.C., Chen, T.H.H., et al., 2010. Absolute numbers of lives saved and overdiagnosis in breast cancer screening, from a randomized trial and from the Breast Screening Programme in England. Journal of Medical Screening 17 (1), 25–30.

Chapter 25

1. The Royal College of Radiologists, 2007. The Role and Development of Brachytherapy Services in the United Kingdom. the Royal College of Radiologists, London http://www.rcr.ac.uk/publications.aspx?PageID=149&PublicationID=254.

2. Guedea, F., Venselaar, J., Hoskin, P., Hellebust, T.P., Peiffert, D., Londres, B., Ventura, M., Mazeron, J.J., Limbergen, E.V., Pötter, R., Kovacs, G., 2010 Dec. Patterns of care for brachytherapy in Europe: updated results. Radiother Oncol 97 (3), 514–520, Epub 2010 Oct 13.

Chapter 26

1. Kelland, L.R., 2005 Chapter 1 Cancer cell biology, drug action and resistance, 3–17, in Brighton, D., Wood, M., 2005 The Royal Marsden's Hospital Handbook of Cancer Chemotherapy, Elsevier Churchill Livingstone, Edinburgh

2. Watson, M., Barrett, A., Spence, R., Twelves, C., 2006. Oncology, second ed. Oxford University Press, Oxford.

3. Saltmarsh, K., De Vries, K., 2008. The paradoxical image of chemotherapy: a phenomenological description of nurses' experiences of administering chemotherapy. European Journal of Cancer Care 17, 500–508.

4. McIlfatrick, S., Sullivan, K., McKenna, H., Parahoo, K., 2007. Patients' experiences of having chemotherapy in a day hospital setting. Journal of Advanced Nursing vol. 59 (3), 264–273.

5. Barr, L., Cowan, R., Nicholson, M., 2004. Oncology, second ed. Churchill Livingstone, Elsevier Limited, London.

6. Tadman, M., Roberts, D., 2007. Oxford Handbook of Cancer Nursing. Oxford University Press, Oxford.

7. Spence, R.A.J., Johnston, P.G., 2001. Oncology. Oxford University Press.

8. Neal, A.J., Hoskins, P.J., 2003. Clinical oncology: Basic principles and practice, third ed. Arnold of Hodder Headline Group, London.

9. Macmillan Cancer Relief http://www.macmillan.org.uk/Cancerinformation/Cancertreatment/Treatmenttypes/Chemotherapy/Chemotherapy.aspx accessed 8.10.11

10. Khan, S., Dhadda, A., Fyfe, D., Sundar, S., 2008. Impact of neutropenia on delivering planned chemotherapy for solid tumours. European Journal of Cancer Care 17, 19–25.

11. Randall, R.J., Ream, E., 2004. Hair loss with chemotherapy: at a loss over its management?. European Journal of Cancer Care 14, 223–231.

12. Cancer Research UK http://cancerhelp.cancerresearchuk.org/about-cancer/cancer-questions/hair-loss-and-wigs accessed 8.10.11

13. Miller, M., Kearney, N., 2004. Chemotherapy – related nausea and vomiting - past reflections, present practice and future management. European Journal of Cancer Care 13, 71–81.

14. Molassiotis, A., Stricker, C.T., Eaby, B., Velders, L., Coventry, P.A., 2008. Understanding the concept of chemotherapy – related nausea: the patient experience. European Journal of Cancer Care 18, 444–453.

15. Ng, W.I., Della Florentina, S.A., 2008. The efficacy of oral ondansetron and dexamethasone for the prevention of acute chemotherapy- induced nausea and vomiting associated with moderately ematogenic chemotherapy – a retrospective audit. European Journal of Cancer Care 19, 403–407.

16. Kyle, G., 2009. Methylnaltrexone: a subcutaneous treatment for opioid – induced constipation in palliative care patients. International journal of Palliative Care vol. 15 (11), 533–540.

17. Wagner, L.I., Cella, D., 2004. Fatigue and cancer: causes, prevalence and treatment approaches. British Journal of Cancer 91, 822–828.

18. Stone, P.C., Minton, O., 2008. Cancer-related fatigue. European Journal of Cancer 44, 1097–1104.

19. Gielissen, M.F.M., Verhagen, C.A.H.H.V.M., Bleijenberg, G., 2007. Cognitive Behaviour Therapy for fatigue cancer survivors: long term follow up. British Journal of Cancer 97, 612–618.

20. Wolf, S., Barton, D., Kottschade, L., Grothey, A., Loprinzi, C., 2008. Chemotherapy induced peripheral neuropathy: prevention and treatment strategies. European Journal of Cancer 44, 1507–1515.

21. Mitchell, T., Turton, P., 2011. 'Chemobrain': concentration and memory effects in people receiving chemotherapy – a descriptive phenomenological study. European Journal of Cancer Care 20, 539–548.

22. Mitchell, T., 2007. The social and emotional toll of chemotherapy – patients' perspectives. European Journal of Cancer Care 16, 39–47.

23. Harrold, K., 2010. Effective management of adverse effects while on oral chemotherapy: implications for nursing practice. European Journal of Cancer Care 19, 12–20.

24. Oakle6y, C., Johnson, J., Ream, E., 2010. Developing an intervention for cancer patients prescribed oral chemotherapy: a generic patient diary. European Journal of Cancer Care 19, 21–28.

Chapter 27

1. Hemminki, A., 2002. From molecular changes to customised therapy. European Journal of Cancer vol. 38 33–338.

2. Godfrey, H., 2004. Understanding the human body: biological perspectives for health care. Churchill Livingstone, Edinburgh.

3. Copier, J., Dalgleish, A.G., Britten, C.M., Finke, L.H., Gaudernack, G., Gnjatic, S., Kallen, K., Kiessling,

R., Schuessler-Lenz, M., Singh, H., Talmadge, J., Zwierzina, H., Hakansson, L., 2009. Improving efficacy of cancer immunotherapy. European Journal of Cancer vol. 45, 1424–1431.

4. Stanford, J.L., Stanford, C.A., O'Brien, M.E.R., Grange, J.M., 2008. Successful immunotherapy with Mycobacterium vaccae in the treatment of adenocarcinoma of the lung. European Journal of Cancer vol. 44, 224–227.

5. Grange, J.M., Krone, B., Stanford, J.L., 2009. Immunotherapy for malignant melanoma – tracing Ariadne's thread through a labyrinth. European Journal of Cancer vol. 45, 2266–2273.

6. Graham, A.H., 2009. Administering rituximab: infusion –related reactions and nursing implications. Cancer Nursing Practice vol. 8 (2), 30–35.

7. Henning, I.M., Twelves, C., 2008. Loading doses for costly biological: a cause for concern or tilting at windmills? European Journal of Cancer vol. 44, 1493–1496.

8. Martini, F.H., Nath, J.L., 2009. Fundamentals of Anatomy and Physiology, eighth ed. Pearson International, San Francisco.

9. Dunlop, R.J., Campbell, C.W., 2000. Cytokines and advanced cancer. Journal of pain and symptom management vol 20 (3), 214–232.

10. Tadman, M., Roberts, D., 2007. Oxford Handbook of Cancer Nursing. Oxford University Press, Oxford.

11. Ward, U., 1995. Biological therapy in the treatment of cancer. British Journal of Nursing vol. 41 (15), 869–891.

12. Causer, L., 2005. Radioimmunotherapy in the treatment of non Hodgkin's lymphoma. Cancer Nursing Practice vol. 4 (9), 27–33.

13. Hull, D., Chester, M., 2008. Management of patient participation in a hepatocellular carcinoma clinical trial. Cancer Nursing Practice vol. 8 (7), 35–39.

14. National Institute for Health and Clinical Excellence, 2009. Sunitinib for the first line treatment of advanced and/or metastatic Renal

Cell Carcinoma. Technology appraised 169. NICE, London.

15. Thomson, N., 2011. Multidisciplinary clinic for patients with metastatic renal cell carcinoma. Cancer Nursing Practice vol. 10 (7), 22–27.

16. Lemmens, L., Claes, V., Uzzell, M., 2008. Managing patients with metastatic colorectal cancer on bevacizumab. British Journal of Nursing vol. 17 (15), 944–949.

17. Boxall, J., Nathan, P., (20060 Renal Cell cancer: causes, prognosis, management and treatments, Cancer Nursing Practice, vol. 5(3), 29-32

18. Davis, C., 2008. Stopping cervical cancer in its tracks. Cancer Nursing Practice vol. 7 (5), 19–21.

19. Panlagua, H., 2006. Knowledge of cervical cancer and the HPV vaccine. British Journal of Nursing vol. 15 (3), 126–127.

Chapter 29

1. Dimond, B., 2002. Legal aspects of radiography and radiology. Blackwell, Oxford.

2. Society of Radiographers, 2008. Code of Conduct and Ethics. Society of Radiographers, London.

3. Health Care Professions Council, 2008. Standards of conduct, performance and ethics. Health Care Professions Council, London.

4. Department of Health, 2001. Good practice in consent implementation guide: consent to examination or treatment. Department of Health, London.

5. Health Care Professions Council, 2009. Standards of proficiency for radiographers. Health Care Professions Council, London.

6. Society and College of Radiographers, 2007. Consent to imaging and radiotherapy treatment examinations: an ethical perspective and good practice guide for the radiography workforce. Society of Radiographers, London.

7. Health Care Professions Council, 2008. Confidentiality: information for registrants. Health Care Professions Council, London.

8. Herring, J., 2010. Medical law and ethics, third ed. Oxford University Press, Oxford.

Index